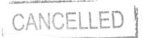

ML

THE CLINICAL HANDBOOK OF
EAR, NOSE AND THROAT DISORDERS

THE CLINICAL HANDBOOK SERIES

THE CLINICAL HANDBOOK OF
EAR, NOSE AND THROAT DISORDERS

WILLIAM R. WILSON, MD

JOSEPH B. NADOL, JR., MD

GREGORY W. RANDOLPH, MD

WITH MEDICAL ILLUSTRATIONS BY ROBERT J. GALLA

The Parthenon Publishing Group
International Publishers in Medicine, Science & Technology

A CRC PRESS COMPANY

BOCA RATON   LONDON   NEW YORK   WASHINGTON, D.C.

**Library of Congress
Cataloging-in-Publication Data**

Wilson, William R.
  Clinical handbook of ear, nose and
  throat disorders / William R. Wilson,
  Joseph B. Nadol, Jr., Gregory W.
  Randolph; with medical illustrations by
  Robert J. Galla.
  p. : cm.
  Includes bibliographical references and
  index.
  ISBN 1-85070-605-0 (pbk. : alk. paper)
    1. Otolaryngology – Handbooks,
  manuals, etc. 2. Clinical medicine –
  Handbooks, manuals, etc. I. Nadol,
  Joseph B. II. Randolph, Gregory,
  III. Title.
  [DNLM: 1. Otorhinolaryngologic Diseases
  – Handbooks. WV 39 W754c 2002]
  RF46.W535 2002
  617.5'1-dc21

                           2002021009

**British Library Cataloguing-in-Publication
Data**

Wilson, William R.
  Clinical handbook of ear, nose and
  throat disorders. – (The clinical
  handbook series)
  1. Otolaryngology
  I. Title II. Nadol, Joseph B.
  III. Randolph, Gregory W.
  IV. Galla, Robert J.
  617.5'1

  ISBN 1-85070-605-0

Published in the USA by
The Parthenon Publishing Group Inc.
345 Park Avenue South
10th Floor
New York, NY 10010, USA

Published in the UK and Europe by
The Parthenon Publishing Group Limited
23–25 Blades Court, Deodar Road
London SW15 2NU, UK

Copyright ©2002
The Parthenon Publishing Group

Typeset by Speedlith Group, Manchester, UK
Printed and bound in the USA

Contents

Preface   vii

List of contributors   ix

Acknowledgements   x

The ear and temporal bone

1   Functional anatomy, physiology and examination of the ear   1
      Joseph B. Nadol, Jr

2   Hearing loss   31
      Joseph B. Nadol, Jr

3   The draining ear   61
      Joseph B. Nadol, Jr

4   The dizzy patient   83
      William R. Wilson

5   Facial paresis and paralysis   113
      Joseph B. Nadol, Jr

6   Pain syndromes in the head and neck   133
      Joseph B. Nadol, Jr

7   Ear emergencies   147
      Joseph B. Nadol, Jr

The nose and paranasal sinuses

8   Anatomy, physiology and examination of the nose and
      paranasal sinuses   165
      William R. Wilson

9   Nasal and sinus congestion and infection   183
      William R. Wilson

10 Nasal and facial emergencies   209
    William R. Wilson

The head and neck

11 Anatomy of the neck, examination of the head and neck
    and evaluation of neck masses   231
    Gregory W. Randolph

12 Sore mouth and throat   265
    Gregory W. Randolph

13 Hoarseness and the larynx   299
    Gregory W. Randolph

14 Dysphagia   341
    Gregory W. Randolph

15 Airway evaluation   353
    Gregory W. Randolph

16 Salivary gland disorders   377
    Gregory W. Randolph

17 Thyroid and parathyroid disorders   395
    Gregory W. Randolph

18 Radiology of the ear, nose and throat for the primary
    care physician   419
    Alfred L. Weber

Appendix 1   Common medications used in otolaryngology   461

Appendix 2   Common instruments used in otolaryngology   469

Index   475

Preface

This handbook is dedicated to all students of clinical otolaryngology, both young and mature. It and its predecessor, *Quick Reference to Ear, Nose, and Throat Disorders* (Philadelphia: J.B. Lippincott Co., 1983) evolved from a syllabus developed for a course for primary care physicians by the Department of Otology and Laryngology of the Harvard Medical School at the Massachusetts Eye and Ear Infirmary.

Although there are certainly many excellent texts of otolaryngology, this clinical handbook was specifically intended for primary care physicians, emergency room physicians and their trainees, and medical students. The symptom-oriented text provides practical algorithms for diagnosis and management. The appendixes describe pharmaceuticals commonly used in otolaryngologic practices and instruments that are necessary for a complete otolaryngologic examination. It is hoped that this text will serve, as its title implies, as a handbook and quick reference for busy clinicians and medical students, and that it will benefit their patients.

William R. Wilson, MD
Joseph B. Nadol, Jr., MD
Gregory W. Randolph, MD

List of contributors

Joseph B. Nadol, Jr., MD
Walter Augustus Lecompte Professor
Department of Otology and Laryngology
Harvard Medical School; and

Chief of Otolaryngology
Massachusetts Eye and Ear Infirmary
Boston, MA

Gregory W. Randolph, MD
Assistant Professor
Department of Otology and Laryngology
Harvard Medical School; and

Assistant Surgeon in Otolaryngology
Massachusetts Eye and Ear Infirmary
Boston, MA

Alfred L. Weber, MD
Professor of Radiology
Harvard Medical School; and

Chief of Radiology (Emeritus)
Massachusetts Eye and Ear Infirmary
Boston, MA

William R. Wilson, MD
Professor Emeritus
George Washington University
Division of Otolaryngology/Head and Neck Surgery
Washington, DC

Acknowledgements

We wish to thank our medical and surgical colleagues, residents in otolaryngology, and medical students, whose comments and questions have inspired and helped to focus the subject matter of this book.

We also wish to thank Carol Ota and Bob Galla, whose attention to details of the manuscript and illustrations have been most helpful, for their tireless efforts to provide a text that we hope will be useful to our readers.

1

Functional anatomy, physiology and examination of the ear

Joseph B. Nadol, Jr

Functional anatomy and physiology
    Auricle and external auditory canal
    Tympanic membrane
    Middle ear and mastoid cell system
    Ossicles
    Inner ear and internal auditory canal
    Facial nerve
Examination of the ear
    Inspection and cleaning
    Otoscopy
    Tests of auditory function
        Tuning fork and whisper tests
    Behavioral audiometry (standard hearing tests)
    Special behavioral tests
        Summary of special behavioral audiometry tests
    Auditory evoked response testing
    Otoacoustic emissions
    Tympanometry
    Tests for functional hearing loss
Vestibular testing
    Caloric tests
    Positional testing
        Aschan classification of positional nystagmus
    Fistula test
Facial nerve tests
    Site-of-lesion testing
    Neurophysiologic tests of neuronal viability
Other office otologic testing

FUNCTIONAL ANATOMY AND PHYSIOLOGY

The ear is divided anatomically into external, middle and inner ear segments (Figures 1.1 and 1.2). The external ear consists of the auricle and the external auditory canal. The middle ear consists of the ossicular chain and air space continuous with the mastoid air–cell system; it is separated from the external ear by the tympanic membrane. The inner ear consists of the bony otic capsule, auditory and vestibular receptor organs and the internal auditory canal containing the seventh and eighth cranial nerves.

Auricle and external auditory canal

The auricle, with the exception of the lobule, contains a cartilaginous skeleton that develops from cartilaginous accumulations, or 'hillocks', derived from the first (mandibular) and second (hyoid) branchial arches. Therefore, congenital malformations of these arches are commonly associated with auricular abnormalities. Disordered embryologic development of the first branchial groove may result in dysplasia (stenosis) or atresia of the external auditory canal. The intrinsic musculature of the auricle allows rotation of the external ear in animals, but this function is vestigial in the human.

The lateral one-third of the external auditory canal is composed of cartilage extending from the auricle and is covered by skin with appendages specialized for cerumen production. The medial two-thirds of the external canal has a bony skeleton derived from the tympanic, mastoid and squamous portions of the temporal bone. The skin here is thin, devoid of appendages and easily abraded by instrumentation of the canal.

Tympanic membrane

The eardrum, or tympanic membrane (Figure 1.3), is divided into two distinct parts. The pars flaccida, or Shrapnel's membrane, lies above the anterior and posterior malleal folds. The pars tensa comprises the rest of the tympanic membrane. Landmarks visible on routine otoscopy include the lateral process of the malleus, which forms a bony prominence at the junction of Shrapnel's membrane and the pars tensa; the manubrium; and the umbo, where the pars tensa is attached to the end of the malleus. In the young, translucent tympanic membrane, the long process of the incus, the suprastructures of the stapes and the chorda tympani nerve

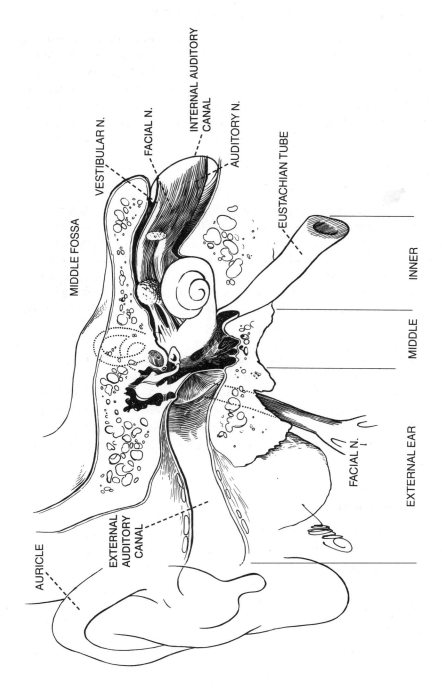

Figure 1.1   Coronal section of the right ear and temporal bone

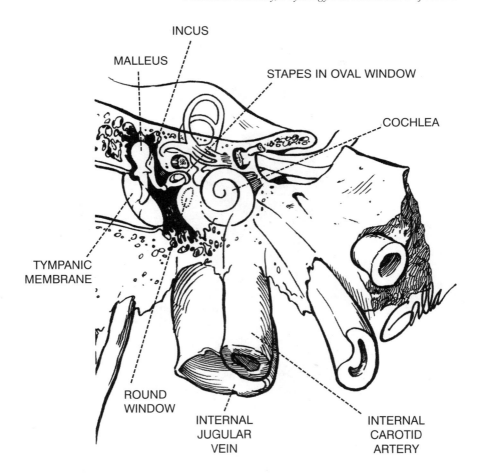

INCUS

MALLEUS

STAPES IN OVAL WINDOW

COCHLEA

TYMPANIC
MEMBRANE

ROUND
WINDOW

INTERNAL
JUGULAR
VEIN

INTERNAL
CAROTID
ARTERY

Figure 1.2   Magnified view of the middle and inner ear

may all be visible. The 'light reflex' is a wedge-shaped reflection of the light seen with the otoscope as originating at the umbo and extending anteroinferiorly to the edge of the tympanic membrane. Although often present, the light reflex does not ensure the absence of disease, nor does its absence signify pathology.

It is important that the examiner visualize both parts of the drum. The pars flaccida is the most commonly overlooked, and it is in this area that the most serious disease processes, such as cholesteatoma, may be located.

The tympanic membrane serves several important functions. First, it closes the middle ear space from the external ear canal. Second, it collects and transmits sound selectively to the oval window of the inner ear via the

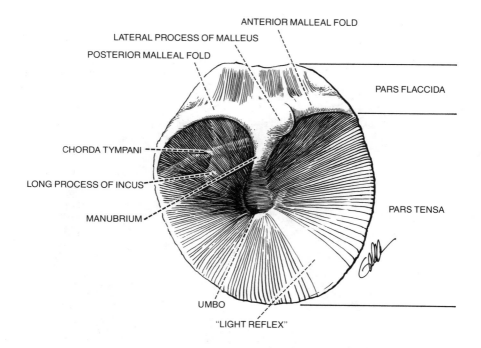

ANTERIOR MALLEAL FOLD

LATERAL PROCESS OF MALLEUS

POSTERIOR MALLEAL FOLD

PARS FLACCIDA

CHORDA TYMPANI

LONG PROCESS OF INCUS

PARS TENSA

MANUBRIUM

UMBO

"LIGHT REFLEX"

Figure 1.3 Otoscopic view of the tympanic membrane, which is divided into the pars flaccida and pars tensa by the anterior and posterior malleal folds

ossicular chain. Third, it protects the round window – the second opening between the middle and inner ear – from sound waves, thus providing an important acoustic phase difference between the oval and round windows.

Middle ear and mastoid cell system

The middle ear and eustachian tube are derived from the dorsal end of the first pharyngeal pouch. The pneumatization of the mastoid is limited at birth to the antrum, the mastoid cell area closest to the middle ear. There is wide variability in the extent of pneumatization, which progresses during the first 2 decades of life.

The medial two-thirds of the eustachian tube is cartilaginous and ends in the nasopharynx. It is normally closed and opens during swallowing, owing to the muscular activity of the tensor veli palatini.

Ossicles

The ossicular chain consists of the malleus, incus and stapes (Figures 1.1 and 1.2). Their function is to transmit mechanical energy from the tympanic membrane across the air-filled middle ear to the fluid-filled inner ear. The malleus is the longest ossicle, but only the manubrium and a portion of the neck are visible by otoscopy. The head of the malleus lies above the level of the tympanic membrane in the epitympanum. There it articulates with the body of the incus, which in turn articulates with the head, or capitulum, of the stapes. The ossicles are suspended within the middle ear by the suspensory, anterior and lateral ligaments of the malleus and the posterior ligament of the incus.

The relative lengths of the malleus and incus and their axis of rotation produce a mechanical advantage, a lever mechanism, which results in a gain of approximately 2.5 db as sound is transmitted through the middle ear. An additional mechanical advantage is achieved through a hydraulic effect that results from the ratio between the effective surface areas of the tympanic membrane (approximately 55 mm^2) and the stapes footplate (approximately 3.2 mm^2). This ratio provides an additional gain of 25 db.

The ossicular chain, with the exception of the stapes footplate, is derived from the first and second branchial arches. Middle ear abnormalities and conductive hearing loss are commonly associated with first and second branchial arch syndromes such as Crouzon's disease and Treacher–Collins syndrome.

There are two middle ear muscles: the stapedius and tensor tympani. The stapedius originates in the bony facial canal, inserts on the capitulum or neck of the stapes and is innervated by the seventh cranial nerve. The tensor tympani originates in a semicanal superior to the eustachian tube, inserts at the neck of the malleus and is innervated by the fifth cranial nerve. It is thought that these muscles decrease the compliance of the ossicular chain and tympanic membrane and may serve a protective role in the presence of intense auditory stimulation.

Inner ear and internal auditory canal

The inner ear is contained in the bony otic capsule. The membranous labyrinth is divided anatomically into two parts: the auditory portion, or cochlea, and the vestibular labyrinth, consisting of the three semicircular canals, the utricle and the saccule (Figure 1.4). The entire membranous labyrinth, both auditory and vestibular, is suspended in perilymphatic

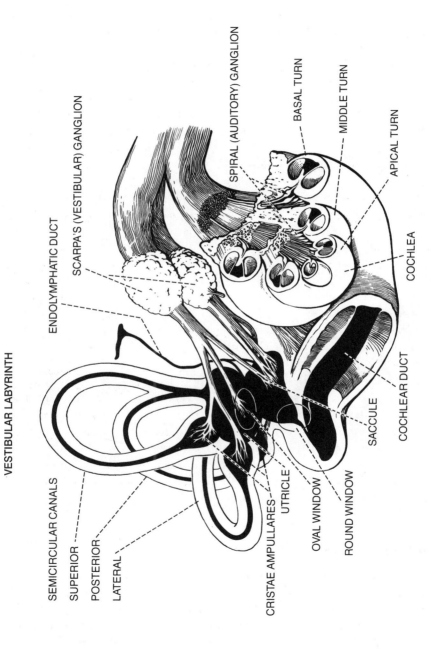

Figure 1.4 Inner ear. The cochlea has been sectioned along the modiolus. The endolymphatic space is shown in black

fluid, which is contained by the surrounding bony otic capsule (Figure 1.5). Perilymph is similar chemically to extracellular fluid and cerebrospinal fluid (CSF). The perilymphatic space surrounds the entire membranous labyrinth and is continuous with the subarachnoid space around the nerves of the internal auditory canal and via the cochlear aqueduct. It is thought that perilymph is produced not only by simple diffusion of CSF into the inner ear, but also as an ultrafiltrate of plasma. The continuity of perilymph and CSF provides a route of infection from the ear to the CSF and vice versa.

The membranous labyrinth, which is suspended like a complex balloon within the perilymph, contains endolymph. This fluid is most similar to intracellular fluid and has a very high potassium level (150 ± 10 mEq). The endolymphatic fluid space of the cochlear system is connected to that of the vestibular system by a narrow duct, the ductus reuniens (Figure 1.5). It is thought that the stria vascularis of the cochlear portion of the membranous labyrinth and the dark cell area of the vestibular portion are responsible for the production of endolymph. The endolymphatic duct and sac, which extends from the utricle and saccule into the posterior fossa, is thought to be at least partly responsible for resorption of endolymph. The exact mechanism for maintenance of the ionic gradients between perilymph and endolymph is not known. The ionic gradient creates a voltage gradient or 'endocochlear potential' within the inner ear. This in turn is important for the transducer function of the cochlea, i.e. transforming mechanical input into electrical responses in the eighth nerve.

The neuroepithelium of both the auditory and vestibular systems lies at an interface between the perilymph and endolymph. The internal and external hair cells, lying in a spiral array on the basilar membrane, are the auditory receptor cells of the organ of Corti (Figure 1.6). The mechanical properties of the basilar membrane allow a maximal point of vibration at a different site along its length for each frequency in the physiologic range. Displacement of the basilar membrane leads to stimulation of the hair cells, which in turn causes depolarization of the first order cochlear neuron and the conduction of an action potential. Thus, the basilar membrane serves as a first order frequency analyzer. High frequency sounds are detected at the basal end of the cochlea; low frequency sounds are detected at the apical end (Figure 1.4). The afferent signals from each ear are transmitted via the auditory nerve to several brain-stem nuclei and to both cerebral hemispheres.

The semicircular canals of the vestibular apparatus lie in the three planes of space (Figure 1.4). The sense organs, or cristae ampullares, are

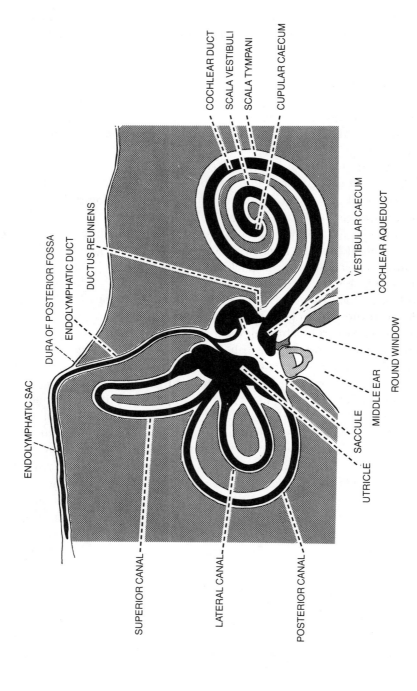

Figure 1.5 Schematic drawing of the fluid spaces of the inner ear. The endolymphatic space is shown in black. The perilymphatic space is shown in white

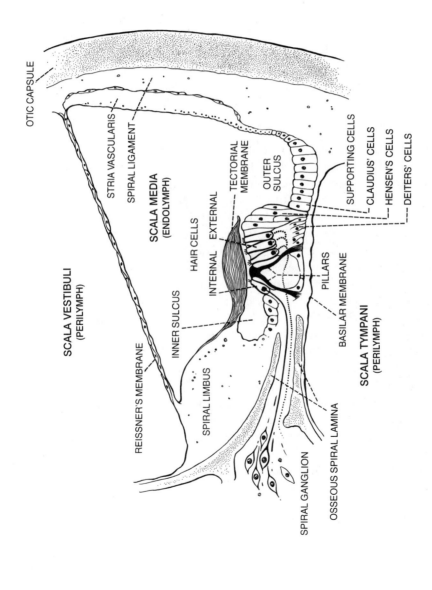

Figure 1.6 Radial section of the organ of Corti

sensitive to angular acceleration in the plane of each canal. Two additional sense organs, the maculae, are contained in the utricle and saccule. The overlying otolithic membrane allows the macula to be sensitive to linear acceleration, or gravitational pull. As in the cochlea, displacement of the inner ear fluid by rotation of the head in the semicircular canals, or in the case of the macules, displacement of the otolithic membrane by gravitational pull, results in stimulation of hair cells, which in turn causes depolarization of first order vestibular neurons. The afferent impulse is then transmitted to the vestibular nuclei in the brain stem. Both auditory and vestibular nerves pass from the inner ear through the internal auditory canal and the subarachnoid space to brain-stem nuclei.

Facial nerve

Because of the anatomical relationships between the facial nerve and other structures of the inner ear, disorders of the facial nerve are often treated by the otolaryngologist. The motor root of the facial nerve originates in the facial nucleus of the pontine brain stem (Figure 1.7). The nerve passes through the anterosuperior aspect of the internal auditory canal, adjacent to auditory and vestibular nerves. The nerve then passes through the geniculate ganglion, which contains the cell bodies of sensory fibers that also travel in the trunk of the nerve. The course of the nerve bends sharply posteriorly at the first genu and then sharply inferiorly at the second genu near the stapes footplate. It then descends in the bony fallopian canal in the most anterior part of the mastoid and exits at the skull base through the stylomastoid foramen. The nerve trifurcates at the pes anserinus shortly after its exit from the stylomastoid foramen and innervates the muscles of facial expression. The motor root of the facial nerve innervates the muscles of facial expression, the stapedius, the occipitalis, the buccinator, the platysma, the stylohyoid and the posterior belly of the digastric. The facial nuclei in the pons receive input via the corticofacial fibers in the pyramidal tract (responsible for voluntary facial movements); via the craniofacial fibers in the extrapyramidal system (responsible for non-voluntary facial movements); and from various brain-stem nuclei (responsible for reflex movements, such as the corneal and blink reflexes). These various inputs are important in evaluating facial paralysis (see Chapter 5).

The nervus intermedius portion of the facial nerve contains somatic sensory, visceral afferent, taste and general visceral efferent fibers. The somatic sensory fibers carry sensation from the posterior aspect of the

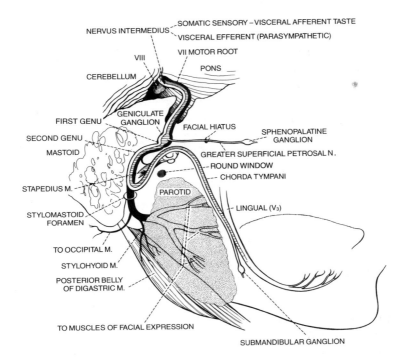

Figure 1.7 Diagram of the course of the facial nerve. The facial nerve has both motor (black) and sensory fibers. The sensory fibers have their cell bodies in the geniculate ganglion and together with the visceral efferent fibers are called the nervus intermedius. The visceral afferent fibers are shown in white, the visceral efferent fibers as striped

external auditory canal and synapse in the spinal tract of the fifth cranial nerve. The visceral afferents carry sensation from the pharynx, nose and palate to the tractus solitarius by way of the greater superficial petrosal nerve. Taste from the anterior two-thirds of the tongue is transmitted to the nucleus of the tractus solitarius by way of the chorda tympani branch of the facial nerve. General visceral efferent fibers pass through the nervus intermedius portion of the facial nerve from the superior salivatory nucleus as preganglionic parasympathetic fibers. These fibers pass peripherally either through the greater superficial petrosal nerve to the lacrimal gland and the glands of the nose and palatine mucosa or through the chorda tympani nerve and submandibular ganglion to the submandibular and sublingual glands.

EXAMINATION OF THE EAR

Inspection and cleaning

Cerumen, which is produced in specialized apocrine glands located in the lateral one-third of the external auditory canal, often accumulates in sufficient quantity to interfere with examination of the canal and drum. Ninety-five per cent of Whites and Blacks have dark, oily wax. Most Asians have dry, light, flaky wax. Wax may be removed by irrigation with water at body temperature or mechanically using either a loop or a ring curette, a handheld speculum and a headlight or mirror. Impacted cerumen may be softened by 3% hydrogen peroxide drops used three times daily for 3 days prior to removal.

Otoscopy

By positioning the seated patient with his head tilted backwards approximately 30°, the examiner has a clear view of the ear canal and tympanic membrane without resorting to contortions of his own head and neck. Retraction of the auricle posteriorly will facilitate insertion of the speculum by straightening the external canal and dilating the meatus. With his dominant hand the examiner straightens the external canal by pulling on the auricle posterosuperiorly in the adult and posteriorly in the child. Once the speculum is inserted, the auricle may be released, and the examiner's dominant hand is freed for other manipulation. The examiner should hold the otoscope in his non-dominant hand to free his dominant hand for manipulation or suctioning of the external canal. In a child or a combative adult the examiner should place the fifth finger of the hand holding the otoscope against the squamous portion of the patient's skull to prevent injury to the skin of the external canal during head movements.

Examination of the ear canal and tympanic membrane should be performed in an orderly fashion, starting with a circumferential inspection of the bony external canal. The most constant landmark in the diseased tympanic membrane is the lateral process of the malleus. The examiner should identify this first, because it will automatically orient him as to the location of the pars flaccida and the pars tensa. The pneumatic otoscopic head allows the examiner to induce movements of the drum and therefore to determine the presence of fluid or masses behind the tympanic membrane. In addition, moving the tympanic membrane may make healed perforations of the tympanic membrane that are almost transparent more visible. Additional magnification may be achieved by using a binocular operating microscope.

The otoscope findings can be summarized by diagramming the tympanic membrane as a circle and the malleus as an obtuse angle formed at the lateral process of the malleus (Figure 1.8). Perforations may be illustrated simply by outlining the location in red. Pathology visualized in the middle ear may be the result of more significant disease in the nasopharynx. Hence, nasopharyngoscopy should be performed routinely in cases of serous otitis media in adults to rule out a neoplastic process.

Eustachian tube function may be evaluated by examining the movement of the tympanic membrane while the patient performs a modified Valsalva maneuver. This is done by filling the patient's oropharynx with air and having him blow out against closed lips and nose or by having the patient blow up a balloon. If there is a perforation, the function of the tube may be evaluated by listening through a small rubber catheter or Toynbee tube placed in the external auditory canal while the patient swallows or performs a modified Valsalva maneuver. With good tubal function, a hiss of air will be heard. If these techniques fail, more forceful insufflation of air into the patient's middle ear may be achieved by

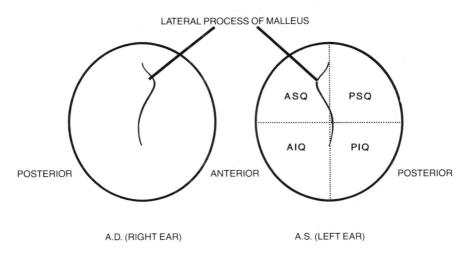

A.D. (RIGHT EAR)   A.S. (LEFT EAR)

Figure 1.8 Schematic representation of both ear drums used to diagram pathology. The principal anatomical landmark is the malleus and its lateral process. The drum may be divided into four quadrants as shown in the diagram of the left ear. ASQ, anterosuperior quadrant; PSQ, posterosuperior quadrant; AIQ, anteroinferior quadrant; PIQ, posteroinferior quadrant

politzerization. This consists of forcing air through one naris of the nose with the other naris occluded while the patient swallows or says 'kick' or 'Coca-Cola' to lift the soft palate and close the nasopharynx. The air source may be a Politzer bag or low-pressure compressed air. Tympanometry, as discussed below, may also be used to supplement clinical evaluation of tubal function.

Tests of auditory function

Tuning fork and whisper tests

It is advisable to perform tuning fork and whisper tests on all patients even though audiology may be obtained subsequently. The Rinne test is based on a comparison of sound conduction by bone with sound transmission through the air of the external auditory canal. A 512-cycle/s fork is best for this purpose. The fork is struck against the examiner's knee or a rubber pad and held firmly against the patient's mastoid bone where the skin is thinnest. The examiner's opposite hand must be used for counterpressure to ensure firm apposition of tuning fork to bone. The tuning fork is then held at the external auditory canal with the two blades of the tuning fork aligned with the axis of the external canal. In most adults and some young children, a modified Rinne test is performed by asking the patient to compare the loudness of the stimulus transmitted by bone and air. If this is confusing to the patient, the classical Rinne test may be performed by holding the base of the fork against the patient's mastoid process until the tone is no longer heard. The fork is then held at the external auditory canal, and the patient is asked whether the tone is still audible. The Rinne test is recorded as positive if air conduction is superior to bone conduction or negative if the converse is true. When the Rinne test is positive, the hearing may be normal or sensorineural hearing loss may be present. A negative Rinne test usually implies conductive hearing loss. However, a 'false-negative Rinne test' may be produced by ipsilateral profound sensorineural deafness and transmission of sound by bone conduction to the opposite ear.

The Weber test is a test of lateralization of sound and is performed with the same tuning fork. The fork is placed on a midline structure such as the patient's forehead or the vertex of his skull. The patient is asked in which ear, if either, the sound is heard to be louder. In sensorineural hearing loss the sound will be heard in the midline or will lateralize to the better hearing ear; in conductive hearing loss it will lateralize to the poorer hearing ear. This test is particularly sensitive if the fork is placed on the central incisors of the maxilla.

Hearing acuity can be estimated by using voice tests. A series of spondaic words, such as 'baseball', 'hot dog', 'earthquake', 'sidewalk', 'mousetrap' and 'greyhound', is spoken at graded intensities at the external canal, and an approximation of threshold is made. A whisper lies in the range of 0–30 db hearing level (HL), normal conversational speech between 40 and 60 db HL and a shout between 60 and 90 db HL. Masking of the opposite ear must be done and is best achieved using the Barany noisemaker, which can achieve masking levels of approximately 80 db (see Appendix 2). Comparison of whisper tests with subsequent behavioral audiometry will, over time, titrate the examiner and provide a check on the audiometry.

Behavioral audiometry (standard hearing tests)

The best test of auditory function in a cooperative child or adult is behavioral audiometry. Thresholds of frequencies between 250 and 8000 cycle/s are measured in db HL (a scale of loudness with 0 db HL being the threshold of normal controls at each frequency). Air conduction and bone conduction are measured separately in each ear. If there is hearing loss, masking may be necessary in the contralateral ear, because sounds of 40 db and greater will be transmitted by bone conduction across the skull to the opposite ear. The various symbols for masked and unmasked air conduction and bone conduction are illustrated in Figure 1.9.

With normal hearing, both air conduction and bone conduction will be superimposed at each test frequency between 0 and 10 db. It is important to realize that 0 db HL is the threshold for both bone conduction and air conduction and that the normal superiority of air conduction over bone conduction is taken into account by the normalization of testing. If air conduction is inferior to bone conduction, a conductive hearing loss is present (Figure 1.9c). A conductive hearing loss is due to a disorder in the external auditory canal, tympanic membrane or middle ear. A sensorineural hearing loss is indicated by a bone curve lying below the 0–10-db threshold at any frequency tested (Figure 1.9d). This implies pathology in the inner ear or auditory neural pathways.

After pure-tone audiometry is performed, the speech reception threshold (SRT) is determined for each ear. Beginning at a level approximately 20 db above the average of the three midfrequencies, two-syllable words of equal stress (spondees) are presented in 2-db decrements. The SRT is defined as the faintest level at which the patient can correctly identify

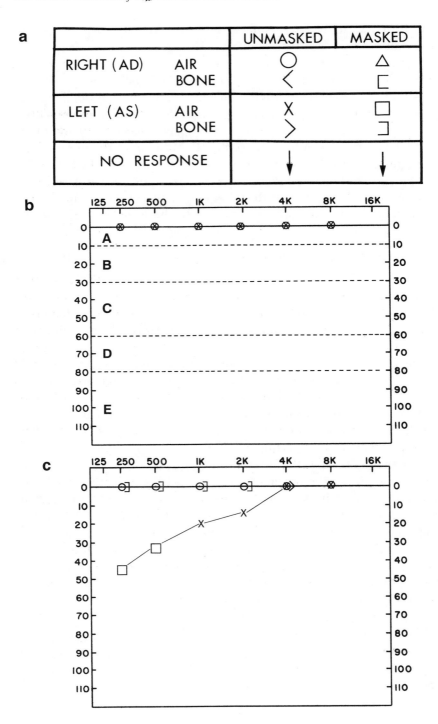

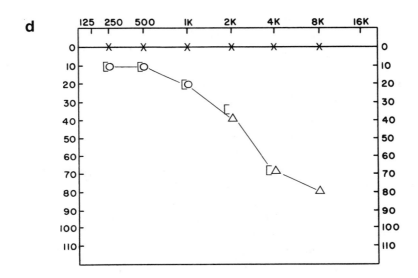

Figure 1.9 *(see also previous page)* (a) Symbols used in behavioral audiometry. (b) A normal audiogram. The hearing threshold for both ears is 0 db HL at each frequency tested. **A** Normal hearing (0–20 db, if both ears hear equally). A small hearing loss relative to the other ear can be detected and still be within the normal range. Perfectly normal hearing should be in the 0–10-db range. Most speech, except for fricatives, falls within the 750–2000 Hz frequency range. **B** Mild hearing loss (20–35 db). The patient is aware of hearing difficulty when there is background noise or when in groups. He must concentrate in school and at meetings. Preferential seating is beneficial. **C** Moderate hearing loss (35–50 db). Impaired communication. The patient hears a loud conversational voice in a one-to-one situation but is confused by background noise. He has difficulty hearing on the telephone. Hearing aid(s) are advisable when discrimination scores are good. Most patients begin to lip-read. **D** Severe hearing loss (50–80 db). Amplification (hearing aids) is mandatory. The value of the hearing aid depends in large part on the patient's ability to understand. Hearing aid use is much better if discrimination scores are greater than 80%. **E** Profound hearing loss (80 db or greater): hearing aids are of adjunctive value only. Many patients cannot hear their own voice and therefore speech may be affected. Powerful body hearing aids are usually employed. Profound hearing losses are usually accompanied by poor discrimination. (c) Normal hearing in the right ear and a low-frequency conductive hearing loss in the left ear. Masking of the right ear with white noise during testing of the left ear is required, because of the large difference in hearing between right and left. The masked bone conduction is normal in the left ear, but air conduction hearing is reduced for the low frequencies, indicating a conductive hearing loss (for explanation of symbols, see (a)). (d) Normal hearing in the left ear and a descending sensorineural hearing loss in the right ear. The masked bone conduction is the same as the air conduction in the right ear, indicating a sensorineural hearing loss. Masking for bone-conduction testing is almost always required. Masking for air conduction is required if a differential of more than 40 db exists between the ears. Because of the slope of this audiogram, one would expect the discrimination score to be affected as well (for explanation of symbols, see (a))

approximately 50% of the words. The purpose of speech-reception testing is twofold. First, it serves to confirm the patient's midfrequency pure-tone responses, and second, it determines the intensity at which subsequent speech discrimination tasks are to be presented. The spondaic words for determination of SRT in Table 1.1 are useful for office whisper testing. Alternatively, a pure-tone average (PTA) may be calculated using thresholds at 0.5, 1, 2 and 3 or 0.5, 1, 2 and 4 kHz.

Pure-tone levels are not a complete indication of how well the patient hears, because comprehension also depends on discrimination ability. The word discrimination test is performed at a level approximately 40 db above the previously determined SRT or PTA for each ear in order to approximate a comfortable level for the comprehension of speech. Masking is used in the contralateral ear, and a list of 50 phonetically balanced, monosyllabic words such as 'yes', 'church' and 'boy' is read to, and repeated by, the patient. The patient's discrimination score is reported as the percentage of words identified correctly. Discrimination testing also provides diagnostic information as to the site of a lesion. In the instance of conductive hearing loss or sensorineural loss with pathology at the cochlear hair cell level, the speech discrimination score will be above 80%. On the other hand, when the primary site of hearing loss is neuronal (retrocochlear), very low discrimination scores are the rule.

Flat hearing losses are usually associated with good discrimination scores. Individuals with flat hearing losses are good candidates for satisfactory hearing-aid usage. In general, the more steeply a hearing loss slopes into the high frequencies, the worse the discrimination scores. Patients with poor speech discrimination complain that they hear, but do not understand. Although amplification is useful, it does not solve this problem.

Table 1.1   Spondaic words for determination of the speech reception threshold

Greyhound	Hot dog
Schoolboy	Padlock
Inkwell	Mushroom
Whitewash	Hardware
Pancake	Workshop
Eardrum	Horseshoe
Headlight	Armchair
Birthday	Baseball
Duck pond	Stairway
Sidewalk	Cowboy

Special behavioral tests

'Recruitment' signifies an abnormally rapid growth of sensation of loudness in a diseased ear. In the clinic, the patient will complain that loud noises are 'too loud' or that they 'irritate' his affected ear. The presence of recruitment is an indication of a cochlear, rather than a retrocochlear, lesion.

A 512-Hz tuning fork can be used to assess recruitment. First, the fork is struck softly, and the patient compares the sound level heard in one ear to the sound level heard in the other. Then the fork is struck sharply, and the process is repeated. In the second instance, if recruitment is present the sound should be perceived in the diseased ear as equal to or louder than in the normal ear.

One specific audiologic test for the measurement of recruitment is the alternate binaural loudness balance test (ABLB). The patient is asked to compare the loudness of two tones of the same frequency that are presented alternately to the unimpaired and impaired ear until the tones are perceived as being of equal relative loudness.

The tone-decay test detects abnormal function of the auditory nerve. In this instance, a constant sound will be perceived as fading out over a 60-second period in the patient's affected ear(s). An objective measurement of tone decay is made by presenting a barely perceptible pure tone and recording the increment in decibels necessary for the patient to sustain perception of the tone for 60 seconds. A positive test (30 db or greater of added sound energy) suggests that the primary site of hearing loss is neuronal and is often interpreted as an indication of retrocochlear (auditory nerve) pathology. In most clinics this test has been superseded by auditory evoked response testing to evaluate the site of a lesion.

Summary of special behavioral audiometry tests to determine the site of a lesion

(1) *Discrimination score* Low score indicates retrocochlear (i.e. auditory nerve) pathology;

(2) *Recruitment* Positive recruitment test indicates cochlear injury;

(3) *Tone decay* Positive test indicates auditory nerve pathology.

Békésy audiometry is an automated audiometric test that compares the test subject's threshold for a continuously presented tone with his threshold for an interrupted tone. Five types of tracings are described. This test is not used routinely. Its principal function is rapid automated screening.

Auditory evoked response testing

Behavioral audiometry may be difficult or impossible to perform in patients under the age of 2.5 years or in adults with emotional or neurologic disorders. In such patients, auditory evoked response techniques may be useful in approximating a threshold and in screening for retrocochlear pathology. This technique is based on computer summation of evoked responses from the cochlea, auditory nerve and brain-stem pathways in response to an acoustic stimulus (click).

Depending on the electrode placement and the time window after the stimulation, one may selectively examine electrical activity at the cochlear, eighth nerve, brain stem or cortical levels. When the parameters of the recording are set up to detect activity in the cochlea and eighth nerve, the testing is called electrocochleography. When set up for waves generated from the auditory pathway within the brain stem, the recording is called a brain stem evoked response (BSER). When set up for the auditory portion of the electroencephalogram (EEG), the recording is called a cortical evoked response. Unlike electrocochleography and BSER, cortical evoked responses are drastically altered by various drugs or varying levels of attention.

The BSER is the most popular of these three techniques, because it can be performed with surface electrodes rather than canal or middle ear electrodes, which are required in electrocochleography. In addition, electrocochleography requires a local anesthetic in the adult and a general anesthetic in the child. Furthermore, the BSER provides information at the level not only of the eighth nerve, but also of the brain stem. The findings of this test are unchanged by state of awareness, pharmacologic levels of drugs or general anesthesia. In addition to approximation of hearing (pure tone) threshold, the BSER has also proved useful in evaluating patients for retrocochlear pathology. The BSER requires no anesthesia in an adult, and in a child it may be performed during natural sleep or under mild sedation.

By means of a summating computer, the BSER measures the electrical response of the auditory system to a series of rapid clicks that can be presented to the ear at different intensities. Once the sounds have exceeded the hearing threshold, a series of waveforms numbered 1 to 7 can be detected within the first 10 ms. The first wave represents the action potential from the eighth nerve, the second is probably generated at the cochlear nucleus and the others have complex origins from progressively higher centers in the brain stem. Each wave peak has an expected latency.

The fifth peak is the largest and most predictable and is therefore used as an indicator of hearing threshold level by the BSER (Figures 1.10a and b). Because of computer averaging, semiautomated recordings of the BSER can be mde in relatively high ambient noise, such as a neonatal intensive care unit where newborns are screened for hearing loss.

Conductive hearing losses and cochlear injuries will raise waveform thresholds but in general will not change the waveforms or interwave latencies. Eighth nerve and brain-stem injuries such as tumors or multiple sclerosis do cause waveform distortions and increased interwave latencies, thus making the test a very sensitive indicator of pathology in these regions (Figure 1.10c).

Otoacoustic emissions

The normal ear emits a faint sound in response to acoustic stimuli. These evoked otoacoustic emissions (EOAE) can be easily detected using a sound source and a microphone in the ear canal. Three classes of EOAE have been described, depending on the acoustic stimulus required to evoke them:

(1) Transient EOAE elicited by acoustic clicks or tone pips;

(2) Stimulus frequency EOAE elicited by sustained pure tone stimulation;

(3) Distortion product EOAE elicited by two simultaneous pure tones.

Transient and distortion product EOAE can be used clinically to screen for hearing loss in neonates. In addition, because EOAE are thought to be generated by outer hair cells, these emissions can theoretically be used for site of lesion (cochlear vs. retrocochlear) testing.

Tympanometry

For tympanometry, or impedance audiometry, the ear canal is sealed and the pressure within the external auditory canal is varied. With the use of a probe tone the impedance, or conversely the compliance, of the eardrum and attached ossicular chain may be measured. This technique may be helpful in the diagnosis of middle ear disorders and is frequently used as an adjunct to audiometry in the screening of schoolchildren, because they have a high incidence of otitis media.

Five types of tympanograms have been identified (Figure 1.11). Type A demonstrates a normal middle ear compliance. Type As demonstrates

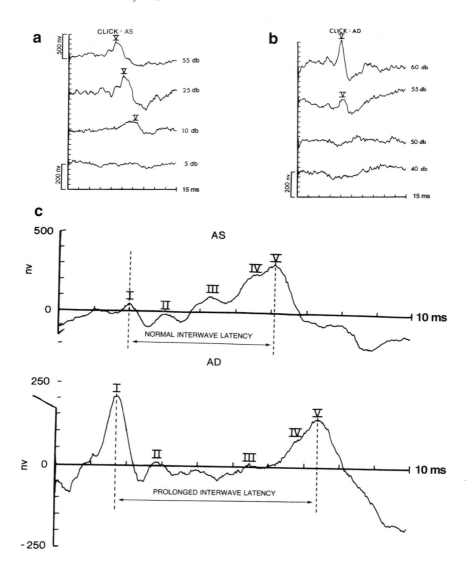

Figure 1.10 Hearing threshold determination using brain-stem evoked response (BSER) audiometry. Wave V is normally detectable at a threshold at or below 10 db. (b) Hearing threshold determination using BSER audiometry. The threshold for wave V is approximately 50 db, suggesting approximately 40 db of hearing loss in the right ear. (c) Waveforms from BSER audiometry in a documented case of vestibular schwannoma in the right ear. The absolute latency of wave V and the interwave latency (I–V) are prolonged in the right ear, suggesting retrocochlear pathology

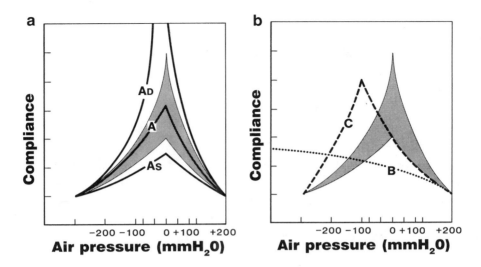

Figure 1.11 (a) Tympanometry patterns. The normal range is indicated by the shaded area. A, normal tympanogram; As, 'stiffness' lesion. Stiffness of the ossicular chain will demonstrate a peak at normal pressures, but decreased compliance. This pattern may be seen in otosclerosis; AD, 'discontinuity pattern'. There is infinite compliance and an extrapolated peak at normal pressure. This is due to a disruption of the ossicular chain or an extremely flaccid tympanic membrane. (b) B, no peak compliance – consistent with middle ear effusion (such as serous otitis or acute otitis media). C, compliance is in the normal range, but a peak at −150 mmH$_2$0 is consistent with negative middle ear pressure. This is a sign of early eustachian tube blockage or otitis media

decreased compliance at each pressure tested, which is consistent with stiffness of the ossicular chain. Type AD shows infinite compliance and is consistent with ossicular discontinuity. Type B shows no point of maximum compliance and very little change in compliance over the range of −200 to +200 mmH$_2$O and is consistent with middle ear effusion. Type C is similar to type A except that the maximum point of compliance is found by applying negative pressure to the external auditory canal, and this is consistent with partial eustachian tube dysfunction and middle ear atelectasis.

Because the contraction of the stapedius muscle results in measurable changes in the impedance of the tympanic membrane, the same equipment may be used for measuring the acoustic reflex threshold (ART) and acoustic reflex decay (ARD). The ART has been used as a somewhat rough but objective measurement of hearing in neonates and in patients who are difficult to test, and as a means of corroborating behavior threshold. In addition, the ART and ARD may be used in conjunction with ipsilateral and contralateral stimuli as a means of evaluating the site of a lesion in sensorineural hearing loss.

Tests for functional hearing loss

In patients suspected of malingering or of having psychogenic deafness, special behavior tests such as the Stenger, Lombard and delayed feedback tests may be used by the audiologist. The BSER may also be used for this purpose in totally uncooperative patients.

VESTIBULAR TESTING

Caloric tests

The single best office test of the vestibular system is caloric testing. This may be performed in an office setting, using Frenzel's lenses to prevent ocular fixation. First, the eyes are examined for spontaneous nystagmus. Second, the ear canal and drum are checked for obstruction or perforation. Third, the minimal caloric test, or Kobrak test, is performed by the instillation of 5 ml water at 80°F (27°C) with the patient in a sitting position and the head inclined backwards 60°. The time of onset and time of termination of nystagmus are noted. After 10 min, the opposite ear is tested. If no response is achieved with water at 80°F, 5 ml iced water is used. The range of normal response to thermal calorics is great; hence, this test is best applied to a unilateral lesion by comparison with the opposite normal side. Nystagmus is more accurately measured with the use of electronystagmography (ENG) (see Chapter 4). When there is a perforation of the tympanic membrane, thermal stimulation can be performed by using 2 ml iced sterile saline or otic drops. For a full discussion of vestibular function tests, see Chapter 4.

Positional testing

If a patient complains of vertigo that occurs in one position only, positional testing should be performed. The patient is placed on an examination table so that his head hangs over the end of the table. The following positions are assumed by the patient with the examiner controlling the patient's head: head hanging; head hanging with left ear down; head hanging with right ear down. Between each position the patient is brought to the fully erect position. The examiner records whether vestibular symptoms are present, whether nystagmus is present, whether the onset of nystagmus is immediate or delayed and whether the nystagmus fatigues by maintaining the provocative position or by repeating the provocative position. The most common form of positional nystagmus is benign positional nystagmus, or vertigo, also called cupulolithiasis. In this disorder the nystagmus is rotatory, demonstrates a latency of several seconds and fatigues; there is an intense feeling of vertigo with the affected ear downward. The Aschan classification of positional nystagmus is commonly used.

Aschan classification of positional nystagmus

(1) *Type I* Nystagmus is non-fatiguable, and direction changes with head position;

(2) *Type II* Nystagmus is non-fatiguable, but direction remains fixed despite change of head position;

(3) *Type III* There is positional nystagmus in any direction but it demonstrates definite latency and fatigue.

Patients with type I findings almost always have a central disorder. Those with type II may have a peripheral vestibular disorder, but again most patients with type II findings have central disorders. Type III findings are almost always peripheral in origin.

Fistula test

In the fistula test, objective nystagmus and a subjective sensation of unsteadiness or shift in body position may be induced by changing the pressure in the external auditory canal. This is most conveniently achieved with a Politzer bag with an olive tip while the examiner observes the patient's eyes with Frenzel's lenses. In the presence of chronic otitis media, a positive test usually implies a labyrinthine fistula due to cholesteatoma. With an intact eardrum, a positive test has been described in congenital syphilis (Hennebert's sign) and Ménière's disease.

FACIAL NERVE TESTS

It is often valuable in cases of facial paralysis to determine first, the sites of involvement of the facial nerve in its anatomical course from the brain stem to the periphery; and second, whether the lesion is caused by degeneration of the nerve fibers (neurotmesis or axonotmesis) or simply a physiologic block (neuropraxia).

Site-of-lesion testing

Because of the mixed nature of the facial nerve, with motor, somatosensory, viscerosensory, taste and visceral efferent components, the site of a lesion may be evaluated in several ways:

(1) *Salivary flow test (chorda tympani)* The submaxillary ducts are anesthetized and cannulated with no. 60 polyethylene tubing. Lemon juice is used to stimulate salivary flow, and the number of drops secreted per minute on each side is compared. A difference of 70% or more between the two sides is considered significant.

(2) *Taste (chorda tympani)* Taste can be compared on the two sides either with physiologic stimuli, such as concentrated salt and sugar solutions, or with an electrogustometer.

(3) *Stapedial reflex* The function of the stapedial branch (motor division) is tested with impedance audiometry techniques.

(4) *Lacrimation (greater superficial petrosal nerve at the level of the geniculate ganglion)* This is evaluated by Schirmer's test.

Neurophysiologic tests of neuronal viability

There are a number of tests, each with limitations, that over time will differentiate between neuropraxia and nerve degeneration. These include the nerve excitability test, electromyography and electroneurography. All of these require special equipment. The major limitation of the neurophysiologic tests is that, even in the case of total transection of a nerve, transmission as tested distal to the site of the lesion will be little affected for approximately 3 days. For a more complete description of facial nerve testing, see Chapter 5.

OTHER OFFICE OTOLOGIC TESTING

Depending on the suspected disease process, elements of the standard neurologic testing (cranial nerve, cerebellar and gait) may be necessary.

Selected readings

Janfaza P, Nadol JB Jr, Galla R, Fabian RL, Montgomery WW. *Surgical Anatomy of the Head and Neck*. Philadelphia: Lippincott Williams & Wilkins, 2001

Schuknecht HF, Gulya AJ. *Anatomy of the Temporal Bone with Surgical Implications*. Philadelphia: Lea & Febiger, 1986

Lonsbury-Martin BL, Martin GK, McCory MJ, Whitehead ML. New approaches to evaluation of the auditory system and a current analysis of otoacoustic emissions. *Otolaryngol Head Neck Surg* 1995;112:50–63

2

Hearing loss

Joseph B. Nadol, Jr

Definitions and history taking
Specific diagnoses
Conductive hearing loss
   Conductive hearing loss secondary to obstruction of the external canal
      Cerumen
      Foreign body
      External otitis
      Developmental defects
      Exostoses and osteomas
   Conductive hearing loss secondary to disorders of the tympanic
      membrane
      Hyalinization and tympanosclerosis
      Perforation
   Conductive hearing loss due to disorders of the middle ear
      Effusions
      Mass lesions within the middle ear
      Malleus fixation
      Incus resorption
      Stapes fixation
Sensorineural hearing loss
   Bilateral sensorineural hearing loss
      Presbycusis
   Genetically determined sensorineural hearing loss
   Congenital, non-hereditary deafness
   Ototoxicity
Unilateral or asymmetrical sensorineural hearing loss
   Otitis media
   Bacterial meningitis
   Direct trauma
   Acoustic trauma

    Perilymph leaks
    Syphilis
    Neurologic disorders
    Neoplasms
        Cerebellopontine angle tumors
    Hearing loss associated with other metabolic or systemic disorders
        Arterial disease
        Other metabolic disorders
    Disorders of unknown or immune-mediated cause
        Ménière's disease
        Collagen vascular diseases
        Immune-mediated sensorineural hearing loss
        Sudden idiopathic sensorineural deafness
Tinnitus
Hearing aids and cochlear implants
    Hearing aids
    Cochlear implants

DEFINITIONS AND HISTORY TAKING

To evaluate hearing loss, the examiner must have in mind a diagnostic strategy in order to establish whether or not the hearing loss requires urgent treatment and which additional diagnostic tests are necessary to determine its cause. Several aspects of the clinical history are critical in this evaluation:

(1) Is the hearing loss unilateral or bilateral? Generally speaking, a unilateral loss, especially sensorineural hearing loss (SNHL), will require more diagnostic work-up.

(2) Is the hearing loss slowly progressive or was the onset sudden? A sudden hearing loss may require emergency treatment. Slowly progressive bilateral symmetrical sensorineural hearing loss suggests such etiologies as genetic causes or the degeneration of aging. Sudden or rapidly progressive SNHL suggests the possibility of infection, trauma, tumor, or toxic or immune-mediated disease.

(3) Are there any associated symptoms that will help differentiate various causes of hearing loss?

(a) Is there tinnitus? Subjective tinnitus, or head noise, is a sound, apparently produced in the hearing centers of the midbrain, that may accompany both sensorineural and conductive hearing loss. Objective tinnitus can be heard by the examiner as well as by the patient by using a Toynbee tube. Pulsatile tinnitus may be due to an arterial–venous malformation, a partial arterial occlusion and bruit, or a vascular tumor, such as a glomus tumor, in or near the ear.

(b) Are there vestibular symptoms? Here, the terminology used in questioning a patient is important. Patients often do not understand the meaning of the term 'vertigo', but do understand 'unsteadiness', 'imbalance' or 'spinning dizziness'. Concurrent vestibular symptoms suggest involvement of the vestibular labyrinth or vestibular nerves.

(c) Is the hearing loss associated with pain in either ear? Pain may suggest infection (viral or bacterial) or tumor.

(d) Is there any history of drainage from the ear canal at the onset of the hearing loss or preceding it?

(e) Is there history of trauma preceding the hearing loss? This is particularly important in sudden SNHL. Trauma may occur as a result of direct injury, such as a blow to the head, skull fracture, slap injury to the external canal, foreign body into the external canal or as a result of barotrauma. Barotrauma implies a sudden change in ambient pressure such as may occur during aircraft descent and scuba diving or because of an explosion. Sudden hearing loss after ear trauma requires consideration of the possibility of 'perilymph leak', ossicular disruption, temporal bone fracture or acoustic injury to the inner ear.

(f) What is the history of drug administration? Ototoxicity may present as a bilateral symmetrical or asymmetrical SNHL which is rapidly progressive or sudden in onset, with or without vestibular symptoms.

(g) Are there other associated medical illnesses, such as neurologic disturbances, either central or peripheral; blood dyscrasias; diseases of bone; a history of neoplasm that might result in metastasis to the temporal bone; or collagen vascular disease?

(h) Is there a family history of hearing loss, vestibular disturbances or other disorders (neurologic, endocrine, visual, etc.)?

(i) Is there an otologic history of similar problems, otologic surgery or other treatment?

The history taking should be followed by examination of the ear, including the auricle, external canal and tympanic membrane. The tuning fork test and clinical approximation of speech reception threshold should be performed. An audiogram or other tests can then be ordered on an emergency basis or can be planned as part of a future evaluation by the primary physician, or the patient may be referred to an otologist for these tests.

SPECIFIC DIAGNOSES

A final or working diagnosis or differential diagnosis should be made after the preliminary evaluation. In the following sections, brief descriptions of several specific disorders as well as the criteria for their diagnosis are given. The usual treatment is outlined, including possible surgical remedies. When surgery is a therapeutic alternative, a brief description of the surgery is given as well as non-surgical alternatives.

CONDUCTIVE HEARING LOSS

By definition, conductive hearing loss has the site of dysfunction in the external canal, tympanic membrane or middle ear space.

Conductive hearing loss secondary to obstruction of the external canal

Obstruction may be the result of simple cerumen accumulation, a foreign body, edema, or neoplastic or congenital obstruction of the external canal.

Cerumen

Cerumen may be removed by irrigation, suction or curettage. Irrigation may be the easiest treatment for both patient and physician, but it should not be used if a perforation of the drum is known or suspected. An additional disadvantage of irrigation is that irritation of the tympanic membrane may occur and make any further diagnosis difficult at that time. When irrigation is done, it should be performed with water maintained at body temperature to avoid a caloric response. This is best achieved with a cerumen syringe (see Appendix 2). The stream of water is directed towards the posterior canal wall so that a plane of cleavage is created between skin and wax and the full force of the water does not strike the tympanic membrane. Care should be taken to avoid a tight seal in the external canal, with resulting damage to the drum. Thermostatically controlled ear irrigation devices are available for office use.

If there is soft wax or mucopurulent debris in the external canal, suction is essential. Depending on the consistency of the obstructing material, a no. 5 or no. 20 French suction tip is used (see Appendix 2). Suction is performed using a hand-held speculum with headlight and mirror or through an otoscope or microscope.

For practiced hands, simple curettage is performed with a ring or wire curette, Hartmann's forceps (see Appendix 2), handheld speculum, and headlight and mirror. The forceps may also be used through an otoscope. Hard or particularly deep wax impactions may be removed by first being softened with a glycerol and hydrogen peroxide mixture (Debrox®, GlaxoSmithKline) three times a day for several days prior to irrigation or aspiration.

Foreign body

Foreign bodies in the ear canal are common in children and occasionally may be seen in adults. Several guidelines of therapy are in order. First and foremost, a non-emergency situation should not be made into an emergency by pushing a foreign body further into the canal and possibly damaging the drum or middle ear structures. Local or general anesthesia should be used if necessary to remove the object. Non-spherical objects may be simply grasped with alligator forceps and lifted straight out of the external canal. For spherical objects, a hook placed behind the object or a suction tip may be useful. Living insects should be drowned in mineral oil to prevent unpleasant footfalls on the tympanic membrane and then are removed *in toto* or piecemeal with ear forceps (Hartmann's or alligator) or suction. In general, irrigation should be avoided as it may cause deeper impaction of the foreign body or swelling of vegetable matter. After the foreign body has been removed, the tympanic membrane is carefully inspected to ensure that no perforation of the drum has occurred. Vestibular symptoms and signs should be sought, and the patient's hearing should be tested clinically.

External otitis

External otitis is an inflammatory process involving the skin and occasionally the cartilages of the external canal. This is often accompanied by cerumen impaction within the canal. The treatment of external otitis is outlined in Chapter 3.

Developmental defects

Atresia or dysplastic stenosis of the external auditory canal may occur alone or in association with other abnormalities of the first and second branchial arches or with other auricular deformities. Atresia of the external auditory canal is commonly associated with middle and inner ear abnormalities. Surgical correction is possible in selected cases, based on assessment of inner ear function and the severity of the malformation. In general, surgery is deferred until age 18 or older in a patient with unilateral atresia of the external canal with a contralateral normal ear. In bilateral cases with significant hearing loss, a bone-conducting hearing aid is fitted until age 5, when reconstructive surgery can be considered. In cases of atresia, surgical risks include damage to inner ear function and to the facial nerve, because it often runs an aberrant course. Consultation with an otologist should answer the following questions. What are the risks in this particular case? What is the expected gain in hearing? Is a hearing aid a reasonable option?

When auricular deformities are present and reconstruction is planned, this should be carefully coordinated with the surgery to the external canal and middle ear.

Exostoses and osteomas

Exostoses in the bony external canal usually appear as two or three bony white excrescences covered by skin. These are asymptomatic unless progressive stenosis of the bony canal results in entrapment of water or other material between the exostoses and the tympanic membrane. An osteoma presents as a singular rounded, bony protuberance, originating in the bony canal. Surgery, usually performed either through the ear canal or through an incision behind the ear, involves removal of the exostoses or osteoma with a drill or curette, followed by skin grafting of the external canal. General anesthesia is usually required, and the major risks include possible damage to the tympanic membrane or ossicular chain during the course of the surgery.

Conductive hearing loss secondary to disorders of the tympanic membrane

Hyalinization and tympanosclerosis

As a result of repeated infections of the middle ear space, hyalin may be deposited within the drum and middle ear. It appears as white plaques in the tympanic membrane and may result in hearing loss due to ossicular fixation or stiffening of the ear drum. Isolated hyaline deposits within the drum rarely produce significant hearing loss unless associated with ossicular fixation. Some patients with this form of conductive hearing loss are surgical candidates. The suitability for surgery as determined by an otologist is based on a number of considerations, including hearing on the contralateral side, the age of the patient and eustachian tube function.

Perforation

Perforations may be either marginal or central. A marginal perforation is one in which the perforation extends to the tympanic annulus. A central perforation is one that is surrounded by a remnant of normal tympanic membrane. An acute central perforation is likely to heal without intervention; a marginal perforation is less likely to do so. Furthermore, squamous epithelial ingrowth into the middle ear with subsequent cholesteatoma formation is much more common with a marginal perforation (see Chapter 3). A posterior perforation, either central or marginal, especially over the round window area, may result in a conductive hearing loss of up to 40 db. Acute perforation of the drum may result from direct trauma or barotrauma and constitutes an otologic emergency if there is evidence of injury to the ossicular chain or to the inner ear (see Chapter 5). Chronic perforations may be the result of a large, unhealed traumatic perforation or, more commonly, of chronic otitis media.

Treatment   The treatment of a chronic, dry perforation consists of myringoplasty or tympanoplasty. Repair of a perforation of the tympanic membrane may be done to correct the conductive hearing loss and because the patient desires to avoid the annoyance of water precautions during showering and swimming. Even so, surgical repair of an uncomplicated perforation, with or without conductive hearing loss, must be considered elective. Office treatment of an uncomplicated perforation by an otologist might include mechanical abrasion of the margins of the perforation and application of a small cigarette-paper patch. With this method, a perforation may close over a period of a week to several months. All patients with a perforated tympanic membrane should take precautions against recurrent middle ear infections due to water entering the middle ear. Silicone or wax ear plugs (which can be purchased in a pharmacy) are generally satisfactory for showering, but most will leak to some degree if put under the stress of swimming. In addition, perforations, especially of the marginal type, should be observed by an otologist to ensure that there is no ingrowth of squamous epithelium into the middle ear space (forming, for example, cholesteatoma).

Surgical correction of a small perforation (up to 2 mm) may be performed as an outpatient procedure under local anesthesia, using a fat graft. Surgical correction of an anterior perforation behind an anterior canal-wall bulge, a perforation associated with large conductive loss, or a perforation in which squamous epithelial ingrowth is possible, is generally performed as an ambulatory surgical procedure under local or general anesthesia. Small posterior perforations with or without a hearing loss are usually corrected by a transcanal technique similar to the approach used for stapes surgery under local anesthesia. Larger perforations or anterior perforations require endaural, or post-auricular, incisions that open the canal widely and permit the surgeon to visualize the entire drum. Temporalis fascia is the most common graft material used to repair the drum.

The overall success rate of tympanoplasty is approximately 85%. Therefore, the greatest risk of this surgery is a 15% chance of failure. Other complications include those from anesthesia and a very small risk of damage to the ossicular chain, facial nerve or inner ear. Treatment of a perforation with drainage is discussed in Chapter 3. The treatment of an acute perforation is discussed in Chapter 5.

Conductive hearing loss due to disorders of the middle ear

Hearing loss resulting from disorders of the middle ear may be caused by middle ear effusions, stiffness lesions or discontinuity of the ossicular chain.

Effusions

Serous otitis media   Serous otitis media is recognized by the presence of an air–fluid level in the middle ear or of a golden-to-bluish discoloration of the drum and lack of compliance of the drum as tested by pneumo-otoscopy or tympanometry. Serous otitis media is the most common cause of conductive hearing loss in children. It is much less common in adults, but may be seen as a complication of upper respiratory infection or allergy. In an adult, the presence of serous otitis media must initiate a search for neoplastic obstruction of the nasopharyngeal end of the eustachian tube. This is done by indirect or direct nasopharyngoscopy, soft tissue radiography of the nasopharynx, computerized tomography (CT) of the skull base in selected cases and nasopharyngeal biopsy if indicated. There is a relatively higher incidence of nasopharyngeal carcinoma in Chinese men.

In children, the treatment of serous otitis media involves a preliminary search for a medically treatable cause of eustachian tube dysfunction. For example, questions concerning allergic symptoms may lead to a formal allergic evaluation. Examination of the nasopharynx, either by mirror examination or with a lateral X-ray view, may demonstrate adenoid hypertrophy sufficient to cause stasis within the nasopharynx and eustachian tube dysfunction. Craniofacial abnormalities, either gross or relatively subtle, particularly those involving the mandible and occlusion, are associated with a relatively high incidence of ear disease secondary to eustachian tube dysplasia or dysfunction. There may be a positive family history of such disorders.

Palatal abnormalities, particularly cleft palate, may be associated with serous otitis media. The eustachian tubes are opened during swallowing and yawning by the contraction of the tensor veli palatini muscles. This muscle pair meets at the median palatal raphe. In the child with a cleft palate the eustachian tubes have a compromised mechanism for opening. Hence, most of these children require long-term otologic care for recurrent serous otitis media and chronic otitis media.

There is evidence that the intermittent mild-to-moderate impaired hearing associated with serous otitis media, which can range up to 45 db, will result in a deficit in language acquisition among preschool and school-aged children. Hearing screening programs in school, as well as the increased awareness of hearing problems by physicians and parents, have helped reduce this problem. Untreated serous middle ear effusions may eventually lead to the development of dense fibrous tissue (adhesive otitis media) and permanent conductive hearing loss.

If the preliminary search for an identifiable cause of eustachian tube dysfunction is unrewarding, a trial of decongestants and antihistamines is usually tried. Self-inflation through the use of a modified Valsalva maneuver, the blowing up of balloons by the patient or the use of a Politzer bag may also help. If the fluid is persistent, and is causing a significant hearing loss, myringotomy and the insertion of a ventilating tube constitute a reasonable temporizing maneuver. In an adult, this can be performed under local, or topical, anesthesia and, in a child, under general anesthesia. A myringotomy is made in the anterior-inferior quadrant of the drum, the fluid is aspirated and a ventilating tube is inserted. The tube does not serve as a drain, but as an alternative means for air to enter the middle ear. Drainage from a ventilating tube other than during the first few days after insertion usually means that there is an infection in the middle ear or mastoid. Risks of myringotomy are minimal, but include possible production of a permanent perforation or surgical damage to the ossicular chain. The patient with tubes in place must not allow water to enter the external canal during showering or swimming. The patient or parent should understand that drainage from the ear may be the only indication of acute infection because the usual pain associated with acute suppurative otitis media may not occur with a tube in place. For children with recurrent serous otitis media and adenoid hypertrophy, myringotomy may be combined with adenoidectomy (placement of a tube is a temporizing maneuver). In addition to reduced inflammation from proper middle ear ventilation, improved eustachian tube function will result from growth of the head, allergic treatment and, if indicated, adenoidectomy. A ventilating tube usually remains in place for 8–12 months. However, in ears in which tubes have been inserted so many times that the fibrous layer of the drum has been compromised, the tube may be lost within a few weeks.

Other effusions   Blood or cerebrospinal fluid within the middle ear may also produce conductive hearing loss. Hemotympanum in the presence of significant head injury implies a basilar skull fracture despite negative radiologic evaluation, including tomography. The hemotympanum need not be treated, because the blood will be resorbed spontaneously within several days. A hemotympanum may also result from barotrauma during airplane descent or scuba diving. Cerebrospinal fluid may enter the middle ear from the middle or posterior fossa secondary to trauma or, in rare cases, to spontaneous leakage through dural defects.

Mass lesions within the middle ear

Variants in anatomy, such as a high-riding and dehiscent jugular bulb, an aberrant internal carotid artery, an aneurysm of the carotid artery or neoplastic growths such as glomus tumors, may present as a conductive loss but are usually visible as a mass behind the tympanic membrane. For such lesions, otologic and radiographic consultation is needed.

Malleus fixation

The malleus may be fixed to the bone of the epitympanum by new bone or fibrous tissue as a result of inflammatory changes or bone dysplasias. Fixation of the malleus may be detected by pneumo-otoscopy or by depression of the malleus handle.

Incus resorption

As a result of trauma or septic or aseptic necrosis, the incudostapedial articulation may be disrupted. The long process of the incus is most commonly affected because of the relatively poor blood supply to this portion of the ossicle. Total discontinuity in the presence of an intact drum will produce a characteristic hearing loss of 60 db and a characteristic discontinuity pattern on tympanometry. Lesser degrees of disruption, such as subluxation of the incus or a fibrous union between the incus remnant and the capitulum of the stapes, will result in lesser degrees of loss. If the drum becomes retracted against the stapes head in conjunction with resorption of the incus – a situation called myringostapediopexy – very little, if any, hearing loss may be detectable. Disorders of the malleus, the incus and the ossicular articulations can usually be corrected by transcanal ossiculoplasty (Figure 2.1). In an adult, this is carried out under local anesthesia. Rearrangement of ossicles, autologous bone grafts or substitution with alloplastic materials may result in elimination of the conductive hearing loss. The risks of these procedures are minimal and consist of those attendant to anesthesia and surgical trauma.

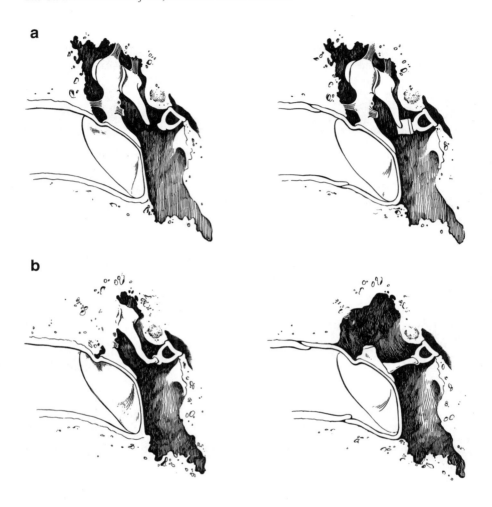

Figure 2.1 (*see also following page*) (a) Ossiculoplasty, type II. A conductive loss caused by discontinuity of the incudostapedial joint (left). This is corrected by a bone interposition (right). (b) Ossiculoplasty, type IIIa (minor columella). The conductive hearing loss is caused by fixation of the head of the malleus and the body of the incus (left). This is corrected by interposition of a bone graft or alloplastic implant between the malleus handle and stapes capitulum (right). (c) Ossiculoplasty, type IIIb (major columella). A conductive hearing loss is caused by loss of the superstructure of the stapes and the long process of the incus (left). This is corrected by an interposition of a bone graft or alloplastic implant between the malleus handle and the stapes footplate (right). (d) Stapedectomy. The conductive hearing loss is caused by ankylosis of the stapes footplate (left). This is corrected by fenestration of the footplate and replacement of the stapes superstructure with a Teflon® wire or other prosthesis from the incus to the oval window (right)

c

d

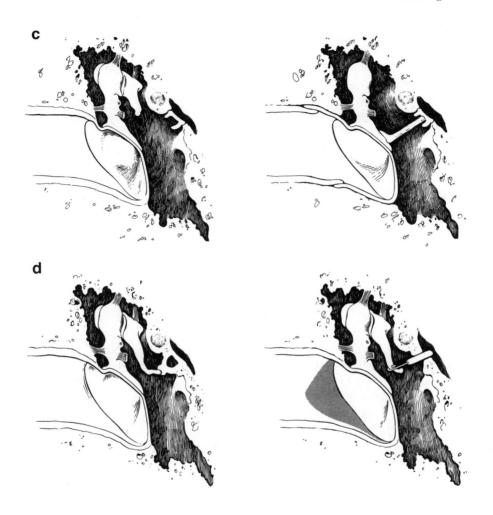

Stapes fixation

Stapes fixation may occur as the result of congenital fixation in association with a branchial arch syndrome, or it may occur as an isolated congenital abnormality. Fixation of the stapes may also occur as a result of bone dysplasias and hyaline or fibrous deposition at the stapediovestibular joint due to recurrent, acute or chronic middle ear infection. However, the most common cause of stapes fixation is otosclerosis. Otosclerosis is inherited as an autosomal dominant disorder with variable penetrance. The prevalence of conductive hearing loss due to otosclerosis ('clinical otosclerosis') is approximately 1 in 100 among Whites and 1 in 1000 among those of African or Asian extraction. Hearing loss results from disordered bone growth at the stapediovestibular joint, causing fixation. Conductive loss occasionally may be caused by bony closure of the round window niche. The disorder is usually bilateral, but the stage of progression is different in each ear, and otosclerosis may present as a unilateral conductive loss. The natural history of otosclerosis is slow progressive hearing loss, but it is rare that a conductive hearing loss will exceed 50 db. Otosclerosis may also cause a concomitant SNHL loss by invasion of the cochlear otic capsule.

Diagnosis   The diagnosis is presumptive, based on the presence of a normal ear canal and tympanic membrane, normal motion of the malleus and the presence of a conductive loss. A CT scan in some cases may show a characteristic 'halo' around the cochlea. The ultimate diagnosis is made during surgical exploration of the middle ear.

Treatment   When the hearing loss becomes handicapping, usually when the threshold reaches 30 db or worse in the better hearing ear, treatment may consist of either amplification with a hearing aid or surgical correction. Amplification is recommended for individuals with an 'only hearing ear' and for those who cannot or will not take the risks involved in surgical correction.

A stapedectomy is usually performed under local anesthesia and requires approximately 1 hour (Figure 2.ld). The posterior drum is turned forward, and the stapes is either partially or totally removed. Most often, a pros-thesis made of Teflon® (Du Pont) or stainless steel and shaped like a miniature piston is fitted into an opening in the footplate and fixed to the long process of the incus, thus replacing the stapes. The success rate, as measured by closure of the air–bone gap to within 10 db, is approximately 96%. The risks of surgery include a 2% incidence of SNHL that may be profound and preclude the subsequent use of a hearing aid in that ear. In such cases, vertigo, usually temporary, may also occur. The most common complication is impaired taste on the ipsilateral anterior tongue due to an injury to the chorda tympani nerve. Perforations of the drum or damage to the facial nerve are rare complications. Relative contraindications include a mixed hearing loss in which the degree of SNHL will still require amplifications despite a successful stapedectomy. On the other hand, with severe mixed cases, stapedectomy may permit successful amplification by elevating the air conduction threshold to levels more suitable for a hearing aid. Surgery for otosclerosis should never be performed in an only hearing ear. Age is not a contraindication.

SENSORINEURAL HEARING LOSS

A presumptive diagnosis of the cause of a SNHL is made largely on the basis of history and audiometric pattern. Usually, a unilateral hearing loss requires further evaluation in the form of vestibular or radiographic evaluation and will be discussed separately.

Bilateral sensorineural hearing loss

Presbycusis

Approximately 30% of the adult population over 70 years of age has a handi-capping SNHL ascribable to no other cause than the cumulative effects of the aging process. Diagnosis is made by history and audiometric pattern.

Diagnosis   The hearing loss caused by presbycusis is slowly progressive and bilaterally symmetrical. Four patterns of presbycusis have been described by Schuknecht[1] (Figure 2.2):

(1) *Sensory presbycusis*   The usual audiometric pattern in this form of degeneration is a bilateral high-frequency SNHL starting at 2–3 kHz. Discrimination scores are good, and recruitment may be present. The histopathologic correlate is loss of hair cells in the basal turn of the cochlea with preservation of cochlear neurons.

(2) *Neural presbycusis*   The typical audiometric pattern in this form of degeneration is a gradually descending threshold curve with reduced discrimination scores. The histopathologic correlate is primary degeneration of nerve elements of the inner ear and probably higher auditory pathways.

(3) *Metabolic presbycusis*   The audiometric pattern is bilateral 'flat' thresholds (i.e. with equal decrement of threshold at all frequencies). The discrimination score is usually good, except in severe hearing losses. The histopathologic correlate is degeneration of the stria vascularis, an epithelial component in the inner ear involved in homeostasis of fluids of the inner ear.

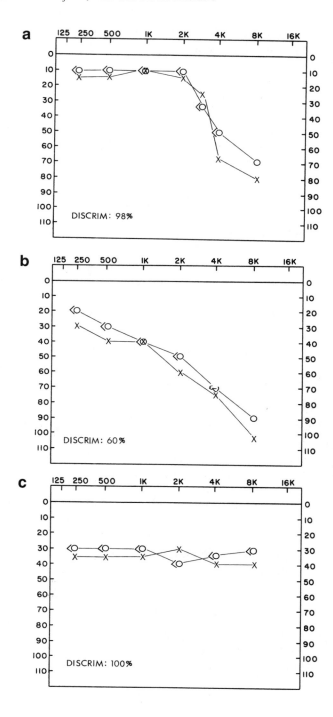

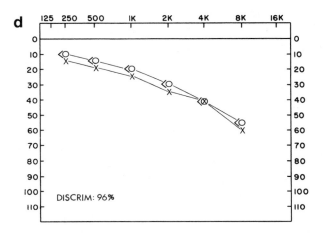

Figure 2.2 (*see also previous page*) (a) Patterns of presbycusis, sensory: bilateral sensorineural hearing loss with sharp onset and good discrimination, consistent with loss of hair cells in the basal turn. Discrimination remains good, because there is little loss of cochlear neurons. For definitions of the symbols, see Figure 1.9a in Chapter 1. (b) Patterns of presbycusis, neural: bilateral, down-sloping sensorineural hearing loss with poor discrimination, consistent with degeneration of first-order cochlear neurons of the auditory nerve. (c) Patterns of presbycusis, metabolic: bilateral, flat sensorineural hearing loss with good discrimination, consistent with atrophy of the stria vascularis. (d) Patterns of presbycusis, mechanical: bilateral, down-sloping sensorineural hearing loss with sharp onset and good discrimination, consistent with an inner ear 'stiffness lesion'

(4) *Mechanical presbycusis* The usual clinical finding is a symmetrical, descending audiometric pattern but with good discrimination, unlike in the neural type. Histologically, there is no loss of hair cells, neurons or striae to correlate with the hearing loss, and disorders of mechanical elements of the inner ear, such as the basilar membrane, have been postulated.

Slow progression is common in all forms of presbycusis. Patients may be told that the average rate of deterioration is approximately 5 db of speech reception threshold in 3–5 years. However, this rate varies considerably from patient to patient. In a patient with the usual onset of hearing loss in the third to fifth decade of life, a typical audiometric pattern, bilateral symmetry and no complicating medical factors, no further investigation is needed to make this diagnosis.

Some families have a strong tendency towards progressive hearing loss beginning in the fifth and sixth decades. Early in the course of presbycusis, many older persons deny or fail to recognize this hearing loss, attributing their difficulties to mumbling or background noise, until it is pointed out by others. As with other forms of hearing loss, the first symptom of presbycusis is often tinnitus. Another complaint is increased inability to hear at meetings or difficulty hearing someone in the next room. Very commonly, poor discrimination accompanies hearing loss, and for such patients loud sounds and voices are irritating, yet comprehension is poor. As the hearing loss progresses, the patient has increasing difficulty hearing the ring of the telephone and doorbell. In order to communicate with the patient, others may have to begin speaking loudly, a source of irritation to both the patient and his family. Most patients acquire some self-taught lip-reading skills; many become frustrated and tend to withdraw, not wishing to suffer the embarrassment of not hearing well in social situations. Patients with presbycusis, like all hearing-impaired persons, hear better when spoken to directly in quiet surroundings. Speaking slowly and clearly is more helpful than shouting. For patients with presbycusis the act of listening requires concentration, but many have slowed cognitive functions as well, compounding their difficulties.

Treatment　Presbycusis is usually treated with hearing aids or, in severe to profound sensorineural loss, with cochlear implantation.

Genetically determined sensorineural hearing loss

Diagnosis　Dominant forms of inheritance constitute approximately 25% of genetically determined SNHL. The onset is typically after birth and is progressive. Recessive forms constitute 75% of the total, are typically present at birth and may be non-progressive. Hearing loss of both the dominant and recessive types may be associated with defects in other systems that may be used as markers to identify the hearing loss as genetically determined. A partial listing of known genetically determined syndromes involving hearing loss is presented in Table 2.1, and the reader is referred to the selected readings at the end of the chapter for further description of the clinical presentation, progression and diagnosis of individual entities. More than 50% of all hereditary deafness is not associated with other defects.

Table 2.1   Hereditary nerve deafness

I. Dominant (25% of total); onset of hearing loss typically after birth and progressive)
  A. Without associated defects
    1. Congenital severe deafness
    2. High-tone deafness
  B. Inborn errors of metabolism and deafness
    1. Amino acids
      a. Tyrosine
        (1) Tietze's syndrome (albinism and deafness)
        (2) Waardenburg's syndrome: 1% of total hereditary deafness; 20% of dominant types
      b. Proline
        (1) Hereditary mental retardation, prolinemia and deafness
      c. Methionine
        (1) Hereditary mental retardation, homocystinemia, deafness, dislocated lenses and fatty degeneration of liver
  C. Nephropathies and deafness
    1. Alport's syndrome (1% of hereditary deafness)
      a. Hereditary nephritis and deafness
    2. Hereditary nephritis, urticaria, amyloidosis and dominant nerve deafness
      a. Progressive sensorineural hearing loss from youth
    3. Hereditary nephritis, mental retardation, epilepsy, diabetes and dominant nerve deafness (Hermann's syndrome)
  D. Ectodermal defects and deafness
    1. Ectodermal dysplasia, anhidrotic type and deafness
    2. Bilateral acoustic tumors and deafness (neurofibromatosis-2)
  E. Degenerative disease of nervous system and deafness
    1. Huntington's chorea
  F. Skeletal defects and deafness
    1. Craniofacial dysostosis (Crouzon's disease)
    2. Cleidocranial dysostosis
    3. Mandibulofacial dysostosis

II. Recessive (75% of total; typically congenital and non-progressive)
  A. Without associated defects (50% of hereditary deafness)
    1. Recessive congenital deafness
    2. High-tone deafness
    3. Mid-tone deafness
  B. Inborn errors of metabolism

continued on following page

continued

1. Amino acids
    a. Tyrosine
        (1) Albinism and deafness
        (2) Photophobia and nystagmus
        (3) Deafness (congenital)
2. Carbohydrates
    a. Mucopolysaccharides
        (1) Gargoylism (Hurler's syndrome)
        (2) Morquio's disease (osteochondrodystrophy)
        (3) Onychodystrophy
3. Lipids
    a. Ganglioside lipidoses
        (1) Tay–Sachs disease
4. Minerals
    a. Copper
        (1) Wilson's disease (hepatolenticular degeneration)
C. Degenerative diseases of the nervous system
    1. Friedreich's ataxia
    2. Schilder's disease
    3. Unverricht's epilepsy
D. Skeletal defects
    1. Generalized defects
        a. Osteopetrosis (Albers–Schönberg disease)
    2. Defects of vertebrae
        a. Klippel–Feil syndrome
E. Congenital heart disease and deafness
    1. Electrocardiogram (ECG) abnormalities (Jervell–Lange–Nielsen syndrome)
F. Endocrine abnormalities
    1. Thyroid
        a. Non-endemic goiter and deafness (Pendred's syndrome; 10% of hereditary deafness)
G. Eye abnormalities
    1. Retinitis pigmentosa (Usher's syndrome; 10% of hereditary deafness)
    2. Retinitis pigmentosa, mental retardation, dwarfism (Cockayne's syndrome)

III. Trisomies
   A. Trisomy 13
   B. Trisomy 18

The estimated incidence of profound hereditary deafness is approximately 1 in every 2000 live births in the USA. The genes involved in the development of the ear number in the thousands, and either single or multiple gene dysfunction may result in abnormalities. Several genes causing SNHL have been mapped. For example, in Usher's syndrome the genetic defect has been mapped to the 11q13,11p, 14q32, 1q32–41 regions, suggesting considerable genetic heterogeneity. In Waardenburg's syndrome, the defect has been mapped to at least the 2q35–37 region. The diagnosis of a genetically determined hearing loss is often presumptive and based on the pattern of onset and progression, the exclusion of other causes of hearing loss and a family history consistent with the diagnosis. Further laboratory investigation may include tomography of the temporal bone to diagnose forms of dysplasia involving the bony otic capsule. This carries little therapeutic significance, however. Chromosomal studies are not useful except in severe and multiple associated congenital defects.

Treatment   In cases of partial hearing loss, an attempt should be made to place the disorder into the known varieties of genetically determined loss, so that a probable natural history may be determined. A hearing aid is usually prescribed when the hearing threshold in the better ear is greater than 30 db. In congenitally severe-to-profoundly deaf children, rehabilitation may include cochlear implantation and is usually best coordinated with education programs specifically designed for the hearing-impaired child.

Congenital, non-hereditary deafness

Not all congenital deafness is genetically determined. Known cases include ototoxic drugs, anoxia and birth injury. Early onset of deafness may be secondary to bacterial meningitis, and inner ear damage may be due to measles and mumps.

Ototoxicity

The list of drugs known or thought to be ototoxic continues to grow. The most common include the aminoglycoside antibiotics, loop diuretics, quinine and its derivatives, salicylates and chemotherapeutic agents such as cisplatin. The hearing loss caused by ototoxicity is usually bilateral and symmetrical. Ototoxicity may be increased by concurrent renal disease, genetic predisposition or multiple drug therapy such as diuretics and aminoglycoside antibiotics. Although in most cases ototoxicity is secondary to parenteral administration, in some cases it may follow oral or even topical administration, such as topical neomycin in extensive burns. The vestibular system may be selectively affected before the auditory system by some drugs, such as streptomycin and gentamicin.

UNILATERAL OR ASYMMETRICAL SENSORINEURAL HEARING LOSS

Otitis media

Chronic and, rarely, acute otitis media may be complicated by suppurative labyrinthitis with resultant destruction of the inner ear. The diagnosis is based on associated signs of infection. Hearing can rarely, if ever, be saved once suppurative labyrinthitis has occurred.

Bacterial meningitis

Partial or complete bilateral or unilateral SNHL occurs as a sequela in approximately 21% of cases of bacterial meningitis. This is due to damage to the cochlear nerve in the infected subarachnoid space or to spread of the suppurative process into the inner ear via the perilymphatic space and the cochlear aqueduct. In addition, transient hearing loss may occur as a result of metabolic dysfunction in the inner ear. Hearing loss is more common when there has been a delay between the onset of meningitis and treatment, when the infecting organism is pneumococcus or meningococcus and when there is concurrent development of other neurologic sequelae.

Direct trauma

Temporal bone fractures, particularly transverse fractures, may result in total profound SNHL and are commonly associated with injuries to the vestibular and facial nerves. Hearing loss may occur without fracture as a result of transmission of acoustic energy to the inner ear from a blow to the head. This usually results in an abrupt high-tone hearing loss that is worse in the ear closest to the site of injury. Penetrating wounds, such as those resulting from pencil or cotton tip applicator, may result in perilymphatic leakage and SNHL (see Chapter 5).

Acoustic trauma

Exposure to loud noise may result in a unilateral or bilateral SNHL. This may result from one exposure to intense noise, or it may be cumulative over years of exposure to high-intensity industrial noise. The audiometric pattern demonstrates abrupt loss in the 3–4 kHz area in cases of single exposures to high-intensity sound and a gradually down-sloping pattern with long-term exposure to loud but less intense noise. The diagnosis is made by the typical audiometric pattern and a history consistent with noise exposure. For an example of hearing loss from acute noise trauma, see Chapter 5.

Perilymph leaks

Leakage of perilymph from the inner ear into the middle ear may be caused by blunt or penetrating trauma to the head, by severe acoustic (noise) trauma, by blast injuries or, in rare cases, it may occur spontaneously. The presenting symptoms and signs include SNHL with or without a conductive hearing loss and with or without vestibular complaints. The SNHL may be fluctuant or progressive and usually has a down-sloping pattern. Clinical signs may also include spontaneous nystagmus, nystagmus and vertigo induced by placing the affected ear downward in a head-hanging position (positive Hallpike positional testing) or nystagmus induced by changing the pressure in the external auditory canal (positive fistula test). Surgical exploration may be necessary for diagnosis. The most common sites for fistula are the oval or round windows. Surgical treatment consists of repairing the fistula with free tissue grafts.

Syphilis

Syphilis, either congenital or acquired, may produce SNHL. This may be symmetrical, but usually one ear is more affected than the other. Routine serology such as the Venereal Disease Research Laboratory (VDRL) and rapid plasma regain (RPR) card tests may not be positive in late-latent syphilis, and hence a fluorescent treponemal antibody absorption (FTA-ABS) test should be performed in suspected cases. Cerebrospinal fluid serology is usually negative. The SNHL may be sudden in onset, rapidly progressive or fluctuating (similar to the hearing loss in Ménière's disease). Discrimination scores are characteristically low, and severe vestibular hypofunction, as determined by caloric testing, and vestibular symptoms are usually present.

Treatment with oral corticosteroids and intramuscular antibiotics over a period of several months has proved effective in some patients (see Chapter 4).

Neurologic disorders

Loss of hearing or vestibular function may be a presenting symptom of a demyelinating disease such as multiple sclerosis. The usual pattern of SNHL is a progressive, high-frequency type, although it may be sudden and unilateral and may recover to a degree. Speech discrimination is usually decreased. The BSER may suggest a retrocochlear lesion. A magnetic resonance imaging (MRI) scan may be diagnostic. Central vascular insufficiency or stroke may also cause hearing loss, as discussed below.

Neoplasms

Rarely, primary tumors of the temporal bone may invade the inner ear and cause SNHL. Metastatic lesions may demonstrate no local manifestation with the exception of hearing and vestibular dysfunction. The most common sources of metastatic lesions to the temporal bone in order of frequency are carcinomas of the breast, kidney, lung, stomach, larynx, prostate and thyroid. Temporal bone, CT scans and/or MRI in suspected cases may be diagnostic.

Cerebellopontine angle tumors

Vestibular schwannoma (acoustic neuroma) and other tumors of the cerebellopontine angle, such as meningiomas, may cause unilateral or auditory and vestibular dysfunction.

Diagnosis The hearing loss may be slowly to rapidly progressive, although cases of sudden or fluctuant hearing loss have been described. Audiometric criteria that raise the suspicion of a cerebellopontine angle tumor include poor discrimination, positive tone decay and acoustic reflex decay. Caloric testing with or without electronystagmography (ENG) will detect severe ipsilateral vestibular hypofunction in the majority of cases. Often these patients have little or no vestibular symptoms despite marked loss of caloric function. Also, brain-stem evoked response audiometry has proved to be a sensitive test for the presence of cerebellopontine angle tumors. Interwave latency prolongation, either I–III or I–V, suggests the diagnosis. MRI with gadolinium enhancement will reliably detect tumors over 5 mm in diameter and CT scanning with contrast enhancement will reliably demonstrate tumors over 1.0 cm in diameter. Bilateral vestibular schwannomas may occur in neurofibromatosis-2.

Treatment   Most tumors of the cerebellopontine angles are benign and grow slowly. No treatment may be indicated in the aged or debilitated individual. For patients who are surgical candidates, it is usually best to remove the tumor when it is first discovered, because the morbidity and mortality of surgery are correlated with tumor size. The surgical approach depends on the size of the tumor, the presence of usable hearing and the necessity of preserving this hearing. A tumor under 2 cm in diameter, in a patient with no usable hearing, may be removed through a transmastoid–translabyrinthine approach, which requires little retraction of intracranial structures. For larger tumors or in cases in which the decision has been made to attempt to preserve hearing, a combined neurosurgical and otologic procedure by way of the suboccipital route is most popular.

Complications of tumor removal are significant. Temporary or permanent facial paresis or paralysis occurs in at least 30% of cases. Other complications include cerebrospinal fluid leak, meningitis or stroke in rare cases. In aged and debilitated patients who require surgery because of the progression of symptoms, intracapsular subtotal removal is often indicated to limit the morbidity. In tumors with documented enlargement, radiotherapy using stereotaxic gamma irradiation or proton irradiation may arrest the growth of the tumor.

Hearing loss associated with other metabolic or systemic disorders

Arterial disease

Although the concept of hearing loss due to involvement of the end-arterial blood supply of the inner ear by arteriosclerotic cardiovascular disease is intuitively attractive, there is little evidence to support such a hypothesis. Hemorrhage into the inner ear or certain well-described vascular insufficiencies of the posterior circulation are rare but do occur. These include the lateral medullary syndrome and occlusion of the anterior-inferior cerebellar artery. The lateral medullary syndrome, or Wallenberg's syndrome, is caused by occlusion of the vertebral or posterior inferior cerebellar artery. Symptoms consist of headache, vertigo, vomiting, diplopia and dysphagia. Findings include ipsilateral fascial analgesia, ipsilateral ptosis and miosis, contralateral trunk analgesia and thermanesthesia, and ipsilateral paralysis of the soft palate, pharynx and larynx. Occlusion of the anterior inferior cerebellar artery may be suspected with the sudden onset of vertigo, SNHL, facial paralysis and cerebellar and sensory signs including ipsilateral loss of pain and temperature sensation on the face, including corneal hypesthesia. Partial loss of pain and temperature sensation on the contralateral side may occur.

The syndrome of vertebrobasilar ischemia is probably invoked more often than it occurs. Usually, SNHL and vertigo are associated with other sensory and motor disturbances such as diplopia, blurred vision, transient hemianopsia, dysarthria and hemiparesis.

Other metabolic disorders

SNHL has been tentatively associated with diabetes mellitus, although convincing evidence is lacking. The same is true of thyroid disease with the exception of Pendred's syndrome, a coincidentally inherited syndrome of thyroid and auditory dysfunction.

Disorders of unknown or immune-mediated cause

Ménière's disease

In Ménière's disease, the SNHL is usually unilateral, although it may be bilateral in 20% of cases. A characteristic low-frequency SNHL is often present. Hearing loss is commonly fluctuant early in the disease and is associated with acute attacks of prostrating vertigo and tinnitus and a feeling of fullness within the affected ear. Variant forms are recognized. For example, the cochlear variant of Ménière's disease consists of fluctuating low tone SNHL, tinnitus and aural fullness, without vestibular symptomatology. In uncomplicated cases the diagnosis is made by history and audiometric patterns. In cases of severe sensorineural loss, exclusion of a cerebellopontine angle tumor may be necessary (see above, Cerebellopontine angle tumors).

Collagen vascular diseases

Unilateral or bilateral SNHL and vestibular symptoms have been described as complicating Wegener's granulomatosis, polyarteritis nodosa, temporal arteritis, Cogan's syndrome and a relapsing polychondritis.

Immune-mediated sensorineural hearing loss

Rapidly progressive bilateral or unilateral SNHL may be immune mediated in the absence of systemic symptoms. The characteristic audiometric pattern is a down-sloping loss, often with decreased speech discrimination. Vestibular symptoms may be present. Blood studies for immunologic disease, such as anti-nuclear antibodies and rheumatoid factor, are usually negative. The erythrocyte sedimentation rate and Raji cell test may be positive. The most useful diagnostic test is a western blot analysis for circulating antibody against inner ear protein. Treatment consists of high-dose steroids (prednisone, 60 mg/day) for a minimum of 4 weeks and often a much longer period. In recalcitrant cases, immune suppression with cyclophosphamide or methotrexate, or rarely plasmapheresis, may be useful to stabilize or improve hearing.

Sudden idiopathic sensorineural deafness

Sudden idiopathic sensorineural deafness is diagnosed after other causes of sudden SNHL have been excluded. The disorder is most commonly unilateral but in rare cases may be bilateral or sequential. Vestibular complaints may accompany the hearing loss. The precise etiology is uncertain, although many authors believe it to be related to viral disease. Although a number of treatments have been recommended, to date only steroid therapy in selected patients has proved to be efficacious. This disorder is more fully discussed in Chapter 7.

TINNITUS

Tinnitus auris, defined as a sound in the ear, may be described by the patient as a ringing, hissing, engine-like or pulsating noise. It is important to distinguish subjective from objective tinnitus. Subjective tinnitus can only be heard by the patient and is usually an epiphenomenon associated with the presence of hearing loss. Objective tinnitus is defined as tinnitus that can be heard by the patient and the observer. Common causes of objective tinnitus include vascular sounds caused by tumors (e.g. glomus tumors), or turbulence in the blood stream caused by stenosis, high flow states (e.g. anemia) or other vascular abnormalities such as carotid aneurysm or kinking of the jugular vein. Work-up for objective tinnitus will include careful ear and neck examination and often radiographic evaluation such as CT, MRI, magnetic resonance angiography or invasive angiography. Subjective tinnitus requires only a clear diagnosis of the cause of hearing loss. Treatment of subjective tinnitus includes careful explanation of the benign course to the patient, habituation regimens and tinnitus maskers.

HEARING AIDS AND COCHLEAR IMPLANTS

Hearing aids

A hearing aid is a miniaturized electronic amplifier and can effectively be used for conductive and most forms of SNHL. One or two hearing aids are usually prescribed when the speech-reception threshold exceeds 30–35 db in the better-hearing ear. It is a common misconception that a hearing aid is not useful in SNHL. Nothing could be further from the truth in most cases, although several factors will influence the success of amplification. For instance, patients with low discrimination scores will have more difficulty using their hearing aid than will those with normal scores, but even patients with discrimination scores of under 10% may obtain useful information with amplification. Also, the presence of recruitment and a sharply down-sloping audiometric pattern may make amplification difficult. Patients with a flat SNHL with good discrimination (that is, those with the metabolic type of presbycusis) almost always do extremely well with amplification.

There are several types of hearing aid. In air-conduction hearing aids the amplification system may be contained in a mold within the ear ('in the ear (ITE) aid') or it may be suspended behind the auricle ('behind the ear (BTE) aid') or worn in a pocket or harness at the chest or belt level. This last type of hearing aid is usually reserved for severe-to-profound SNHL where high gain is necessary, such as in children with severe congenital SNHL, or in adults with severe presbycusis. The amplification system may be incorporated into eyeglass frames. However, this combination may prove inconvenient if either hearing aid or lenses become non-functional. A more sophisticated hearing aid is the contralateral-routing-of-signals (CROS) aid, designed for individuals with unilateral deafness. A microphone in the deafened ear reroutes sound to a receiver in the hearing ear. A further variant is the BICROS aid for individuals with bilateral hearing loss in which only one ear is able to process amplified sound. In this situation, microphones are placed at each ear, and both signals are routed to the ear with usable hearing. A bone-conduction hearing aid transmits sound to the skull rather than through the external canal. This may be necessary in cases of atresia of the external canal or in cases in which chronic ear discharge cannot be controlled.

The frequency gain can be tailored to the pattern of hearing loss. Some aids are 'programmable', i.e. the response characteristics may be changed by the user, depending on the listening conditions. With the burgeoning variety of design and gain characteristics, a hearing-aid fitting should be carried out with the guidance of an audiologist in a hearing and speech center. Optimal use of a hearing aid requires training, and courses for patients to learn to use their instrument should be provided at such centers. Inadequate training and motivation, rather than the impracticability of amplification, is the most common cause of failure to use a hearing aid. The principal drawback of a hearing aid is that it will not return hearing to a normal state as eyeglasses restore normal vision in cases of myopia. It helps, but does not overcome the problem of poor speech discrimination. Hearing aids amplify ambient noise (wind, traffic, kitchen noises) as well as more useful sounds and require frequent adjustment because of changing sound levels. Another drawback is the initial cost and the cost of replacement batteries. Also, small hearing aids are difficult to use by the elderly with arthritic fingers or severe tremor.

Cochlear implants

When SNHL reaches severe to profound levels with very poor or absent speech discrimination, a hearing aid is of little or no use. In such cases, a cochlear implant may be considered. A cochlear implant consists of an implantable electrode usually surgically implanted in the inner ear via the round window and a coupling device at the skin level designed to receive signals from an external 'speech processor' that transduces acoustic signals into electrical impulses. These electrical signals bypass the damaged inner ear and directly stimulate the auditory nerve. Speech perception achieved by use of a cochlear implant varies widely among users. Some achieve only sound awareness, while a minority achieve 'open set' speech discrimination allowing speech understanding without lip-reading. Progress in speech processor design may be expected to increase the utility and application of these devices in the future.

Selected readings

Gorlin RJ, Toriello HV, Cohen MM Jr. *Hereditary Hearing Loss and Syndromes*. New York: Oxford University Press, 1995

Nadol JB Jr. Hearing Loss. *N Engl J Med* 1993;329:1092–102

Nadol JB Jr. Pathoembryology of the middle ear. In Gorlin RJ, ed. *Fifth International Conference on Morphogenesis and Malformation of the Ear*. New York: Alan R Liss, 1980: 181–209

Wilson WR, Byl FM, Laird N. The efficacy of steroids in the treatment of idiopathic sudden hearing loss. *Arch Otolaryngol* 1980;106:772–6

Moscicki RA, San Martin JE, Quintero CH, Rauch SD, Nadol JB Jr, Bloch KJ. Serum antibody to inner ear protein in patients with progressive hearing loss. *J Am Med Assoc* 1994;272: 611–16

Bibliography

1. Schuknecht HF. Disorders of aging. *Pathology of the Ear*. Philadelphia: Lea & Febiger, 1993

3

The draining ear

Joseph B. Nadol, Jr

External otitis (swimmer's ear)
  Diagnosis
  Treatment
    Systemic antibiotics
    Topical antibiotics
    Analgesia
  Malignant external otitis
    Diagnosis
    Treatment
  Chondritis of the auricle
  Bullous myringitis
  Herpes zoster oticus (Ramsay Hunt syndrome)
  Chronic fibrosing external otitis
Acute suppurative otitis media
  Diagnosis
  Role of paracentesis
  Treatment
  Follow-up
  Complications
    Rupture of eardrum
    Acute mastoiditis
    Bezold's abscess
    Facial paresis
    Role of mastoidectomy
Chronic otitis media
  Chronic active otitis media without cholesteatoma
    Diagnosis
    Treatment
  Chronic active otitis media with cholesteatoma
    Diagnosis

Treatment
Complications of chronic active otitis media
Labyrinthine fistula
Facial nerve paresis
Petrositis
Brain abscess and meningitis
Phlebitis and thrombosis of the lateral venous sinus
Surgery of the infected ear
Risks of surgery
Expectations of surgery

Drainage from the external auditory canal in the absence of trauma implies infection in the external canal or middle ear and mastoid. There are three entities, and variations of these, that need to be considered: external otitis, acute suppurative otitis media and chronic otitis media.

EXTERNAL OTITIS (SWIMMER'S EAR)

Dermatologic conditions that affect the rest of the body, including eczema, may also affect the squamous epithelium of the external auditory canal, and the treatment for a dermatologic condition involving the ear is similar to the treatment for the condition in general. These conditions rarely cause drainage, but they may cause itching, flaking and the accumulation of desquamated epithelial debris, which requires periodic cleaning.

Infectious external otitis causes drainage, intense pain, tenderness and hearing loss due to obstruction of the external canal.

Diagnosis

The usual clinical setting includes precedent maceration of the external canal resulting from water retained during swimming or showering or resulting from trauma caused by an attempt to clean the external canal. Often the accumulation of cerumen or debris in the canal may result in infection by causing retention of water in the canal and by prompting the patient to manipulate the ear.

It is important to differentiate external otitis from otitis media. Both cause pain, and both may cause drainage from the canal. Although the external auditory canal is usually normal in cases of otitis media, it may be somewhat macerated, especially if perforation of the drum has occurred and the ear is draining. The attribute that best distinguishes external otitis from otitis media is tenderness. External otitis causes intense tenderness over the tragus and pain when the auricle is displaced, whereas uncomplicated otitis media does not.

External otitis and otitis media may coexist. For example, untreated acute suppurative otitis media with perforation and drainage may cause secondary inflammatory changes in the external canal. In such cases both disorders should be treated; oral antibiotics should be administered for otitis media and topical antibiotics for otitis externa.

Treatment

The ear canal must be cleaned in order to diagnose external otitis and exclude middle ear pathology and to initiate proper treatment for external otitis. When the debris within the canal is loose or liquid, cleaning is best accomplished with a no. 5 Barron or no. 70 Pilling suction tip (see Appendix 2). Suction aspiration of the ear canal is performed with a headlight and hand-held speculum, through an otoscope or with a microscope. The drum is examined for perforation and evidence of middle ear pathology. In external otitis, the squamous epithelium of the lateral surface of the drum may be macerated and inflamed in the absence of middle ear pathology. Once the canal is cleaned, a screening hearing evaluation should be performed with a tuning fork and whisper tests. In general, tuning fork tests are normal in otitis externa. Evidence of a conductive hearing loss is strongly suggestive of concomitant middle ear disease.

Systemic antibiotics

Oral antibiotics are generally not useful in the treatment of external otitis and are not used unless there is evidence of early cellulitis at the meatus or of significant adenopathy in preauricular or infra-auricular areas. Culture of the drainage is usually not performed in uncomplicated cases. The usual causative organisms are *Staphylococcus aureus* or *Pseudomonas aeruginosa*, but external otitis may also be caused by fungi. Fungal otitis is usually recognized by the appearance of spores or mycelia in the external canal.

Topical antibiotics

Commercially available antibiotic or acidic eardrops combined with hydro-cortisone are essential in the treatment of external otitis. These include Cortisporin® (Monarch Pharmaceuticals, Bristol, TN, USA), Pyocidin® (Forrest Pharmaceuticals, St. Louis, MO, USA) and Vosol HC® (Wallace Laboratories, Cranbury, NJ, USA). Cortisporin is available as a suspension or solution. The suspension is said to be less likely to cause pain in an inflamed ear, but it has the disadvantage of causing accumulation of suspended ingredients in the ear canal. There is little reason to differentiate between these drugs, although Vosol has the advantage of not containing an antibiotic. Any of these solutions may be used in the presence of a perforation, but some otologists prefer not to use an ototoxic antibiotic, such as neomycin, with an open middle ear. Also, neomycin may cause contact dermatitis in sensitive individuals.

In special situations non-otic topical solutions may be useful in the management of uncomplicated external otitis. For example, 0.1% tobramycin ophthalmic solution may be useful in cases in which the offending organisms include *P. aeruginosa* or *Proteus*, or in patients with a history of allergy to more conventional otic drops. Similarly, Vasocidin® (CIBA Vision, Basel, Switzerland), a sulfa-based antibiotic ophthalmic solution, may be used. For fungal external otitis, Lotrimin® (Schering Plough, Kenilworth, NJ, USA) or 1% tolnaftate solution may be effective.

If the ear canal is swollen shut, it may be necessary to insert an ear wick to act as a conduit for topical drops. Wicks may be obtained commercially (Merocel® Pope® wick, Merocel Corp., Mystic, CT, USA) or may be made from a neurosurgical patty or simply a segment of 4 × 4 sponge. The wick is inserted into the ear canal using Hartmann's or bayonet forceps. It is usually premoistened with otic drops, and the patient continues to apply three drops to the lateral aspect of the wick three times a day. The patient is usually asked to remove the wick in 2 days. Drops should be continued for a minimum of 1 week at the same dosage. Follow-up for uncomplicated external otitis is usually not necessary, but patients are instructed to return if the symptoms do not resolve after this course of treatment. Also, if it was impossible to examine the eardrum, follow-up after edema has subsided is necessary to assess the drum, middle ear and hearing.

Analgesia

Otitis externa causes intense pain, and narcotic analgesics may be required for the first 2–3 days.

Malignant external otitis

Simple external otitis in diabetics may progress to a life-threatening disorder known as malignant external otitis. The infective organism is almost always *P. aeruginosa*, and the usual, but not exclusive, clinical situation involves an elderly diabetic. It is thought that the diabetic angiopathy seen elsewhere in the body also occurs in the skin of the external auditory canal and allows a superficial infection to become invasive. Once the epithelial barrier is broken, the infectious process spreads rapidly anteriorly into the parotid space or, more often, inferiorly into the retromandibular fossa. From there the cellulitis may then spread to the stylomastoid foramen, causing facial paresis and paralysis, and to the jugular foramen, causing lower cranial nerve paresis and thrombosis of the sigmoid sinus. This may lead to the spread of the process along vascular and fascial planes of the skull base. Late in the course of this disease, osteomyelitis of the mastoid tip, skull base and petrous apex may occur.

Diagnosis

External otitis in an elderly diabetic should always raise the question of malignant external otitis. If the usual course of treated external otitis does not occur (i.e. gradual improvement of symptoms starting on the second or third day, resulting in complete resolution within 7–10 days), malignant external otitis should be considered. The earliest presenting sign is breach of the epithelial barrier, usually on the floor of the cartilaginous external canal, with granulation tissue replacing lost epithelium. Later, there may be exposed cartilage or tympanic bone in the ear canal. Facial and lower cranial nerve paresis must be considered late signs, and morbidity and mortality are directly related to the stage reached prior to treatment. Plain mastoid films or tomography of the temporal bone are negative until late in the disease, when osteomyelitis has occurred. Furthermore, radiographs may lag several weeks behind the stage of disease. It is important to recognize the difference in pattern of spread of infection in malignant external otitis as compared to chronic otitis media. In the latter, cranial neuropathy occurs as a complication of the infectious process spreading from the pneumatized spaces of the temporal bone; hence, computerized tomography (CT) of the temporal bone will be abnormal. In malignant external otitis, cranial neuropathy is secondary to cellulitis of the caudal surface of the skull base and usually precedes clinical and radiographic involvement of the pneumatized spaces of the temporal bone.

Treatment

Until recently, long-term intravenous antibiotic treatment was considered essential in malignant external otitis. The usual regimen is a combination of carbenicillin and tobramycin, the drug selection being based on culture and sensitivities. Surgical intervention is necessary if the canal is occluded by granulation, and simple office curettage may be all that is necessary. Late in the disorder, when osteomyelitis or abscess formation at the skull base has occurred, extensive transmastoid surgery may be necessary for salvage. Antibiotic therapy at our institution is maintained for 4 weeks when there is no evidence of osteomyelitis and for 6 weeks when there is evidence of bone involvement. More recently, the introduction of oral ciprofloxacin has dramatically altered the need for parenteral therapy. Ciprofloxacin is now used initially in cases uncomplicated by cranial neuropathy or radiographic evidence of osteomyelitis.

Chondritis of the auricle

Cellulitis of the auricle and subsequent chondritis of the auricular cartilage may occur as a sequela of external otitis or as a complication of an injury to the auricle.

The most common causative organisms of cellulitis and chondritis are *S. aureus* and *P. aeruginosa*. Intravenous antibiotics are usually required and are selected by culture if drainage is present. Empirical treatment should include coverage for both organisms. If a hematoma is present, it must be drained. If the cellulitis responds poorly to antibiotics, debridement of sequestered cartilage may be necessary.

Bullous myringitis

Bullous myringitis may be confused with external otitis. In this disorder, thought to be caused by a virus, the ear canal is normal. However, the layers of the drum are separated by bullae that contain serosanguineous fluid. This is usually extremely painful but does not produce systemic signs. Puncture of the blebs with a myringotomy knife may be necessary for control of pain.

Herpes zoster oticus (Ramsay Hunt syndrome)

Herpes zoster oticus is a herpetic disorder that is often heralded by intense pain in the ear before the herpetic vesicles appear. Hearing loss, vertigo and facial paralysis may also occur.

Treatment consists of oral corticosteroids, such as a 10-day tapering course of prednisone, acyclovir and analgesics. Because the herpetic vesicles may become superinfected, prophylactic antibiotics are often used. *S. aureus* is a frequent offender.

Chronic fibrosing external otitis

Chronic fibrosing external otitis is relatively rare, and is due to chronic or repeated episodes of external otitis in which subepithelial fibrosis causes stenosis of the external canal, thickening of the drum and eventually a conductive hearing loss. Surgical treatment is required for correction. The skin of the external canal and lateral aspect of the drum are removed, the bony ear canal and meatus are enlarged and the lateral surface of the drum and ear canal are covered with split-thickness skin grafts.

ACUTE SUPPURATIVE OTITIS MEDIA

Acute suppurative otitis media, an infection of the middle ear space, is a common complication of serous otitis media in children and may be a sequela of an upper respiratory infection in children or adults. The most common organisms include pneumococcus, *Streptococcus* and *Hemophilus influenzae* infection. The incidence of *H. influenzae* infection is higher in children under 5 years of age. *S. aureus* may also occasionally cause otitis media. Virus and microplasma organisms have been implicated in a minority of cases of otitis media, based on the clinical finding that a percentage of cultured middle ear exudates show no growth.

Diagnosis

Although the tympanic membrane is usually intact early in the course of acute suppurative otitis media, it may rupture very early with streptococcal infections or if a thin neomembrane from a previous perforation is present. Within the first few hours of infection, the only physical finding may be erythema in the posterosuperior quadrant of the eardrum. Shortly thereafter, bulging and widespread erythema of the tympanic membrane occur. A slight conductive hearing loss may be produced, and adults may complain of a slight sense of unsteadiness. There should be no tenderness of the external canal or auricle or over the mastoid cortex. In the absence of signs of complication, no X-ray films are necessary. Culture may be performed if perforation has occurred.

Role of paracentesis

Paracentesis for the drainage and culture of purulent material is usually not indicated except in extenuating circumstances, such as in an immuno-suppressed individual, a patient with concurrent meningitis, mastoiditis or facial nerve paresis, or in a neonate. Paracentesis can be accomplished with a local anesthetic injected into the skin of the posterior canal wall, using 1%

Xylocaine® with 1 : 100 000 epinephrine (adrenaline), the use of ion-tophoresis or a drop of phenol solution on the eardrum. Needle aspiration or myringotomy should be performed in the anterior inferior quadrant of the drum to avoid damage to the facial nerve or ossicular chain.

Treatment

In the adult the drug of choice is penicillin. The usual dosage is 250–500 mg by mouth, four times a day for 10 days. Erythromycin is a reasonable alternative to penicillin in the presence of penicillin allergy. Treatment of acute otitis media in children up to 7 years of age requires an antibiotic effective for both pneumococcus and *H. influenzae*. The choice for an effective therapy might be amoxicillin (20 mg/kg per day) divided into three doses, or ampicillin (50 mg/kg per day) in four doses for 10 days. If the child is allergic to penicillin, erythromycin (40 mg/kg per day) plus sulfisoxazole (100 mg/kg per day) divided into four doses can be used. Decongestants (e.g. Actifed®, Pfizer, New York, NY, USA and Dimetapp®, Whitehall-Robinson, Madison, NJ, USA) probably have little direct effect upon otitis media, but they may be useful in patients with an associated blocked nose and rhinorrhea. Pediatric nose drops, such as xylometazoline (Otrivine®, CIBA Consumer Pharmaceuticals, Edison, NJ, USA), are also useful in this regard.

Follow-up

All patients with acute otitis media should be re-examined in approximately 2–3 weeks. They should be told that pain associated with otitis media should resolve within hours of the initiation of antibiotic treatment. If persistent pain or drainage occurs, the patient should return for further examination. It is important to recognize that coalescent mastoiditis may occur in the presence of otoscopic improvement of the eardrum while on antibiotics. Thus, persistent or worsening pain, fever after the first 2 days of treatment or facial paresis requires radiographic evaluation of the mastoid, despite otoscopic improvement of the middle ear component. Especially in children, serous otitis media may persist for some weeks after an acute episode of suppurative otitis media and should be treated in the same fashion as uncomplicated serous otitis media (see Chapter 2).

Occasionally, a child will develop recurrent otitis media of one or both ears despite apparently proper antibiotic therapy. It is likely that this is the same infection, which is suppressed but not eliminated by the course of antibiotics and continues to recur. In cases with a history of recurrent acute suppurative otitis media, following a 10-day course of ampicillin or erythromycin and sulfisoxazole for an acute infection, the patient should be placed on prophylactic antibiotics, such as ampicillin (125 mg) or sulfisoxazole (500 mg), each morning for 3–6 months. This long-term therapy is very effective for this problem, rarely leads to the growth of resistant bacteria or antibiotic allergy and avoids the hazards of recurrent infections and fever.

If prophylactic antibiotics fail to prevent recurrent acute otitis media, the placement of a ventilating tube, even without evidence of persistent serous otitis, may be effective.

Adults often complain of a sense of fullness or a slight ache in the ear even in the absence of serous otitis for 3–6 weeks after a bout of acute otitis media. A follow-up clinical evaluation of hearing should be carried out, and if an abnormality is suspected, audiometry should be performed. Persistent serous otitis media in an adult should result in a search for a cause of eustachian tube dysfunction, such as nasopharyngeal carcinoma.

Complications

Rupture of eardrum

An eardrum may rupture rapidly with streptococcal infections or in the presence of an organism, often *S. aureus*, not sensitive to the prescribed antibiotic. If rupture has occurred, the drainage should be cultured, and topical antibiotics should be used in addition to oral antibiotics. Some otologists hesitate to use otic drops containing neomycin in the presence of a perforation. Rupture of the tympanic membrane due to an otherwise uncomplicated suppurative otitis media usually heals spontaneously within a few weeks after the drainage has subsided. Occasionally a perforation will persist and may require tympanoplasty.

Acute mastoiditis

Acute mastoiditis was common in the preantibiotic era and still occurs today occasionally, even if there has been no delay in treatment of acute suppurative otitis media. Pathognomonic signs of mastoiditis include persistent pain after initiation of antibiotic treatment, tenderness or periosteal elevation over the mastoid cortex, displacement of the auricle anteriorly caused by periosteal elevation and sagging of the posterosuperior external canal wall. The diagnosis is confirmed by CT of the mastoid. This will show loss of the normal bony trabecular pattern of the mastoid cells in addition to fluid density. The treatment of acute mastoiditis includes intravenous antibiotics and a myringotomy for culture, drainage of purulent material and, usually, the placement of a ventilating tube. Intravenous antibiotics are continued for 7–10 days based on Gram stain and culture.

The most common pathogens in acute mastoiditis include *Streptococcus pneumoniae*, *H. influenzae*, *S. aureus*, *Proteus mirabilis*, *Staphlococcus epidermidis*, *P. aeroginosa* and *Moraxella catarrhalis*. Mixed flora including aerobic and anaerobic organisms are common.

Bezold's abscess

If the treatment of mastoiditis is delayed, or if a loculation of pus develops in the mastoid tip, an abscess may occur below the mastoid tip in the neck, owing to erosion of the lateral mastoid cortex. Because the sternocleidomastoid muscle originates on the lateral surface of the mastoid cortex, this abscess is medial to the muscle, and hence fluctuance may not be palpated. CT or magnetic resonance imaging (MRI) of the neck may be helpful in making this diagnosis. A Bezold's abscess requires immediate drainage and a simple mastoidectomy for drainage of the loculated purulence within the central mastoid tract in order to prevent spreading of the infectious process to the carotid space and beyond.

Facial paresis

Facial paresis may occur in the presence of mastoiditis; it does not require additional treatment unless the paresis progresses despite antibiotic treatment and paracentesis. If total paralysis and evidence of neuronal degeneration occur, exploration of the mastoid and facial nerve may be necessary.

Role of mastoidectomy

Simple mastoidectomy for treatment of acute mastoiditis was the most common otolaryngologic procedure in the preantibiotic era. It is now rarely performed. It is necessary when the infection has not been responsive to intravenous antibiotics and paracentesis, or in the face of complications such as facial paralysis, Bezold's or subperiosteal abscess, thrombosis of the lateral venous sinus or intracranial complication.

CHRONIC OTITIS MEDIA

Chronic otitis media may be defined as a chronic inflammatory process in the middle ear and/or mastoid. Several clinical subtypes are recognized:

(1) *Chronic active otitis media without cholesteatoma* The presence of a perforation of the ear drum with chronic suppurative drainage;

(2) *Chronic active otitis media with cholesteatoma* The presence of a cholesteatoma in the middle ear and/or mastoid, usually with a perforation and with or without suppurative drainage;

(3) *Chronic inactive otitis media* The presence of chronic suppurative otitis media without cholesteatoma in the past which has now resolved, leaving sequelae such as perforation of the eardrum, ossicular resorption or fixation;

(4) *Chronic inactive otitis media with frequent reactivation* A history of chronic intermittent drainage without cholesteatoma.

Chronic active otitis media without cholesteatoma

A variety of bacterial species have been cultured from chronically draining ears. Gram-negative organisms predominate. The most common pathogens are *P. aeruginosa*, *Streptococcus*, *Escherichia coli*, *S. aureus* and *Proteus*. Often multiple organisms are cultured. Anaerobes may be pathogenic in 30–60% of cases.

Rarely, *Mycobacterium tuberculosis* may cause chronic drainage from the ear. Rapid progression and presence of abundant granulation tissue helps to differentiate tuberculosis from other forms of chronic otitis media. The facial nerve and inner ear may be involved and demonstrate dysfunction relatively early compared to chronic bacterial otitis media. Also, multiple perforations of the drum are thought to be pathognomonic of tuberculous otitis media. Wegener's granulomatosis must be differentiated from this disorder.

Diagnosis

The diagnosis is based largely on the history and otologic findings. Roentgenograms may be useful if cholesteatoma, or complications, is suspected. In chronic active otitis media, the usual radiographic report includes mention of 'underdeveloped or under-pneumatized mastoid with sclerosis'. This does not usually help in guiding treatment and is not needed to make the diagnosis.

Treatment

The first consideration in treatment is to determine whether chronic active otitis media can be transformed into chronic inactive otitis media with medical treatment only. Medical treatment includes the use of topical drops, which has been previously discussed in connection with otitis externa; periodic cleaning of the ear; and instruction to the patient not to allow water to enter the ear canal. Oral antibiotics play little role in the treatment of chronic active otitis media, although oral ciprofloxacillin may be effective in some cases. Occasionally, parenteral antibiotics may be beneficial for treating particularly active purulent drainage.

If the suppurative drainage ceases with this treatment, further treatment becomes elective. The patient may become a candidate for tympanoplasty or ossiculoplasty to repair the drum and ossicular chain, or he may choose to live with the perforation and hearing loss. If the suppurative drainage persists, surgery is recommended in the form of a mastoid-tympanoplasty to remove chronic infection from mastoid air cells and to repair the tympanic membrane and reconstruct the ossicular chain, if necessary.

Chronic active otitis media with cholesteatoma

Diagnosis

A history of perforation, usually with chronic, foul-smelling drainage and the finding of keratin debris within the middle ear – most often in the pars flaccida area – is sufficient for the otologist to make a diagnosis of cholesteatoma. Pathologic verification is seldom necessary at this stage. Roentgenograms may be useful to define the limits of the cholesteatoma or to provide evidence of destruction of ossicles or thinning of the otic capsule.

Treatment

Cholesteatoma requires surgical treatment unless there are extenuating circumstances in the medical history. The surgical procedure is tailored to the extent of the cholesteatoma. For example, a small cholesteatoma may be removed by the transcanal route; a larger one in the attic may be removed by 'atticotomy', but usually mastoid tympanoplasty is required. A description of mastoid surgery is found later in this chapter under 'Surgery of the infected ear'.

Complications of chronic active otitis media

Long-standing suppuration within the mastoid air-cell system, especially with concurrent cholesteatoma, may produce a number of complications.

Labyrinthine fistula

A labyrinthine fistula is caused by resorption of the bone of the otic capsule by the action of enzymes associated with cholesteatoma or chronic active suppurative osteitis. The most common site for a fistula is the lateral semicircular canal in the mastoid antrum. However, any of the canals may be involved, and a cochlear fistula may occur in the middle ear or epitympanum. Untreated, fistulae may progress to bacterial labyrinthitis with destruction of auditory and vestibular end organs and may cause bacterial meningitis. The presence of a fistula is indicated by subjective episodes of unsteadiness, progressive or sudden sensorineural hearing loss and a positive fistula test, in which a nystagmus is elicited by the application of positive or negative pressure to the external canal. The presence of a fistula with chronic active otitis media constitutes an urgent indication for surgery to prevent labyrinthitis and meningitis.

Facial nerve paresis

Bone resorption and chronic active infection may uncover the facial nerve, usually in its horizontal or descending segments. This may result in facial paresis and destruction of a segment of the facial nerve if untreated. Paresis in the presence of chronic active otitis media is an urgent indication for surgery.

Petrositis

Petrositis involves an extension of the suppurative process to the apex of the petrous bone. With acute suppurative otitis media, this occurs as a rare complication called Gradenigo's syndrome. More commonly, it occurs in the clinical situation of chronic active otitis media in the face of an immune deficiency or debilitation.

The diagnosis is suggested by deep head pain, perceived as temporal or retro-orbital, secondary to trigeminal nerve inflammation. Also, there is often ipsilateral sixth nerve paresis, meningismus and white blood cells in the cerebrospinal fluid on spinal tap. Profound sensorineural hearing loss and vertigo can occur with inner ear involvement. Temporal bone CT may demonstrate osteomyelitis or abscess formation in the petrous apex. If the patient is medically stable, surgery to drain the petrous apex should be performed immediately, before septic involvement of the temporal portion of the carotid artery or contamination of the subarachnoid space have occurred.

Brain abscess and meningitis

Bone erosion from chronic infection or cholesteatoma may eventually produce dehiscences in the tegmen of the mastoid and middle ear, dural plate or posterior fossa. In addition, dehiscences in these locations may be an occasional variant of normal anatomy. The suppurative process may extend through such bony defects. Infection may also spread to the intracranial space by a retrograde phlebitis without any bony dehiscence to the dura and subarachnoid space.

Intracranial complication occurs in less than 1% of cases of chronic otitis media. A subdural empyema or brain abscess is usually in direct continuity with the point of entry from the temporal bone. It is rare that the abscess will occur with intervening normal brain tissue between it and the diseased temporal bone. Symptoms suggesting the development of an intracranial abscess include headache, nausea, vomiting, drowsiness and fever – none of which are seen in uncomplicated chronic otitis media. More advanced disease may result in seizures, neck rigidity, aphasia, papilledema and coma. Cerebellar abscess may be accompanied by ataxia and nystagmus. The most common bacteria found in cerebral abscesses are *S. aureus, Streptococcus pyogenes, Streptococcus pneumoniae, Diplococcus pneumoniae, E. coli, Proteus* and *Pseudomonas*. Mixed infections are not uncommon.

CT and/or MRI are currently the most valuable modalities for demonstrating an abscess. Lumbar puncture is performed only if there is no evidence of marked elevation of intracranial pressure. Management usually involves treatment with meningeal levels of intravenous antibiotics followed by drainage of the brain abscess either before or concurrently with mastoidectomy. The mortality rate, despite antibiotic treatment and surgical drainage, approaches 20%.

Phlebitis and thrombosis of the lateral venous sinus

Sequestrated suppuration with or without cholesteatoma may progress posteriorly to involve the lateral venous sinus within the folds of the posterior fossa dura and cause phlebitis or septic thrombosis. The presence of high, spiking fevers, with chills, septicemia, sweating and tachycardia in the presence of either acute or chronic ear infection, should raise the suspicion of lateral venous sinus thrombosis. The fever course has been described as similar to a picket fence, in that the patient's temperature may go up to 105 °F (40.5 °C) and then drop to normal, presumably corresponding to showers of septic emboli and intervals between them.

Diagnosis The clinical signs are most important in diagnosis. The white blood cell count is usually elevated. Lumbar puncture in the absence of otitic hydrocephalus is usually normal. The Tobey–Ayer test will be positive only if thrombosis has already occurred. With extensive thrombosis, otitic hydrocephalus and papilledema may occur. Plain roentgenograms are non-specific. A CT scan or MRI will show absence of flow in the involved venous segment and at times ipsilateral cerebral edema.

Treatment Broad-spectrum antibiotics are used intravenously until the specific organism is identified, on the basis of blood cultures, ear canal drainage or purulence obtained at mastoid surgery. With adequate blood levels of antibiotics, the mastoid should be explored on an emergency basis. Necrotic bone and purulence are removed. The lateral venous sinus is explored with a needle. If an intraluminal empyema is found, the sinus is opened and drained into the mastoid. An uninfected thrombus need not be removed. Rarely, ligation of the internal jugular vein is performed, usually to prevent recurrent emboli. Anticoagulation is used with evidence of progressive thrombosis of intracranial venous channels.

SURGERY OF THE INFECTED EAR

Several surgical procedures are employed, depending on the findings. A simple mastoidectomy involves removal of the pneumatized air cells of the central mastoid tract without entering the middle ear space (Figure 3.1d). This is performed most often for acute mastoiditis that does not respond rapidly to parenteral antibiotics or when the bony trabeculation of the mastoid has undergone osteolysis, as detected by radiography.

For chronic otitis media, various forms of tympanomastoidectomy are currently used (Figure 3.1). The goals of mastoid surgery in order of importance should be first, the elimination of disease and the establishment of a safe ear; second, the rearrangement of anatomy to minimize recurrent disease; and third, the reconstruction of the ear to allow useful hearing if

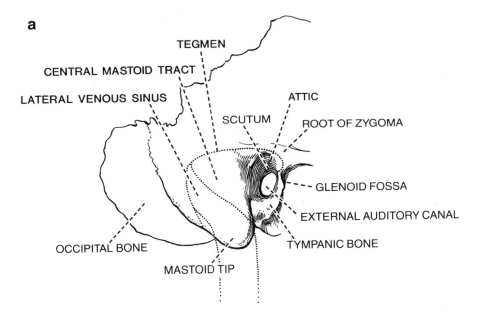

Figure 3.1 (*see also following page*) (a) Surface anatomy of the lateral aspect of the temporal bone. The approximate locations of pertinent internal structures are also indicated. (b) The dotted line indicates the area of bone removal for an antrotomy, used to investigate the possibility of a cholesteatoma or granulations in the mastoid antrum. This procedure is performed following an exploratory examination of the middle ear that identifies disease that could extend into the mastoid antrum. (c) The dotted line indicates the area of bone removed to open the attic and antrum (atticoantrotomy), used to remove a cholesteatoma or granulations limited to these areas. Once the disease and affected ossicles are removed, the ear is reconstructed according to one of the methods illustrated in Figure 3.2. (d) The dotted line indicates the area of bone removed for a simple mastoidectomy, used to explore and drain the mastoid in such cases as antibiotic-resistant mastoiditis. The middle ear and hearing are usually unaffected by this surgery. (e) The dotted line indicates bone removed for a 'canal-wall-up' mastoidectomy, used to remove chronic disease from the mastoid and middle ear space. The posterior wall of the external auditory canal is preserved. (f) The dotted line indicates bone removed for a 'canal-wall-down' mastoidectomy. This procedure includes removal of the posterior wall of the external auditory canal to gain wider exposure and to exteriorize the mastoid into the external canal

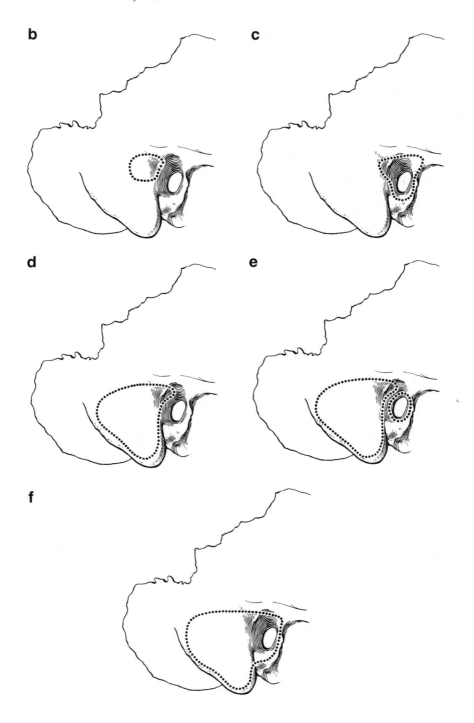

possible. Preservation or removal of the posterior canal wall that separates the ear canal from the mastoid determines whether the procedure will be a 'canal-wall-up' or 'canal-wall-down' mastoidectomy. In the presence of cholesteatoma, most surgeons at this time prefer canal-wall-down mastoidectomy to achieve better exposure. Once the air cells and cholesteatoma that are present are removed, a tympanic graft is placed, to close the middle ear. The usual grafting material is fascia taken from the lateral surface of the temporalis muscle.

Depending upon which ossicles remain, various forms of tympanoplasty are possible. For example, in type I tympanoplasty, all ossicles are preserved. When combined with a canal-wall-down mastoidectomy, this would be called a 'Bondy modified' mastoidectomy. The forms of tympanoplasty most often combined with mastoidectomy are types III, IV and V (Figure 3.2). The type III tympanoplasty, combined with canal-wall-down mastoidectomy, involves placement of a graft directly on the capitulum of the stapes. In type IV, the graft has been placed on the footplate of the stapes. In type V tympanoplasty, the footplate has been removed and replaced with fat underlying the fascial graft.

Risks of surgery

The usual risks that should be explained to the patient include anesthesia of 1–4 hours, risks to auditory and vestibular function and risks to the facial nerve and of recurrent disease. These are all relatively low in incidence. In essence, surgery involves the same types of risks caused by chronic otitis media itself, but the incidence of these complications is much lower with surgery.

Expectations of surgery

The vast majority of chronic draining ears should be rendered dry, and all should be rendered safe. This implies alteration of the anatomy or the exteriorization of pathology to the point that complications are no longer likely. With modern techniques, the patient with mastoidectomy can usually swim and shower without protection, and hearing results are often in the 30-db range if there is reasonable eustachian tube function. The hospital stay is usually overnight. Postoperative care involves removal of sutures, outer mastoid dressing and packing after 1 week, removal of inner packing after 2 weeks and follow-up cleaning and perhaps delayed skin grafting

a

b

c

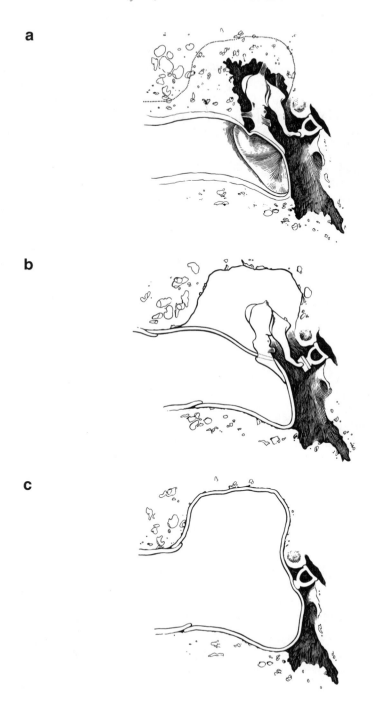

d

e

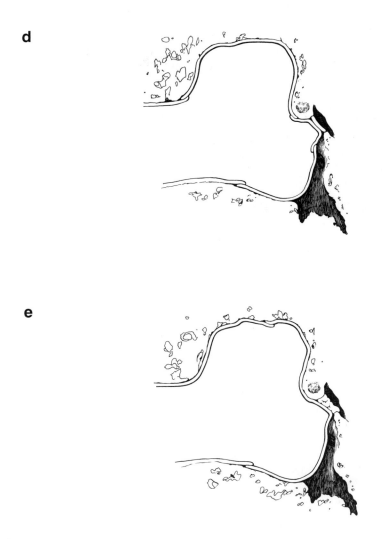

Figure 3.2 (*see also previous page*) (a) The dotted line indicates the area of bone removed in atticotomy or mastoidectomy. (b) Type II tympanoplasty. The mastoid air-cell system has been removed, a fascial graft replaces the drum, and a bone chip reestablishes continuity between the incus and stapes. (c) Type III tympanoplasty. A fascial graft has been laid down on the capitulum of the stapes. (d) Type IV tympanoplasty. The drum has been replaced by temporalis fascia, and a split-thickness skin graft has been placed on the footplate. No other ossicles remain. (e) Type V tympanoplasty. No ossicles, including the stapes footplate, remain. The temporalis fascial graft is laid over a fat graft placed in the oval window

during the next 4–6 weeks. Thereafter, in an asymptomatic ear, all that is required is semiannual cleaning of the ear canal and mastoid bowl to prevent accumulation of wax and keratin debris.

Selected readings

Nadol JB Jr, Eavey RD. Acute and chronic mastoiditis: clinical presentation, diagnosis and management. In Remington JS, Swartz MN, eds. *Current Clinical Topics in Infectious Disease (15)*. Cambridge, MA: Blackwell Science, 1995:204–29

Nadol JB Jr. Histopathology of pseudomonas osteomyelitis of the temporal bone starting as malignant external otitis. *Am J Otolaryngol* 1980;1:359–71

Doroghazi RM, Nadol JB Jr, Hyslop NE Jr, Baker AS, Axelrod T. Invasive external otitis: a report of 21 cases. *Am J Med* 1981;71:603–14

Nadol JB Jr. The chronic draining ear. In Gates GA, ed. *Current Therapy in Otolaryngology–Head and Neck Surgery-3*. Philadelphia, PA: BC Decker, 1987:18–22

4

The dizzy patient

William R. Wilson

Evaluation of vertigo
  Clinical history
  Examination
    Ear canal and tympanic membrane
    Spontaneous vestibular nystagmus
    Positional tests
    Caloric test
    Electronystagmography
    Other tests of vestibular function
Vertiginous disorders involving the inner ear and vestibular nerve
  Ménière's disease
    Variants of Ménière's disease
    Treatment
    Surgery
    Streptomycin and gentamicin therapy
  Acute viral labyrinthitis
    Vestibular neuritis
    Sudden idiopathic sensorineural hearing loss with vertigo
    Ramsay Hunt syndrome (herpes zoster oticus)
    Perilymph fistula
Vertiginous disorders involving the inner ear and vestibular nerve – no
    hearing loss
  Cupulolithiasis
Vertiginous disorders involving the inner ear and vestibular nerve as part
    of a larger syndrome
  Vestibular toxicity
  Acoustic neuroma
  Dysequilibrium of aging
  Multiple sclerosis
  Syphilis: congenital and late latent

Rare disorders
  Waldenström's macroglobulinemia
  Relapsing polychondritis
  Cogan's syndrome
Vertigo resulting from head and neck injury (flexion–extension injury)
Vertigo of brain stem origin
  Vascular disease
  Transient basilar artery ischemia
  Wallenberg's syndrome (lateral medullary syndrome)
  Anterior inferior cerebellar artery syndrome (labyrinthine infarction)
    Cerebellar infarction
  Subclavian steal syndrome
    Migraine-equivalent (atypical migraine)
  Brain stem tumors, paraneoplastic syndrome and metastatic carcinoma
Treatment of vertigo
  Mild to moderate (V1–V2) vestibular attacks
  Marked vertigo (V3) associated with nausea and vomiting
  Chronic positional imbalance and mild to moderate vertigo (V1–V2)
    Exercises
    Vestibular physical therapy

EVALUATION OF VERTIGO

Clinical history

The history is a very important part of the evaluation of dizziness, and it must be taken in a manner that is succinct and useful to the physician. To the layman, dizziness is a general term that encompasses not only vertigo, but also the various forms of lightheadedness, and at times syncope as well. The physician, therefore, must establish that the patient does indeed have vertigo. The patient should have the sensation that the world is spinning (eyes open) or that he is spinning (eyes closed). A sense of imbalance, as if the floor were moving like a rocking deck, is also a form of vertigo. Vestibular disturbances are associated with a visceral response of pallor and, at times, nausea and vomiting. Occasionally a patient will become frightened and may hyperventilate as well, sometimes to the point of tingling and muscular cramping. Hyperventilation serves to enhance vestibular symptoms. Patients with vestibular disorders do not suffer a loss of consciousness, nor do they experience an aura such as that associated with epilepsy or migraine.

Other forms of dizziness may be due to postural hypotension, hypertension, hypoglycemia, medications and neurological, cardiac and vascular disorders, and should be separated by the history and physical examination and the appropriate laboratory work. During the history taking, it is helpful to establish the date of the first attack, the date of the last attack and the frequency with which attacks occur within the following intervals: daily, weekly or monthly. The patient should describe the first attack. The history should contain pertinent information, such as the patient's activity at onset; the intensity of the vertigo; the duration of the attack; the presence or absence of associated symptoms or hearing loss; and the presence of other physical symptoms.

An assessment of the patient's activity at onset is important, because positional vertigo may not be recognized as such by the patient. Complaints may include vertigo that occurs only during head movements, for instance, when washing dishes, hanging clothes or rolling over in bed. Positional vertigo is most commonly associated with cupulolithiasis, post-concussion syndrome, whiplash injury and, rarely, posterior fossa tumors.

The intensity of vertigo can best be measured in terms to which the patient easily relates. Mild vertigo (V1) can be defined as an attack of spinning or imbalance that is not sufficiently severe to cause the patient to discontinue what he is doing. Moderate vertigo (V2) requires the patient to stop his current activities and sit quietly until it clears, usually in less than half an hour. Severe vertigo (V3) is characterized by a marked, spinning sensation with nausea and vomiting that requires the patient to take to bed.

Vestibular falling attacks, or the otolithic crises of Tumarkin, come without warning and last a few seconds. They represent an unusual form of vestibular symptomatology and are distinguished from a faint or seizure by the fact that there is no loss of consciousness. The patient often describes a sensation of being pushed to the ground. The attack is generally over within seconds with little residual symptomatology.

Patients suffering from vertigo may be incapacitated for varying periods of time. Attacks of vertigo can last for a few seconds or for several days. They may recur daily or, more commonly, at irregular intervals. The frequency of the subsequent attacks should be noted, and the intensity of the first should be compared to the intensity of the last. This information provides a guide for the physician as to the progress of the disorder.

Hearing changes are the most frequent symptom associated with vertigo. Even when there is no hearing loss present, patients may be able to determine the involved ear because of the sensation of pressure or discomfort. In other patients, hearing loss may have been present unilaterally or bilaterally for many years prior to the first episode of vertigo. Hearing loss is often associated with tinnitus and a blocked sensation of the ear. Not uncommonly, vertigo is associated with sudden hearing loss.

Vertigo associated with fluctuating hearing suggests increased volume of the endolymphatic fluid of the inner ear (cochlear hydrops). For example, the hearing in one ear may decrease for several days and then return, only to decrease again, and so on. These fluctuations most often occur in the low frequencies that are important for the understanding of speech. In addition, patients complain of noise recruitment, a characteristic finding if hearing losses are due to cochlear injury. In this condition, loud noises are perceived in the affected ear as being irritatingly loud. Cochlear hydrops is associated with Ménière's disease and chronic syphilitic labyrinthitis.

Most vestibular disorders are short-lived and amount to a minor medical problem. However, occasionally they result in a significant alteration of lifestyle or, in unusual cases, total disability. Treatment, medical or surgical, should be carefully selected to be appropriate for the symptoms and the patient with consideration of other medical problems, age and occupation. An example of a form used in the evaluation of vertigo is shown in Table 4.1.

Examination

Ear canal and tympanic membrane

In almost every vestibular disorder, the tympanic membrane is normal. The exceptions are vertigo associated with a painful vesicular eruption involving the pinna, canal or drum, suggestive of herpes zoster oticus, or vertigo associated with tympanic membrane perforation, with or without drainage in chronic otitis media.

The fistula test should be performed in all patients with vertigo. In patients with chronic ear disease, a positive test suggests a fistulous tract between the middle ear and inner ear. When a positive fistula test is

Table 4.1   Form used in the evaluation of vertigo

Evaluation of vertigo

Clinical history

Age:	Sex:	Weight:
Description of vertigo:		Hyperventilation?:

Review of symptoms:

Alcohol, cigarettes, caffeine, others:

Other illnesses:

   Ophthalmologic (oculomotor, astigmatism)

   Neurologic

   Cardiovascular

     Arrhythmias

     Hypertension

     Stroke, transient ischemic attack

     Diabetes

     Psychiatric (anxiety, phobias, panic attacks, secondary gain)

Medications used regularly or recent exposure to ototoxic medications:

Symptoms other than vertigo or hearing loss:

Detailed description of first attack: Date:

   Type of vertigo: imbalance, mild (V1), moderate (V2), severe (V3):

   Duration:

   Associated hearing loss, and other ear symptoms (fullness, pressure, tinnitus):

     Other symptoms:

     Treatment:

Subsequent attacks: Date of last attack:

   Frequency of attacks:

   Usual type of vertigo:

   Ear symptoms and hearing loss:

   Treatments tried and effects:

   Estimated degree of disability:

present in patients with an intact tympanic membrane, it suggests the presence of adhesions in the inner ear, most commonly secondary to chronic luetic labyrinthitis or Ménière's disease, or, rarely, the presence of a perilymph leak between middle and inner ears. A fistula test may elicit one of two abnormal signs. The positive fistula sign implies the presence of true nystagmus in response to positive or negative pressure applied to the external auditory canal, and implies a true fistula between the inner and middle ears as can be seen in chronic otitis media. A positive Hennebert sign may be induced in the same manner, but implies ocular deviation and a few compensatory beats of nystagmus. In general, the ocular movements will continue for several seconds after cessation of the stimulus in the fistula sign and immediately in the Hennebert's sign. A positive Hennebert sign implies the presence of endolymphatic hydrops or abnormal adhesions between the medial surface of the footplate and the vestibular labyrinth.

One method of performing the fistula test is to face the patient and ask him to look directly ahead. The tragus is pressed firmly into the ear canal to create a positive pressure, and released. If the patient feels a sense of turning with this maneuver, it is a positive test. There may be a few beats of nystagmus, best seen if the patient is wearing magnifying (Frenzel's) glasses. An alternative method of performing the fistula test is presented in Chapter 1.

Nystagmus Vestibular nystagmus is known as 'jerk nystagmus' because there is a slow deviation of the eye in the horizontal plane and then a very rapid, or jerk-like, recovery. The direction of nystagmus, by convention, is identified by the fast phase. For instance, if the jerks were to the right, the nystagmus would be named right-beating horizontal nystagmus. However, it is the slow phase of nystagmus that is controlled by the vestibular system; the fast phase, called a saccade, is a recovery movement of the eye controlled by the central nervous system. A disorder producing jerk nystagmus may be located at any point in the vestibular system: the end organ, nuclei or central vestibular tracts.

A second, less common form of vestibular nystagmus is rotatory nystagmus. In this form the eye moves in the horizontal plane and rotates relative to the vertical axis as well. This form is usually induced by positional testing.

On the other hand, jerk nystagmus in a vertical plane, or torsional nystagmus, is indicative of central vestibular dysfunction and requires thorough neurological evaluation. Other varieties of nystagmus, such as pendular nystagmus, congenital nystagmus and searching nystagmus are associated with disorders of the neuro-ocular system.

In general, central nystagmus is more likely to be vertical or torsional, less affected by visual fixation and more likely to be direction-changing as compared to peripheral (vestibular) nystagmus.

Spontaneous vestibular nystagmus

Most often, vestibular nystagmus will be suppressed by visual fixation when the eyes are open. There are several maneuvers used to unmask it.

Jerk nystagmus, characteristic of vestibular dysfunction, will be enhanced when the eyes are turned in the direction of the fast phase. In other words, if the rapid phase of the nystagmus is beating to the right, the nystagmus will be strongest, and in some cases only present when the eyes are turned right. First degree nystagmus is present only with the eyes turned in the direction of the nystagmus; second degree nystagmus is present in midgaze as well; third degree nystagmus is present in all fields of gaze.

The patient is asked to watch the examiner's finger at a distance of 2–3 feet (0.5–1 meter). The finger is moved a short distance to the right or left in order to avoid end-position nystagmus, which is normally present near the limits of gaze. Frenzel's glasses (see Appendix 2), goggles with +20 diopter lenses and small lights within, to illuminate the eyes, are useful for vestibular system diagnostics. In a darkened room, the patient is unable to see out, and hence, cannot visually fixate, but the examiner has an excellent view of the patient's eyes and nystagmus.

Nystagmus that is not present in the light will often be noticeable in the absolute dark during examination of the fundus with an ophthalmoscope. This is an excellent way of determining the presence of spontaneous nystagmus that otherwise would be suppressed by visual fixation. During examination of the retina, the direction of the fast phase will be opposite to that noted by direct observation of the eyes.

Positional tests

Vertigo and nystagmus can often be elicited by placing patients through positional changes. In the first positional test the patient is asked to sit on the examination table with his eyes open, preferably wearing Frenzel's glasses, and facing the examiner. The head is turned as far as it will go to the right and left. If this stimulus elicits vertigo or nystagmus, a proprioceptive muscular disorder of the neck – as might be seen after whiplash injury – is suspected. Also, transitory vascular compromise can be induced when pathology of the carotid or vertebral arteries is present.

The Dix–Hallpike maneuvers are illustrated in Figure 4.1. The patient sits on the examination table so that, when lying supine, his head will extend over the table edge. The examiner should support the patient's head between his hands and observe the eyes for nystagmus throughout. If the patient has a history of vertigo when lying on one side, the examiner should begin by bringing the patient's head back to that side. Each head-hanging position should be held for about 10 seconds before the patient begins to sit upright again. Right, left and straight head-hanging positions should all be tested. The type, direction and duration of the nystagmus should be noted.

There are several responses that the examiner might expect from this test. Direction-fixed positional nystagmus is directed to one side only throughout all the position changes. It often fatigues after a few moments and most often represents a vestibular end-organ disorder. Direction-changing positional nystagmus takes several forms. The first type consists of a rotatory nystagmus that begins after a 1–2-seconds delay upon the patient's assuming the head-hanging position and is directed towards the lowermost ear. Upon the patient's sitting upright, the rotary nystagmus reverses direction for a few seconds and ceases. Subjectively, the patient has a frightening sense of whirling vertigo and is certain that he will roll off the table. These findings are pathognomonic of benign paroxysmal vertigo. This condition is the result of loose otoconia that are free to tumble about in the inner ear (cupulolithiasis).

The second type of direction-changing nystagmus is jerk nystagmus that changes direction with different head-hanging positions. For example, with the right ear down, left-beating nystagmus may be visible. This

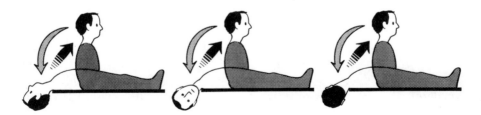

Figure 4.1 The positional testing (Dix–Hallpike) maneuvers. The patient is seated so that his head will hang over the end of the examination table. The maneuver (to the right or to the left) indicated by the history to cause symptoms should be used first. The patient's head is held in the examiner's hands, brought quickly into position and held for approximately 10 seconds before being returned to the upright position. The patient must be instructed to look straight ahead at all times and to keep his eyes open

nystagmus changes to right beating in the head-hanging and left head-hanging positions. Direction-changing nystagmus of this type is seen with unilateral or bilateral vestibular end-organ disorders, but it may occasionally indicate central vestibular dysfunction.

A third form of direction-changing nystagmus is jerk nystagmus that changes direction randomly during a single positioning. For example, the patient might have left-beating nystagmus, then right-beating, followed by left-beating nystagmus over a 30 second period, all while maintaining the right head-hanging position. This nystagmus may be coarse and irregular and is not associated with vestibular symptoms. This type of response is most suggestive of a central vestibular disorder involving the brain stem.

Caloric test

The horizontal semicircular canal can be stimulated by placing warm or cool water against the tympanic membrane. With the patient's head in the supine position, so that there is a vertical axis between the lateral canthus and external auditory canal, the horizontal semicircular canal is placed in a vertical plane. The temperature changes following irrigation of the external canal result in convection currents in the fluids of the horizontal semicircular canal that stimulate the end-organ. After the use of cold water, the nystagmus beats towards the opposite ear, after warm water, it beats towards the same ear. This fact can be remembered using the acronym 'COWS': cold, opposite; warm, same.

The office caloric test is a rough measure of vestibular function, but even so it is very useful. The most important parameter is the speed of the slow phase, which is difficult to judge. Normally, both ears have a similar response. If there is a large difference in amplitude or duration of nystagmus between the two ears, the less responsive one is the affected ear.

The technique for office caloric testing requires Frenzel's glasses, a stopwatch and a syringe. It should be ascertained that the tympanic membrane is intact and the canal is clear of wax. With the use of 5 ml tap water at room temperature 80 °F (27 °C), the patient's ear is irrigated over a 10–20-second period. The nystagmus should be observed for direction of the fast phase, amplitude and duration. Another technique is to use a tuberculin syringe with a 1.5-in 20-gauge needle filled with 0.4 ml iced water. After positioning, the iced water is injected through the speculum of an otoscope against the tympanic membrane. This method elicits approximately the same vestibular response as the first. If there is no response to the above tests in one or both ears, the examination is repeated using 5 ml iced water, the maximum stimulus employed. A form for use in the office examination for vertigo is illustrated in Table 4.2.

Electronystagmography

Electronystagmography (ENG) is vital to a thorough evaluation of vertigo. The test is used to separate nystagmus of central origin from that of peripheral origin, as well as to determine which ear is impaired in cases of

Table 4.2 Form used in the office examination for vertigo

Office examination for vertigo
General
BP: sitting   standing
Pulse:
Respiration:
Heart: Lungs:
Otolaryngology examination
Tuning fork and voice testing
  AD:
  AS:
                        256 Hz   512 Hz
  Rinne AD:
  Rinne AS:
  Weber Test: R   Midline   L
  Fistula Test: AD: AS:
  Neck examination (for masses, bruits):
Vestibular system testing
1. Ask the patient to perform any maneuver that in his experience elicits vertigo.
2. Head shaking. With the patient's eyes closed, move his head briskly from side to side for 1 s.
3. Ask the patient to walk and turn 180° rapidly, making repeated turns.
4. Head turning maneuver. Turn the patient's head to the far right and left, and extend it upwards for 20 s in each position.
5. Dix–Hallpike positional tests (in the light, with the patient's eyes open).
   Upright (U):   Straight down: AD down: AS down:
6. Minimal caloric test:
   Water temperature and amount:
   Response (duration, speed, amplitude):

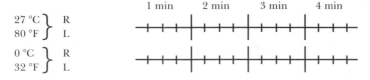

7. Hyperventilate (up to 3 min)

continued on following page

Table 4.2   *continued*

8. Neurologic and funduscopic examination
   Cranial nerves
      I:
      II:
      III, IV, VI: EOMs, pupil
      VII:
      IX, X:
      XI:
      XII:
      Cerebellar tests: Romberg:
                          Rapid movements:
                          Past pointing:
      Gait: Normal or abnormal heel to toe
      Muscle strength:
      Tendon reflexes:
Audiologic studies
      Pure-tone audiometry with air- and bone-conduction levels, speech discrimination scores
      Brain stem auditory response (if indicated):
      Electronystagmography (ENG):
Blood tests
CBC, VDRL or MHA-TP, glucose and 5-h GTT, and thyroid-function studies
Radiologic studies (if indicated)
Cervical spine films
CT scan, MRI
EEG
ECG
Summary of impressions:

---

peripheral dysfunction. It provides a permanent record of the signs of vestibular dysfunction.

An ENG is performed in a specially equipped laboratory and requires approximately 1 hour. The equipment permits recording with the patient's eyes closed, thereby eliminating unwanted visual suppression of the diagnostic eye movements. Electrodes are placed around the patient's eyes to record eye movements by the measurement of changes in the corneal–retinal potentials. The examiner establishes the presence or absence of horizontal or vertical spontaneous nystagmus and any deficiencies in eye-tracking ability. Attempts are made to induce nystagmus by means of head shaking, hyperventilation and positional testing. Last, the Hallpike caloric tests are used. Warm and cool water, 7 °C above and below body temperature, in a prescribed amount and flow rate (approximately 250 ml over a

30–40-second period), is used to irrigate the external canals. The recorded response (nystagmogram) is used to measure the vestibular function of each ear. In the event that there is no response, the test is repeated with 5 ml of iced water.

Measurement of the slow phase of the nystagmus permits an accurate assessment to be made of lateral semicircular canal function.

Other tests of vestibular function

In addition to ENG, vestibular testing laboratories will commonly employ a variety of other tests including the vestibulo-ocular reflexes (VOR) using the rotating chair to achieve bilateral stimulation of the lateral semicircular canals in the vertical axis, visual tracking tests and computerized dynamic posturography, which attempts to segregate non-vestibular dysfunction (visual, somatosensory, vestibulospiral) as a cause of imbalance.

VERTIGINOUS DISORDERS INVOLVING THE INNER EAR AND VESTIBULAR NERVE

Ménière's disease

Ménière's disease or syndrome is a disorder of the peripheral vestibular system. It is due to failure of the endolymphatic resorptive system to keep pace with fluid production, resulting in increased fluid volume in the endolymphatic compartments of the inner ear (endolymphatic hydrops). Whether this failure occurs spontaneously or is secondary to an injury, such as previous viral labyrinthitis, is not certain. However, several facts are known. With a few exceptions, Ménière's disease is not inherited. Endolymphatic hydrops can be created in animals by surgical injury to the endolymphatic sac, the site of resorption. Also, the onset of increased inner ear volume may require many years. Chronic inflammatory conditions, such as long-standing luetic labyrinthitis, will produce endolymphatic hydrops as an end stage. Endolymphatic hydrops causing Ménière's syndrome can thus be caused by a variety of insults to the inner ear such as syphilis, some immune-mediated diseases such as Cogan's syndrome or polyarteritis nodosa, or it may be idiopathic (Ménière's disease).

The term Ménière's disease should not be used interchangeably with labyrinthitis. The disorder has a clear pattern of symptomatology. As described in 1861 by Prosper Ménière, it consists of vertiginous spells associated with hearing loss, tinnitus, nausea and vomiting. The spells of vertigo or hearing loss may precede one another by a matter of years, but they generally present simultaneously. The condition is unusual in children; the incidence climbs until the fifth and sixth decades, then declines. In the majority of patients, Ménière's disease remains unilateral, but the opposite ear may become affected even many years after the first.

The episodes of spinning vertigo associated with Ménière's disease begin abruptly with little or no warning, reaching maximum intensity often accompanied by nausea and vomiting within a few moments. The marked vertigo usually lasts for several hours, but occasionally may persist for 12–24 hours. Residual imbalance can continue for several days more. The recurrence rate of attacks is highly variable and sporadic. They may occur weekly, monthly, occasionally, after many years or not at all. It is unusual for a patient with Ménière's disease to find it necessary to alter his lifestyle permanently or to be classified as partially or fully disabled.

The hearing loss associated with Ménière's disease often begins with a sensation of pressure in one ear associated with some tinnitus. The tinnitus may represent the first symptom of hearing loss perceived by the patient. In early Ménière's disease, hearing loss occurs in the lower frequencies, which are important in the perception of speech. There are two features that characterize it further. First, the hearing loss will fluctuate, so that the hearing will be depressed for a few days and then improve, usually with a concomitant reduction in tinnitus. The fluctuation may be a single occurrence; however, in some cases the hearing continues to fluctuate over many years, resulting in a gradually progressive sensorineural hearing loss. Second, patients note that the affected ear has an increased sensitivity to loud sounds. This phenomenon, known as recruitment, is characteristic of cochlear, rather than neural, auditory dysfunction. To test for recruitment in the office, a 512-Hz tuning fork is struck softly, the patient listens to it alternately with the right and the left ear, and determines in which ear it is louder. The fork is then struck sharply and the patient is asked to compare his ability to perceive this loud sound with each ear. If the hearing loss in the affected ear is not too great, the loud sound will be perceived as equal between the ears or as greater in the ear with diminished hearing.

Variants of Ménière's disease

The classical presentation of Ménière's disease consists of downward fluctuation in hearing, and an increase in tinnitus and aural fullness, simultaneous with the attack of vertigo. Variant forms are recognized.

Lermoyez's syndrome This is a variant of Ménière's disease in which the hearing loss improves subsequently to the episodes of vertigo, nausea and vomiting.

Otologic crisis of Tumarkin These attacks may complicate Ménière's disease, particularly late in its course. In such an attack, the patient is propelled to the ground without warning and without the usual protective vestibulospinal protective reflexes. Thus, facial or shoulder fractures are common. Following the attack, which lasts only seconds, the patient has little or no vestibular symptoms.

Cochlear or vestibular Ménière's disease Although not officially accepted as variants of Ménière's disease, it is true that isolated cochlear symptoms (fluctuant hearing loss, aural fullness, tinnitus) or isolated vestibular symptoms (episodic vertigo) may precede the development of the classical Ménière's disease.

In the office examination of patients with Ménière's disease, the middle ears are normal. There is usually no positional nystagmus. Examination of the eyes, particularly with Frenzel's glasses or in the dark with an ophthalmoscope, will often reveal direction-fixed horizontal nystagmus, most often directed away from the involved ear. Head shaking or hyperventilation can help elicit nystagmus. The whisper and tuning-fork tests will usually demonstrate a hearing loss and recruitment. A minimal cool caloric test will often demonstrate a unilateral reduced response. The neurological evaluation will be negative except for a disturbance of balance and gait that should be appropriate for the degree of vestibular upset.

Further laboratory studies should include an audiogram consisting of pure tones, discrimination scores and reflex delay testing. Also, an ENG should be performed following the attack, to determine the extent of injury to vestibular function and to assess residual spontaneous nystagmus.

Treatment

The medical treatment of vertigo and imbalance associated with Ménière's disease is similar to the generic medical regimen for vertigo discussed on pages 107–111. In addition, in some cases, a diet with no added salt or low salt, or a diuretic may be helpful. The Cawthorne–Cooksey exercises may be of benefit in stabilized Ménière's disease with residual imbalance or slight vertigo.

Surgery

Medical management and the passage of time will adequately control the vestibulopathy of Ménière's disease in the great majority of cases. A variety of surgical treatments are used for Ménière's disease that is not responsive to medical management. They are listed below so that the referring physician will be familiar with the recommended procedures and their relative merits or limitations. Surgery or further medical therapy must be considered only when the patient is truly incapacitated by vertigo. Because of the highly unpredictable frequency of attacks and propensity for long, spontaneous remissions, the assessment of any treatment for Ménière's disease is difficult.

In the Fick operation, a needle is passed through the footplate to create a fistula between the endolymphatic and perilymphatic spaces. There are frequent relapses and a high risk to hearing. This is no longer recommended.

The tack operation is a procedure similar to a Fick operation that implants a tack permanently through the footplate. This operation has only limited success and a high hearing risk. It is now of historical interest only.

The endolymphatic sac operation uses a simple mastoidectomy to expose the endolymphatic sac and drain it into the subarachnoid space or mastoid. Whether drainage actually occurs has not been established. The success rate in control of vestibular symptoms is said to be approximately 60–70%.

In severe cases of Ménière's disease which have been unresponsive to medical management, selective section of the vestibular nerves via the posterior fossa (suboccipital or transmastoid–retrolabyrinthine approaches) or the middle fossa (subtemporal craniotomy) can be performed to ablate vestibular function and preserve hearing in the affected ear.

Labyrinthectomy is a transtympanic or transmastoid procedure to destroy the vestibular end organs that has a very high success rate for the control of vertigo. Because this procedure results in a total loss of hearing, it should be reserved for patients with no usable hearing in the affected ear and unilateral involvement. Postoperative imbalance persists for several weeks.

Labyrinthotomy (endocochlear shunt, round window labyrinthotomy) is a procedure similar to the Fick operation, except that the fistulization of the endolymphatic and perilymphatic spaces is performed through the round window membrane. Control rates of vestibular symptoms have been reported in the 60% range. Further loss of hearing occurs in approximately 20% of cases.

Streptomycin and gentamicin therapy

Use of streptomycin and gentamicin for the treatment of Ménière's disease takes advantage of the fact that the vestibular portions of the inner ear are more sensitive than the cochlea to the ototoxic effects of these drugs.

Gentamicin can be administered by transtympanic injection to induce unilateral vestibular hypofunction. Recurrence of vestibular symptoms may require repeated treatment. Sensorineural hearing loss secondary to the ototoxic effect may occur in up to 25%.

Intramuscular streptomycin treatment is reserved for patients with bilateral severe Ménière's disease or Ménière's disease in an only hearing ear. It requires the administration of vestibulotoxic levels of streptomycin for 2–4 weeks. The treatment protocol may be continued to total ablation (no response to iced water caloric) or alternatively a titration protocol may be used, i.e. continuing treatment until the first signs of vestibular ototoxicity occur (unsteadiness, spontaneous nystagmus) and repeating the regimen if necessary to control vestibular symptoms. Either regimen can be used in an outpatient setting with monitoring of renal, auditory and vestibular function. The titration protocol is less likely to result in chronic ataxia and oscillopsia, which may complicate the ablation protocol.

Acute viral labyrinthitis

Vestibular neuritis

Vestibular neuritis is best defined by a constellation of characteristic clinical symptoms and signs including sudden severe vertigo lasting days; absence of auditory findings; marked reduction in caloric response in one ear; and absence of other neurological symptoms or findings. This disorder affects both sexes equally and is most prevalent in middle age. Because of a frequent association with recent or concurrent upper respiratory infection, a viral infection of the vestibular nerve is suspected, and the term 'epidemic vertigo' is a synonym.

Rarely, the disorder may be recurrent in either the same or the opposite ear. The differential diagnosis includes other peripheral vestibular disorders such as Ménière's disease, acoustic neuroma, perilymph fistula, or even central disorders, such as multiple sclerosis, cerebellar infarction, Wallenberg's syndrome, atypical migraine attack or a central paraneoplastic syndrome.

Clinical examination will reveal normal tympanic membranes, symmetrical hearing, spontaneous nystagmus in the acute phase, usually with the fast component away from the affected side, unilateral reduced or absent caloric response and otherwise normal neurological testing.

Treatment is supportive. Complete resolution of vestibular symptoms within weeks occurs in the majority of cases.

Sudden idiopathic sensorineural hearing loss with vertigo

Sudden idiopathic sensorineural hearing loss may be accompanied by acute onset of vertigo, which clinically is similar to vestibular neuritis other than the presence of a hearing loss. The hearing loss may be treated with oral corticosteroids (see Chapter 2). The vestibular symptoms are treated as in vestibular neuritis.

Ramsay Hunt syndrome (herpes zoster oticus)

Ramsay Hunt syndrome is characterized by deep ear pain and a vesicular eruption of the ear canal and auricle. Frequently, there is associated facial paralysis, hearing loss and vertigo, all of which may be mild or severe. The disorder is due to a regional herpes zoster polyneuritis.

Recovery is dependent upon the magnitude of the original injury. There is evidence that improvement in facial function and hearing is enhanced by corticosteroid therapy. Acyclovir has been used empirically.

Perilymph fistula

Membrane ruptures involving the round window and the annular ligament of the stapes may occur as a result of abrupt changes in atmospheric pressure or cerebrospinal fluid pressure, or as a result of blunt or penetrating trauma to the ear. For example, a typical history might involve a scuba diver who noted a 'pop' in his ear followed by tinnitus and dysequilibrium during an ascent or descent, or a weight lifter might notice similar symptoms while straining. The hearing loss, if not complete initially, may progress over the next few hours or may fluctuate, improving in the morning but worsening during the day. Dysequilibrium is present, and positional vertigo can often be elicited with the injured ear down. The 'fistula test' may be positive. It is theorized that purely intracochlear ruptures of Reissner's membrane can occur as well.

Examination may demonstrate the effects of barotrauma upon the tympanic membrane including a small hemorrhage within the tympanic membrane. Audiology demonstrates a cochlear type of sensorineural loss.

Spontaneous and positional nystagmus may be present, especially with the involved ear down.

The patient should be put at bed rest with the head elevated 30–45°, keeping the affected ear uppermost. When cases with a very clear history of abrupt pressure change show no improvement after a week or so of conservative management, surgical exploration of the middle ear and repair of the leak is suggested.

VERTIGINOUS DISORDERS INVOLVING THE INNER EAR AND VESTIBULAR NERVE – NO HEARING LOSS

Cupulolithiasis

Benign paroxysmal positional vertigo (BPPV), or cupulolithiasis, is a relatively uncommon, but very distinctive form of vertigo that should be known to all primary care physicians (Figure 4.2). The patient describes the acute onset of vertigo each time he assumes the provocative position usually by extension or rotation of the neck. There is usually no associated hearing loss, although BPPV may complicate skull fracture or Ménière's disease, both of which may cause a sensorineural hearing loss. It is caused by free-floating otoconia from the utricular or saccular end-organs. This disorder occurs spontaneously, especially in the elderly – although it may affect any age group, particularly after head trauma.

Examination will demonstrate normal ears. Dix–Hallpike positional tests (Figure 4.2) should be carried out, preferably with Frenzel's glasses. The patient should be reassured that he will not be allowed to fall and reminded that he must keep his eyes open and look straight ahead. His head should be in the examiner's hands and should be placed briskly to the head-hanging position on the symptomatic side. In the characteristic response there is a delay of several seconds before the onset of the sensation of spinning vertigo and the fear of falling. At that time, the examiner will note the horizontal or rotatory nystagmus directed towards the undermost ear. The vertigo and nystagmus will crescendo in a few seconds and then gradually disappear within 30 seconds. Upon the patient's briskly resuming the upright position, the nystagmus reappears but is reversed, becoming horizontal or rotatory in the opposite direction. Repeated attempts at provoking the vertigo will demonstrate fatiguing of the vestibular response.

BPPV will usually resolve spontaneously in a matter of weeks or months. If the condition persists for more than a few weeks, a canalolith

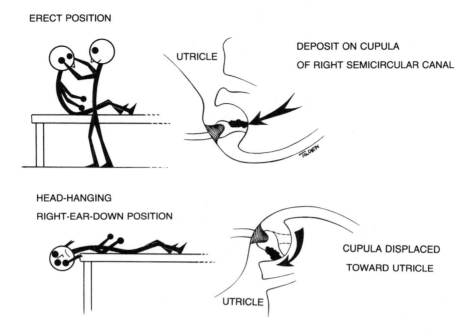

ERECT POSITION

UTRICLE

DEPOSIT ON CUPULA
OF RIGHT SEMICIRCULAR CANAL

HEAD-HANGING
RIGHT-EAR-DOWN POSITION

CUPULA DISPLACED
TOWARD UTRICLE

UTRICLE

Figure 4.2 Benign paroxysmal positional vertigo is the result of otoliths striking the cupula of the ipsilateral posterior (cupulolithiasis) semicircular canal. The canal is stimulated in the head-hanging position when the affected ear is downward. When the test is positive, the patient will experience a frightening sensation of falling, associated with the onset of rotatory and horizontal nystagmus towards the undermost ear, that clears within a minute. On his assuming the erect position, the rotatory nystagmus reverses direction for a few seconds

repositioning maneuver (Epley maneuver) may be used to eliminate free-floating otoliths from the posterior semicircular canal. Because the symptoms are so severe and sudden in onset, vestibular suppressive medications are not useful. Only in rare patients will surgical therapy be advised.

VERTIGINOUS DISORDERS INVOLVING THE INNER EAR AND VESTIBULAR NERVE AS PART OF A LARGER SYNDROME

Vestibular toxicity

Most ototoxic drugs affect both the cochlea and the vestibular labyrinth. There are, however, substances and drugs that affect primarily the vestibular labyrinth. Among the common ones in daily use are caffeine, nicotine, alcohol, quinine and certain tranquilizers and sleep preparations. Tranquilizers, barbiturates and alcohol affect the vestibular system centrally as well. Their overuse may result in a sense of chronic imbalance or, if they have been used to an extreme, in vestibular ataxia.

Of the commonly used antibiotics, the aminoglycosides must be carefully monitored for ototoxicity. Streptomycin and gentamicin are primarily vestibulotoxic; tobramycin, kanamycin and amikacin are more cochleotoxic. It is important to obtain an audiogram prior to beginning treatment with any of these antibiotics. Serum peak and trough drug levels are useful guides to proper dosage. The earliest and best indication of ototoxicity from streptomycin and gentamicin is the onset of imbalance. However, this symptom will not be noticed until the patient attempts to walk. At this point the dosage should be sharply reduced, or the medication should be discontinued. The vestibular effect is characterized by the onset of imbalance, not vertigo, because both end-organs are suppressed simultaneously. The other cochleotoxic aminoglycosides are monitored by audiograms and serum drug levels.

Ototoxic effects are exacerbated by renal failure, the combined use of more than one ototoxic medication, advanced age, previous inner-ear disease and high fever. Certain diuretics, primarily ethacrynic acid and furosemide, are well-known ototoxic drugs that primarily affect the cochlea. Although ototoxic effects are most commonly seen following parenteral administration, they may complicate oral or even topical use in rare cases. Cisplatin has been recognized as cochleotoxic. Aspirin and intravenous erythromycin can cause reversible sensorineural loss.

Acoustic neuroma

An acoustic neuroma (vestibular schwannoma) arises from the Schwann cell sheath, most commonly of the superior vestibular nerve. It is often found in the internal auditory canal extending into the posterior fossa. The tumor will cause a progressive compression or degeneration of cranial nerve VIII and is therefore associated with the gradual onset of tinnitus and sensorineural hearing loss, as well as with intermittent unsteadiness or positional vertigo. Abrupt attacks of vertigo are only rarely seen. Any patient with unilateral progressive sensorineural hearing loss must be evaluated for an acoustic neuroma. The evaluation includes an ENG, auditory brain-stem response, a CT scan with contrast or MRI with contrast enhancement. Bilateral acoustic neuromas are sometimes seen in patients with neurofibromatosis-2.

Dysequilibrium of aging

Dysequilibrium may be caused by the aging process as a result of gradual deterioration of the vestibular system; it is the vestibular equivalent of presbycusis.

Some patients in the eighth and ninth decades of life develop an instability when walking that causes them to walk with short shuffling steps. These symptoms are very troublesome even to patients who are otherwise alert and vigorous. Falls are frequent and may result in fracture or other injury. Medications for vertigo are of no benefit and in fact may worsen the disorder by reducing mental alertness. Patients are benefited most by good light and a stabilizer, such as a cane or handrail. Vestibular rehabilitation therapy may be helpful.

Multiple sclerosis

Vertigo and nystagmus occur in over one-third of the cases of multiple sclerosis. Hearing losses are not nearly so common; they are usually unilateral and may be of a sudden, profound nature. They may recover spontaneously. Vertigo is most probably due to areas of demyelinization located in the middle cerebellar peduncle of the flocculonodular lobe. The diagnosis is based on the finding of multiple, focal neurologic deficits. MRI of the brain may be diagnostic. The age of onset is generally in the fourth and fifth decades.

Syphilis: congenital and late latent

Syphilis, either congenital, or acquired in the late latent phase, may cause auditory and vestibular dysfunction. Auditory and vestibular manifestations of congenital lues usually become evident in the third and fourth decades of adult life. The otologic symptoms include a progressive sensorineural hearing loss that is usually bilateral but progresses at different rates in each ear. The hearing loss may be slowly progressive or may occur suddenly in one ear.

All patients with congenital syphilis develop symptoms of either spinning vertigo or imbalance at some point in the course of the disease and will develop a marked reduction in the function of the vestibular end-organs on caloric testing. The treatment consists of benzathine penicillin G, 1.2 million units intramuscularly weekly, for approximately 12 weeks. In addition, patients are placed on alternate day prednisone therapy, approximately 40 mg, for 1 month. The rationale for this therapy is that after the *Treponema pallidum* has been sequestered in the cochlear tissues for a long period of time, replication occurs only very slowly – approximately once every 90 days. Because penicillin is effective only at the time of bacterial cell division, it is necessary to keep adequate concentrations of the antibiotic available in the cochlear tissues for that entire period of time. Cortisone is used to reduce the inevitable inflammatory response that accompanies the presence of *T. pallidum* in the cochlear tissues. The use of these medications will improve hearing significantly in approximately 15% of patients. In over half the patients it will have a beneficial effect upon the vestibular symptoms.

The otologic effects of late latent syphilis are similar to those of congenital syphilis. The disorder is often confused with Ménière's disease, because there may also be fluctuating hearing and episodes of sudden hearing loss associated with vertigo or marked imbalance. Patients being evaluated for hearing loss and imbalance should always have a microhemagglutination test for *Treponema pallidum* (MHA-TP) drawn in order to rule out either congenital or late latent syphilis, since the Venereal Disease Research Laboratory (VDRL) may be negative.

Rare disorders

Waldenström's macroglobulinemia

Waldenström's macroglobulinemia is a rare cause of vertigo that is due to hyperviscosity of the serum secondary to an excess of monoclonal IgM. This in turn may result in decreased perfusion of the inner ear resulting in hearing loss and vertigo. Treatment of hyperviscosity by plasmapheresis will correct the condition and control the vertigo and hearing loss.

Relapsing polychondritis

Relapsing polychondritis is due to an inflammatory process involving the cartilaginous tissues of the body, most probably the result of anticartilage autoantibodies. The usual presenting signs and symptoms include non-infectious inflammation of the cartilaginous auricle, the cartilaginous portion of the nose, the tarsal plates of the eyelids and occasionally the trachea. Vertigo and hearing loss probably result from an inflammatory reaction involving the endochondral bone of the inner ear. The symptoms are sometimes improved by treatment with corticosteroids.

Cogan's syndrome

Cogan's syndrome affects young adults and both sexes equally. Its clinical presentation mimics congenital syphilis. Progressive sensorineural hearing loss, vertigo and interstitial keratitis are found, but serological tests for syphilis, including the MHA-TP test, are negative. Despite treatment with high doses of steroids or other immunosuppressive medications, hearing loss may become severe, and vestibular function may progress to complete loss of response.

VERTIGO RESULTING FROM HEAD AND NECK INJURY (FLEXION–EXTENSION INJURY)

Patients who have suffered a severe neck injury, such as a whiplash, often complain of a sensation of vertigo when holding their head in certain positions. This is a verifiable complaint that can be documented by the presence of nystagmus on the ENG tracing when certain head positions are assumed. It is theorized that this dysfunction is due to injury to proprioceptive nerve fibers to muscles of the neck. These symptoms may require up to 6 months or more to resolve.

Patients who have suffered a severe head injury even without skull fracture, frequently have a sense of imbalance for many months. This is due to traumatic labyrinthitis.

VERTIGO OF BRAIN STEM ORIGIN

Vascular disease

Vertigo may be caused by compromise of the vascular supply to the inner ear or to the brain stem. The blood supply of the inner ear is supplied by the anterior inferior cerebellar artery, which is a branch of the basilar artery. The labyrinthine artery is the midportion of the anterior inferior cerebellar artery as it loops near the internal auditory meatus. The labyrinthine artery supplies the nerves of the internal auditory canal and then divides into the anterior vestibular artery and the vestibulocochlear artery. The anterior vestibular artery supplies a major portion of the vestibular end-organ; the posterior vestibular artery from the vestibulocochlear artery supplies the remainder.

Transient basilar artery ischemia

Transient basilar artery ischemia can result in a sudden loss of balance without loss of consciousness as a result of reduced blood supply to the vestibular nuclei in the brain stem. Vertigo may be the only symptom or may accompany other neurologic findings related to the posterior cerebral circulation.

Wallenberg's syndrome (lateral medullary syndrome)

Wallenberg's syndrome is characterized by a sudden onset of marked vertigo, usually accompanied by nausea and vomiting, hoarseness, aspiration and cough, and further voice changes secondary to hypernasal speech from palatal dysfunction. The patient may complain of double vision. On examination, there is ipsilateral analgesia of the face, ptosis and myosis of the ipsilateral eye, and ipsilateral paresis or paralysis of the palate, pharynx and larynx. On the body trunk, there is a contralateral loss of pain and temperature sensation. These symptoms are related to either partial or complete occlusion of the ipsilateral vertebral artery or its largest branch: the posterior inferior cerebellar artery.

Anterior inferior cerebellar artery syndrome (labyrinthine infarction)

Anterior inferior cerebellar artery syndrome presents with sudden onset of vertigo, hearing loss, facial paralysis and cerebellar and sensory signs (see Chapter 2).

Cerebellar infarction

Cerebellar infarction without brain-stem infarction is usually embolic. The presenting symptoms include vertigo, ataxia and vomiting, and may be confused with an acute peripheral vestibular disorder. Truncal ataxia and directional changing nystagmus present in cerebellar infarction is absent in peripheral vestibular disorders. MRI will be diagnostic.

Subclavian steal syndrome

Subclavian steal syndrome results in intermittent brain stem ischemia, secondary to an occlusion of either the right or the left subclavian artery proximal to the take-off of the vertebral artery resulting in reversal of blood flow in the vertebral artery. Symptoms of vertigo are associated with exercise of the arm located on the side of the occlusion. The ischemia results from the shunting of blood to the distal subclavian artery on the occluded side through the junction of the two vertebral arteries at the basilar artery. The treatment is surgical correction of the subclavian occlusion in markedly symptomatic patients.

Migraine-equivalent (atypical migraine)

Vertigo may occur as part of a migraine attack. Occasionally vertigo with or without hearing loss may be the only symptoms (atypical migraine). The diagnosis is based on personal and family history of migraine, exclusion of other neurological disorders and the efficacy of prophylactic or symptomatic treatment with antimigrainous medications.

Brain stem tumors, paraneoplastic syndrome and metastatic carcinoma

Vertigo is a relatively common symptom associated with tumors of the brain stem. The most common types are astrocytoma, medulloblastoma, acoustic neuroma and occasionally meningioma and chordoma. Metastatic carcinomas involving the brain stem are most commonly those of the lung, the breast or the bowel. The paraneoplastic syndrome, both cerebellar and bulbar forms, involves multiple neural dysfunction secondary to presumed immune-mediated mechanisms rather than direct tumor invasion.

TREATMENT OF VERTIGO

The treatment of vertigo requires a blend of art and science. The symptoms are frightening and troublesome to patients, though they are usually representative of a benign disorder involving the inner ear. This fact should be used to reassure patients.

One of the most useful devices for treating vertigo is a daily record sheet of symptoms and treatment (Figure 4.3). The form serves several purposes. For one, the patient is reassured of the continuous concern of the physician even though he may be seen at infrequent intervals, such as every 3–4 months. Also, when presented at the next office visit, the daily record establishes at a glance the clinical course of the disorder and the use or misuse of prescribed medications and exercises. Finally, this method incorporates the patient as a partner in his medical care.

Mild to moderate (Vl–V2) vestibular attacks

There are many medications available for the treatment of vertigo. Those that are effective are capable of suppressing mild to moderate vestibular upset. The dosage should be titrated against symptoms, adjusted upward or downward as necessary to keep side effects – usually sleepiness and mild incoordination – to a minimum. Two medications that are effective are meclazine and diazepam. Frequencies of administration are shown in

Table 4.3. A similar sliding scale can be used for proprietary drugs, such as Dramamine® (Pharmacia & Upjohn, Peapack, NJ, USA) and Bonine® (Pfizer, New York, NY, USA). Some physicians use promethazine HCl (Phenergan®, Wyeth-Ayerst Pharmaceuticals, Philadelphia, PA, USA) 6.25–12.5 mg in a similar manner.

Marked vertigo (V3) associated with nausea and vomiting

For treatment of marked vertigo (V3) associated with nausea and vomiting, Tigan® (Monarch Pharmaceuticals, Bristol, TN, USA) is administered 200 mg intramuscularly or as a suppository every 8 hours p.r.n. along with intravenous fluids if necessary. An alternative to Tigan is Compazine® (Smith Kline Beecham Pharmaceuticals, Philadelphia, PA, USA), 10 mg intramuscularly or as a suppository.

Chronic positional imbalance and mild to moderate vertigo (V1–V2)

The vestibular response in the injured system as well as in the intact vestibular system can be suppressed by repeated stimulation. This phenomenon, called habituation, is the mechanism that permits a figure skater to spin in a manner that a non-habituated person could not tolerate. The tolerance of the injured system for motion can be improved by the Cawthorne–Cooksey vestibular exercise program to overcome dizziness:

(1) In order to derive the most benefit, exercises must be done diligently three times a day for at least 5 min;

(2) At each of these times, always start with number 1 in the schedule and proceed to the point at which the exercises cause discomfort from dizziness;

(3) As soon as dizziness occurs, stop and wait for the next exercise period;

Table 4.3 Frequencies of administration of meclazine 12.5 mg (Antivert®) or diazepam 2 mg (Valium®)

Beginning dosage: twice a day
If no response in 24 hours, must continue three times a day
If no response in 48 hours, four times a day.
When vertigo is controlled, reduce the number of pills by one every 5 days

DAILY PATIENT RECORD
VERTIGO AND HEARING LOSS
MARK SYMPTOMS WITH AN X

NAME _____

UNIT # _____

PATIENT # _____

DAY NUMBER	DATE	NO SYMPTOMS	PRESSURE IN EAR	INCREASED EAR NOISE	HEARING CHANGE ↑↓	IMBALANCE C CONTINUOUS I INTERMITTENT	VERTIGO* MILD	VERTIGO* MODERATE	VERTIGO* SEVERE	DROP ATTACK	TIME OF VERTIGO C CONTINUOUS OTHERWISE: HR, MIN, SEC	ACTIVITY AT ONSET	MEDICATION AND NUMBER OF PILLS	CAWTHORNE EXERCISE SCORE	
1															
2															
3															
4															
5															
6															
7															
8															
9															
10															
11															
12															
13															
14															
15															
16															
17															
18															
19															
20															
21															
22															
23															
24															
25															
26															
27															
28															
29															
30															

*VERTIGO MILD: PATIENT MAY CONTINUE ACTIVITIES
MODERATE: CLEARS AFTER PATIENT TAKES A SHORT REST
SEVERE: PATIENT MUST TAKE TO BED; HE EXPERIENCES NAUSEA AND SOMETIMES VOMITING

Figure 4.3 Sample of daily record sheet of symptoms and treatment. The form is quite simple and takes only a few seconds to complete each day. If the patient is symptom-free, 'no symptoms' is checked (ticked), and nothing further is marked for that day. An 'x' is placed in the appropriate space if the patient experiences pressure or noise in the ear. Hearing changes and the sensation of imbalance are similarly indicated. Mild (V1), moderate (V2) and severe (V3) vertigo are noted when present, as well as any drop attacks. The duration of the vertigo, any activity that may have precipitated it and the medications and exercises used for treatment are all recorded

(4) All exercises are started in exaggerated slow time, then progress gradually to more rapid time. The rate of progression – from bed, to sitting, to standing – varies from patient to patient;

(5) A period of 2 months is needed to give the program a fair chance.

Exercises

A. In bed, supine (only if you cannot sit up); otherwise in sitting position without arm rest.
    1. Head immobile, eye movements (at first slow, then quick)
       a. Up and down.
       b. Side to side.
       c. Repeat a and b, focusing on finger.
       d. Focus on finger moving back and forth from about 3 feet (1 m) to 2 inches (5 cm) away from face.
    2. Head mobile, head movements (at first slow, then quick). Later with eyes closed.
       a. Bend forward and backward.
       b. Turn from side to side.
B. Sitting position, without arm rests
  Repeat as in 1 and 2.
    3. Shrug shoulders and rotate upper body.
    4. Bend forward and pick up objects from the ground.
    5. Rotate head and shoulders slowly, then quickly.
       a. Rotate head with eyes open, then closed.
    6. Rotate head, shoulders, and trunk with eyes open, then closed.
C. Standing
    7. Repeat number 1.
    8. Repeat number 2.
    9. Repeat number 5.
    10. Change from a sitting to a standing position with eyes open, and then with them shut.
    11. Throw ball from hand to hand (at eye level).
    12. Throw ball from hand to hand (above eye level).
    13. Change from sitting to standing and turn around in between.
    14. Repeat number 6.
D. Walking
    15. Walk across the room with eyes open, then closed.
    16. Walk up and down slope with eyes open, then closed.

17. Do any games involving stooping or stretching and aiming, such as bowling and shuffleboard.
18. Stand on one foot with eyes open, then closed.
19. Walk with one foot in front of the other with eyes open, then closed.

Vestibular physical therapy

In addition to the Cawthorne–Cooksey exercises, a modern physical therapy department can provide additional therapy designed specifically for vestibular disorders. This is particularly helpful in chronic vestibulopathy such as vestibular ototoxicity, vestibulopathy of aging or following acute injury such as skull fractures or other labyrinthine insults.

Selected reading

Honrubia V, ed. Clinical applications of vestibular science. *Otolaryngol Head Neck Surg* 1995;112:2–188

5

Facial paresis and paralysis

Joseph B. Nadol, Jr

Functional anatomy and physiology of the facial nerve
   Components of the peripheral facial nerve
   Physiology of degeneration
Evaluation of facial nerve regeneration
Sites and subtypes of facial nerve paralysis
History and physical examination in facial paralysis
Electrodiagnostic and topognostic testing for facial nerve dysfunction
   Electrical excitability
   Electroneuronography
   Electromyography
   Topognostic testing
      Schirmer test
      Salivary flow
      Stapedius reflex
Imaging of the facial nerve
Common disease processes affecting cranial nerve VII
   Traumatic facial nerve paralysis
   Iatrogenic injury
   Lyme disease
   Congenital and genetic facial paralysis
   Inflammatory disorders
      Bell's palsy
      Melkersson–Rosenthal syndrome
   Infectious disorders
      Viral disorders
      Bacterial disorders
   Central causes
   Cerebellopontine angle neoplasms
      Acoustic neuroma
Treatment for facial paralysis

Protection of the eye
Therapy for Bell's palsy
Facial nerve decompression and exploration
Surgical rehabilitation of facial paralysis
    Surgical repair of the facial nerve
    Hypoglossal facial anastomosis
    Cross-facial nerve grafting
    Static and dynamic facial slings

FUNCTIONAL ANATOMY AND PHYSIOLOGY OF THE FACIAL NERVE

There are at least three cortical or subcortical neural pathways that innervate the pontine brain-stem nucleus of the facial nerve (cranial nerve (CN) VII). The corticofacial pathway, a part of the pyramidal tract (Figure 5.1), projects from the precentral gyrus to the facial nucleus and mediates voluntary facial motion. Most of the projection is crossed, that is, it originates in the opposite cortex. However, there is an uncrossed input limited to the upper musculature of facial expression. The second major input to the facial nucleus is the thalamofacial pathway, originating in the thalamus. This is both crossed and uncrossed and mediates spontaneous or involuntary (emotional) motion of facial musculature. Other inputs to the facial nuclei arise in other brain-stem nuclei. For example, the corneal (blink) reflex is mediated by input from the nucleus of CN V, and the stapedial reflex (contraction of the stapedius muscle in response to loud noise) is mediated by input from the superior olive. Both the corticofacial and thalamofacial pathways end on a group of facial nuclei in the pontine brain stem (Figure 5.2). The main nuclei are those for the upper and lower facial musculature. In addition, separate nuclei are recognized for the stapedius muscle and for the digastric muscle (accessory facial nucleus).

The lower motor neuron of the facial nerve emanates from the facial nuclei and passes ipsilaterally to the periphery through the cerebellopontine angle, internal auditory canal and temporal bone. Several anatomic segments of the peripheral facial nerve are recognized (Figure 5.3). The pontine segment begins at the facial nuclei and ends at the porus of the internal auditory canal. The meatal segment begins at the porus and ends at the fundus of the internal auditory canal. Within the internal auditory canal, the meatal segment of the facial nerve is located in the anterior-superior quadrant (Figure 5.4). The labyrinthine segment begins at the fundus of the internal auditory canal and ends at the geniculate ganglion. The tympanic segment begins at the geniculate ganglion and ends at the second external genu, which is the beginning of the mastoid descending, or vertical, segment that ends at the stylomastoid foramen.

Components of the peripheral facial nerve

In addition to motor fibers, the peripheral facial nerve carries somatic sensory, visceral afferent, taste and general visceral efferent fibers (Table 5.1, Figure 5.5). Knowledge of the various components of the facial nerve can be employed in site-of-lesion testing in facial paralysis.

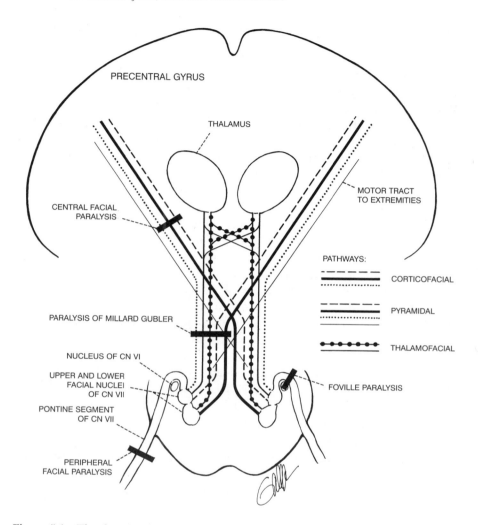

Figure 5.1 The three cortical or subcortical neural pathways that innervate the pontine brain-stem nucleus of the facial nerve include the cortical facial pathway projecting from the precentral gyrus, the thalamofacial pathway originating in the thalamus, and other inputs from brain-stem nuclei including that of cranial nerve (CN) V and from the superior olive

Physiology of degeneration

A classification of nerve injuries has been offered by Sunderland[1]. In nerve injury of the first degree, the perineurial and epineurial nerve sheaths are intact and the nerve fibers are viable, but fail to conduct a neural impulse (neuropraxia). In second degree injury there is degeneration of axons

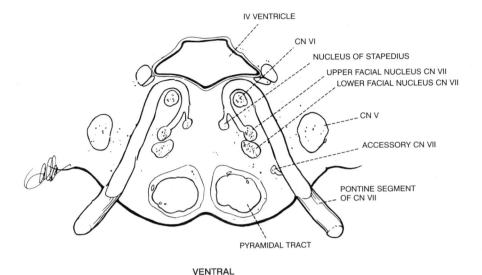

IV VENTRICLE

CN VI

NUCLEUS OF STAPEDIUS

UPPER FACIAL NUCLEUS CN VII

LOWER FACIAL NUCLEUS CN VII

CN V

ACCESSORY CN VII

PONTINE SEGMENT OF CN VII

PYRAMIDAL TRACT

VENTRAL

Figure 5.2 The pontine nucleus of cranial nerve (CN) VII contains a group of facial nuclei, including those for the upper and lower facial musculature, the nucleus of the stapedius and the nucleus for the digastric muscle (accessory facial nucleus)

(axonotmesis), but no disruption of the endoneurial nerve tubes. Since the facial nerve can regenerate and the nerve tubes maintain an appropriate regenerative pathway, recovery is usually nearly complete without synkinesis. In third degree injury, in addition to axonal degeneration, there has been disruption of endoneurial tubes, but not of the perineurium (neurotmesis). Regeneration in such injuries is generally prolonged and results in disordered regeneration (synkinesis). In fourth degree injuries, there has been disruption of axons and endoneurial tubes and partial disruption of the perineurium. In fifth degree injuries, there has been complete transection of the nerve, including axons, endoneurium and perineurium. In fourth and fifth degree injuries, regeneration is incomplete and disordered.

EVALUATION OF FACIAL NERVE REGENERATION

The Facial Nerve Disorders Committee of the American Academy of Otolaryngology – Head and Neck Surgery adopted a grading system for facial nerve recovery subsequently called the House–Brackmann grading system[2] (Table 5.2). It is appropriately used only for facial nerve recovery,

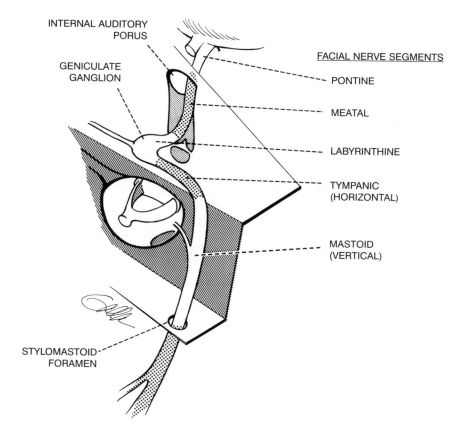

INTERNAL AUDITORY
PORUS

FACIAL NERVE SEGMENTS

GENICULATE
GANGLION

PONTINE

MEATAL

LABYRINTHINE

TYMPANIC
(HORIZONTAL)

MASTOID
(VERTICAL)

STYLOMASTOID
FORAMEN

Figure 5.3 The course and segments of the facial nerve between the pontine brain stem and the facial musculature

not for acute facial nerve injury. A major component of the grading system is the presence or absence of synkinesis, which accompanies recovery rather than the injury itself. In this system, grade 1 represents normal function, that is full recovery, and grade 6 represents total paralysis, or no recovery.

SITES AND SUBTYPES OF FACIAL NERVE PARALYSIS

In general, facial nerve paralysis is described as central if the lesion is proximal to the pontine facial nuclei, and peripheral if it is distal to these nuclei. Subtypes of central facial paralysis are the paralyses of Millard–Gubler and

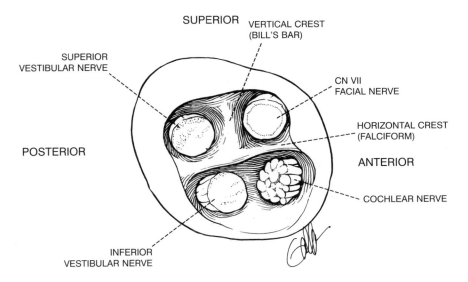

Figure 5.4 The facial nerve occupies the anterosuperior quadrant of the internal auditory canal at its fundus

of Foville. In the paralysis of Millard–Gubler there is ipsilateral facial nerve paralysis, and hemiparesis contralateral to the site of lesion. This is due to the fact that the upper motor neurons of the corticofacial tract cross the pons rostral to the rest of the pyramidal tract (Figure 5.1). In the paralysis of Foville, the clinical picture is that of a lower facial paralysis, except that other nearby brain stem nuclei, usually that of CN VI, are involved and hence, the paralysis is due to a brain stem lesion near the facial nuclei (Figure 5.1).

The differential diagnosis, characteristics of different sites of involvement of the facial nerve, are presented in Table 5.3.

HISTORY AND PHYSICAL EXAMINATION IN FACIAL PARALYSIS

The onset and characteristics of facial paresis and paralysis are extremely important in the differential diagnosis. A complete history includes onset and rate of progression of facial weakness; history of injury or other disease process that may be causative; other otological symptoms such as hearing loss, vertigo or otorrhea; and potentially relevant past medical history such as previous occurrence of facial paralysis, involvement of other cranial nerves and history of tumors elsewhere in the body. A history of multiple

Table 5.1 Components of the facial nerve

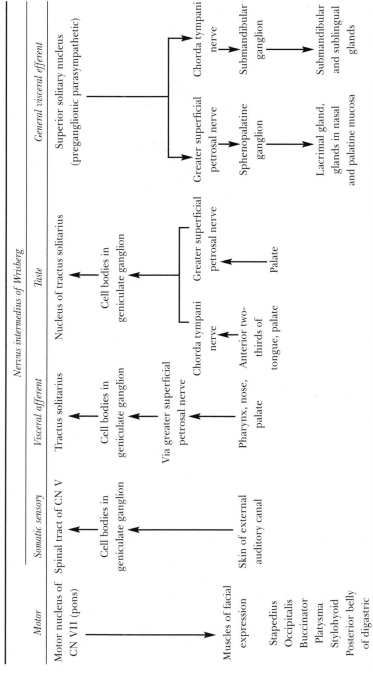

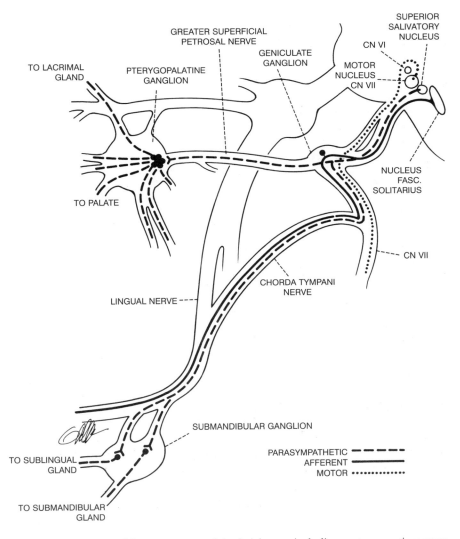

Figure 5.5 Diagram of the components of the facial nerve including motor somatic sensory, visceral afferent, taste and general visceral efferent fibers

sclerosis or tick bite in the recent past is important. The rapidity of progression of facial paralysis is important. For example, in Bell's palsy the evolution of the paralysis is usually complete within 3 days, whereas in neoplastic disorders, facial nerve function may deteriorate over months.

The physical examination should document the degree of facial weakness and divisions affected. A complete head and neck examination should

Table 5.2 Grading system for recovery of facial nerve function. From reference 2

Grade I: Normal
Normal facial function in all areas

Grade II: Mild dysfunction
Gross: Slight weakness noticeable on close inspection. May have slight synkinesis. At rest, normal symmetry and tone
Motion: Forehead: moderate-to-good function. Eye: complete closure with minimal effort. Mouth: slight asymmetry

Grade III: Moderate dysfunction
Gross: Obvious but not disfiguring difference between two sides. Noticeable but not severe synkinesis, contracture or hemifacial spasm, or both. At rest, normal symmetry and tone
Motion: Forehead: slight-to-moderate movement. Eye: complete closure with effort. Mouth: slightly weak with maximum effort

Grade IV: Moderately severe dysfunction
Gross: Obvious weakness or disfiguring asymmetry, or both. At rest, normal symmetry and tone
Motion: Forehead: none. Eye: incomplete closure. Mouth: asymmetric with maximum effort

Grade V: Severe dysfunction
Gross: Only barely perceptible motion. At rest, symmetry
Motion: Forehead: none. Eye: incomplete closure. Mouth: slight movement

Grade VI: Total paralysis
Motion: None

---

be carried out. In particular, an otological examination should be performed and a search made for other cranial neuropathies. The parotid gland and neck should be examined to determine whether there are lesions along the extratemporal course of the facial nerve. The skin of the auricle or external auditory canal may reveal vesicles, suggesting Ramsay Hunt syndrome.

ELECTRODIAGNOSTIC AND TOPOGNOSTIC TESTING FOR FACIAL NERVE DYSFUNCTION

In facial nerve injury electrodiagnostic testing is usually not carried out unless there is complete facial paralysis. The principal value of electrical testing is prognostication concerning degree and timing of recovery. Even after total transection of the facial nerve, the distal fibers retain electrical excitability for 3–5 days. Therefore, these tests are usually of limited value immediately after the injury.

Table 5.3 Differential diagnosis of disorders of the facial nerve

	Structures	*Symptoms*	*Representative disorders*
A.	*Central*		
	Supranuclear (upper motor neuron)	incomplete facial weakness emotional facial response more active than voluntary	stroke, multiple sclerosis, Guillain–Barré syndrome, amyotrophic lateral sclerosis, tumor
		more paralysis in lower than upper face associated neurological involvement	
	Nuclear (brainstem)	complete upper and lower facial palsy	meningitis; tumors including neuroma, meningioma; stroke; metastatic tumor
		associated 6th nerve palsy (failure of lateral gaze)	
B.	*Cerebellopontine angle (CPA)*	lesions may involve auditory and vestibular nerves as well; large lesions can involve 9th, 10th or 11th nerves; the 7th nerve is able to withstand a large amount of stretching without loss of clinical function	acoustic neurinoma, meningioma, congenital cholesteatoma, metastatic cancer to CPA
C.	*Internal auditory canal*	the nervus intermedius is involved before there are clinical signs of 7th nerve palsy; symptoms include decreased tearing, decreased salivary flow or taste changes; subtle changes in motor conduction rates can be measured; associated 8th nerve signs may occur	
D.	*Fallopian canal*	facial weakness at this level may be associated with decreased taste on the ipsilateral anterior tongue or diminished stapedius muscle reflex testing, depending on the location of injury	Bell's palsy, herpes zoster oticus, Melkersson–Rosenthal syndrome, temporal bone fracture, acute or chronic otitis media or tumor; 7th nerve neuroma, glomus jugulare, squamous cell carcinoma
E.	*Extracranial*	the nerve involves only the branches affected by that tumor or traumatic event	trauma, malignant parotid tumor

Electrical excitability

Using an impulse of 0.3 milliseconds, the threshold of nerve excitability is measured by visual inspection of ipsilateral facial motion. Although there is wide variability in threshold from patient to patient, there is usually very little difference from side to side in the same patient. A threshold in milliamperes is determined, comparing the involved versus the uninvolved side. A difference of 3.5 mA is considered evidence of nerve degeneration (axonotmesis or neurotmesis).

Electroneuronography

In this test, a bipolar surface electrode is used – one electrode placed at the stylomastoid foramen and the second placed anterior to the tragus. Using impulses in a square wave at 1 per second and a duration of 0.2 milliseconds, the amplitude of the summating potential is measured. The stimulus voltage is increased until the summating potential is at its maximum. The stimulating voltage is then increased to 110% of that determination to create a 'supramaximal' stimulus. Although the latency, amplitude and duration of the summating potential can be measured, the amplitude is most important clinically. There is an approximately arithmetic relationship between the amplitude of the summating potential and the degree of degeneration of nerve fibers. Thus, in neuropraxia, the summating potential will be equal on the paralyzed and non-paralyzed side, whereas in partial axonotmesis, reduction in amplitude to 50% of the normal side implies degeneration of approximately 50% of nerve fibers of the motor division of the facial nerve.

Electromyography

Degeneration potentials begin approximately 8–10 days after transection of the facial nerve and, hence, electromyography is even less valuable acutely than electrical testing. However, it is particularly useful during a recovery period, in which regeneration potentials may be seen prior to any convincing return of summating potential or visible motion of the face.

Topognostic testing

Schirmer test

This test evaluates the function of the general efferent fibers that pass through the greater superficial petrosal nerve (Table 5.1, Figure 5.5). The conjunctivae of the eyes are anesthetized and strips of blotting paper, 3.5 cm in length and 0.5 cm in width, are folded over the lower lid into the conjunctival sac. The amount of flow of tears is measured after 5 min. Anything over 1.5 cm in 5 min is considered normal, and implies neural integrity.

Salivary flow

Test of salivary flow also evaluates the integrity of general visceral efferent fibers, which pass through the chorda tympani nerve. In this test the mucosa of the mouth is anesthetized and a no. 60 polyethylene catheter is placed in Wharton's duct. The patient is asked to suck on a lemon for 1 min and the salivary secretions are separately collected. Significant diminution of flow implies disruption of the facial nerve above the takeoff of the chorda tympani nerve in its descending segment (assuming that the salivary glands are otherwise normal).

Stapedius reflex

The presence of a stapedius reflex can be evaluated by tympanometry. Absence of a stapedial reflex suggests an injury to the facial nerve above the takeoff of the nerve to the stapedius muscle (descending segment of facial nerve). However, approximately 5% of normal individuals do not have a stapedius reflex.

IMAGING OF THE FACIAL NERVE

Computerized tomography (CT) scans of the temporal bone and magnetic resonance imaging (MRI) of the course of the facial nerve have significantly added to the diagnostic and topognostic capabilities of clinical evaluation. The CT scan is particularly useful when alterations in the bony architecture of the temporal bone are anticipated, such as in chronic otitis media, or temporal bone fracture. MRI is particularly useful in identifying soft tissue lesions along the course of the facial nerve, such as facial schwannoma, acoustic neuroma and infiltrative lesions of the salivary glands.

COMMON DISEASE PROCESSES AFFECTING CRANIAL NERVE VII

Traumatic facial nerve paralysis

The facial nerve, as it passes through the cranial base, may be injured in closed or penetrating injuries. The most common closed injury is a basilar skull fracture. Approximately 50% of transverse fractures of the temporal bone will result in facial paralysis. The management of traumatic facial paralysis secondary to skull fractures is controversial. Some authors feel that, if total facial paralysis is delayed in onset, treatment may be expectant, particularly if CT scans do not show a significant disruption of the fallopian canal. However, some authorities believe that rapid degeneration of the facial nerve, as evaluated by electroneuronography (reduction of summating potential to 10% or less of the normal side within 6 days of onset of complete paralysis), is sufficiently predictive of poor recovery that surgical decompression is warranted.

Penetrating injuries of the face and temporal bone, such as gunshot injuries or lacerations of the face resulting in facial paralysis, suggest neurotmesis and should be surgically explored; the facial nerve should be repaired as soon as the patient is medically stable.

Iatrogenic injury

If the facial nerve has been damaged during the course of a surgical proce-dure, re-exploration of the facial nerve may be necessary, unless the injury to the facial nerve was recognized and evaluated at the first procedure.

Lyme disease

Facial nerve paralysis, including bilateral facial nerve paralysis, has been described as a complication of Lyme disease secondary to tick bite. Antibiotic treatment of Lyme disease will usually result in recovery of facial function.

Congenital and genetic facial paralysis

Facial nerve paralysis at birth may be due to birth injury such as forceps trauma or facial nerve compression against the maternal sacral promon-tory prior to birth. Rarely, there may be agenesis of the facial nerve, most often associated with craniofacial anomalies or the Moebius syndrome.

Inflammatory disorders

Bell's palsy

Bell's palsy is acute facial paralysis of undetermined etiology that each year affects approximately 20 out of every 100 000 persons. Possible causes include viral neuropathy with inflammatory swelling and secondary ischemia due to compression within the fallopian canal. Other possibilities include neural ischemia caused by microvascular disease. There is an 80% good-to-excellent spontaneous (grades I–II) recovery rate, but it is difficult to identify those patients who will recover and those who will not, and to decide upon a subsequent choice of therapy. Opinions regarding methods of testing, interpretation of tests and choice of treatment vary widely and are the source of some controversy in the medical literature. Oral steroids are commonly used in Bell's palsy, although the medical literature differs widely on the efficacy of this treatment.

Presenting symptoms include progressive facial weakness that involves all divisions of the peripheral motor nerve relatively equally. There is sometimes accompanying facial pain and often an antecedent history of viral infection or exposure to a cold air draft. Careful testing may reveal subtle concomitant dysfunction of CN V.

Melkersson–Rosenthal syndrome

Melkersson–Rosenthal syndrome is a recurrent facial paralysis characterized by simultaneous facial palsy and facial edema. Rosenthal noted a fissured tongue in some patients. Decompression of the facial nerve may be recommended in cases with progressive paresis and decreasing evoked summating potentials on electroneuronography.

Infectious disorders

Viral disorders

Herpes zoster oticus is an occasional cause of facial paralysis. It is identified by the associated painful vesicular eruption of the external auditory canal and auricle, as well as by associated sensorineural hearing loss and vestibular injury in some cases. This is a true viral infection, with neural and intraneural round cell infiltration. Treatment includes the administration of oral steroids, unless this is precluded by corneal ulceration. Acyclovir is also usually prescribed.

Rubella and infectious mononucleosis are other viral infections reported to have occurred in association with facial paralysis. Presumably the pathophysiology and therapy would be identical to that for herpes zoster oticus.

Bacterial disorders

Acute suppurative otitis media may cause facial palsy in children and adults. The facial palsy nearly always resolves completely. In addition to the usual oral antibiotic regimen, a myringotomy should be performed in order to drain and culture purulent material. It is presumed that these patients have an area of dehiscence of the bony covering of the nerve in the middle ear. Retrograde infection by way of the chorda tympani is a less likely possibility. Progressive degeneration of the facial nerve, as tested by electroneuronography, may require mastoidectomy and facial nerve decompression, especially if the acute infection is responding slowly to medical management.

Facial paralysis in conjunction with chronic suppurative otitis media, indicated by a chronically infected ear with purulent, foul-smelling drainage, or chronic otitis media with cholesteatoma represents a surgical emergency. Unlike facial paralysis associated with acute otitis media, it will not resolve without surgical intervention. The infected tissue must be removed by mastoidectomy, and the facial nerve is uncovered (decompressed) in the middle ear and mastoid. The success rate for resolution of paralysis is high when surgery is performed within a few days of onset.

Malignant otitis externa is a virulent form of cellulitis and osteitis caused by *Pseudomonas* in diabetics, resulting from an initial superficial otitis externa. Facial palsy is a sign of cellulitis of the skull base or bony involvement. Treatment is predominantly medical.

Central causes

Central causes of seventh nerve paralysis include stroke, multiple sclerosis, Guillain–Barré syndrome, and amyotrophic lateral sclerosis. These are rare forms of facial nerve paralysis involving incomplete as well as complete facial paralysis associated with other neurological complications. The differential findings in central versus peripheral facial paralysis and the subtypes of central paralysis are discussed on pages 118–123.

Cerebellopontine angle neoplasms

Acoustic neuroma

Sensorineural hearing loss and unilateral vestibular dysfunction usually occurs prior to any loss of facial function. In fact, facial nerve paralysis is an unusual finding with acoustic neuroma.

TREATMENT FOR FACIAL PARALYSIS

The treatment for facial paralysis will obviously differ according to the disease process. For example, acute suppurative otitis medial with facial paralysis is managed with drainage of the middle ear and intravenous antibiotics. Facial paralysis due to neoplastic involvement of the facial nerve will often require surgical intervention and resection of the involved nerve segment. However, some general guidelines can be offered for management of facial paralysis including treatments for some specific diagnoses.

Protection of the eye

Because eye closure and lacrimal gland secretion are controlled by the facial nerve, the most urgent management problem in facial paralysis is protection of the eye. Desiccation of the cornea due to a decrease in tear production and a lack of the blink reflex may cause exposure keratitis within a matter of hours. Left untreated, this may lead to severe corneal ulceration and/or scarring and permanent loss of vision. The initial symptoms of exposure keratitis include a red, painful eye. Ophthalmic fluorescein may help demonstrate superficial corneal ulceration. Primary care for facial paralysis should thus include artificial tears used as eye drops every 2 hours or more often, as needed. At night lubricating ointments such as Lacri-Lube® (Allergan Pharmaceuticals, Irvine, CA, USA) are more long-lasting. The eye should be protected at night either by having the lids taped closed or with the use of an eye patch. In cases in which recovery is expected to be prolonged or incomplete, surgical protection of the cornea may be achieved by the use of a lateral tarsorrhaphy or the use of implanted gold weight in the upper lid to allow upper lid closure by gravity. Protection of the cornea is even more acutely indicated in patients with concomitant CN V dysfunction, because loss of sensation to the cornea may preclude the early symptoms of impending exposure keratitis.

Therapy for Bell's palsy

Many physicians use corticosteroids given orally over the course of 7–10 days, although the medical literature is contradictory on the efficacy of corticosteroid treatment. Facial paralysis in Bell's palsy is almost always self-limited, and good if not complete recovery is the general rule. If recovery has not commenced within 6 months of onset, a thorough clinical work-up for other causes of paralysis is warranted. Decompression of the facial nerve is seldom necessary. Possible exceptions include recurrent idiopathic facial paralysis due to Bell's palsy or Melkersson–Rosenthal syndrome.

Facial nerve decompression and exploration

The most common indication for decompression and exploration of the facial nerve is injury, either closed skull trauma or penetrating injuries, or trauma secondary to surgical procedures in the posterior fossa, temporal bone or parotid gland. Occasionally, exploration of the facial nerve is indicated in a patient in whom clinical aspects of the facial paralysis is inconsistent with the usual clinical course of Bell's palsy and in whom radiographic and other clinical tests have not revealed a site or etiology.

Surgical rehabilitation of facial paralysis

Surgical repair of the facial nerve

Surgical repair, either end-to-end anastomosis or autologous cable grafting, is considered preferable to bypass or dynamic sling procedures (to be discussed later). For example, in closed head trauma or penetrating injury of the facial nerve, exploration is warranted once the patient is otherwise medically stable. Surgery within 72 hours will facilitate identification of the facial nerve, because nerve excitability may be preserved for this period of time. Long delays will interfere with the identification of the severed ends of the nerve because of deposition of scar tissue. Repair of facial nerve injuries after delays measured in years may not be successful because of atrophy of the facial musculature and fibrous ingrowth in the remaining distal nerve tube sheaths. In general, an end-to-end anastomosis is considered preferable to interposition grafts. Segments of up to 2 cm may be approximated in an end-to-end fashion by transposition of the facial nerve. End-to-end anastomosis is performed under microscopic control using perineural sutures, collagen vein conduits or biologic adhesives. To replace longer segments of a damaged or resected facial nerve, the greater auricular nerve or sural nerve (both cutaneous sensory nerves, one to the auricular area and the other to the dorsum of the foot) are most commonly used, because of comparable nerve diameters and relatively minor sensory defects.

Hypoglossal facial anastomosis

In cases in which primary end-to-end or cable grafting of the facial nerve cannot be accomplished, a hypoglossal–facial anastomosis may restore tone and motion of the face. For example, in a large acoustic neuroma, a resection of the tumor in the cerebellopontine angle may preclude identification of the pontine segment of the facial nerve and hence preclude nerve grafting. In the hypoglossal–facial anastomosis the ipsilateral hypoglossal nerve is transected or partially transected and sutured to the distal facial nerve in the parotid region proximal to the pes anserinus. This procedure will lead to ipsilateral dysfunction of strap musculature and some hemiatrophy of the tongue. However, after neural ingrowth has occurred, generally in 6–24 months, the patient may have significant improvement in facial tone and may learn to move the face by attempting to move the tongue.

Cross-facial nerve grafting

An alternative to hypoglossal–facial anastomosis is the use of autologous cable grafts ('jump grafts') to allow neural ingrowth from the contralateral normal facial nerve to the distal stump of the damaged facial nerve. This obviously has the advantage of more normal initiation of facial motion, but the disadvantage of paresis on the donor side.

Static and dynamic facial slings

In cases in which permanent paralysis or long-standing paralysis of the face is expected, static or dynamic slings using muscle transfers may provide tone and cosmetic rehabilitation without precluding subsequent facial nerve recovery. The most common sling technique involves strips of the ipsilateral temporalis muscle, innervated by CN V, which are tunneled subcutaneously and imbricated into the orbicularis oris muscle. The masseter muscle may also serve as a source of a muscle sling to the corner of the mouth. Static facial slings may be formed using free grafts of fascia lata and combined with rhytidectomy (face-lift).

In general, the totally paralyzed face can be substantially rehabilitated with a combination of techniques used to achieve corneal protection, facial asymmetry at rest and dynamic motion of selected facial muscle groups.

Bibliography

1. Sunderland S. *Nerves and Nerve Injury*, 2nd edn. Edinburgh: Churchill Livingstone, 1978
2. House JW, Brackmann DE. Facial nerve grading system. *Otolaryngol Head Neck Surg* 1985; 93:146–7

6

Pain syndromes in the head and neck

Joseph B. Nadol, Jr

Causes and clinical implications of primary otalgia
    Acute suppurative otitis media
    External otitis
    Ramsay Hunt syndrome
    Chronic otitis media
    Petrous apicitis or Gradenigo's syndrome
    Neoplasia
Causes of referred otalgia
    Dental pain and the temporomandibular joint syndrome
    Salivary glands
    Nose and paranasal sinuses
    Nasopharynx
    Oropharynx
    Laryngopharynx and esophagus
    Neck
    Neuralgia as a cause of otalgia
        Glossopharyngeal neuralgia (tympanic neuralgia)
        Trigeminal neuralgia
        Sphenopalatine neuralgia
        Geniculate neuralgia
        Eagle syndrome
        Carotidynia
    Follow-up for idiopathic otalgia
Sources of referred head and facial pain
    Ear
    Nose and paranasal sinuses
    Teeth
    Neck
    Orbit
    Other sources of referred pain

Recurrent or chronic pain is one of the most challenging diagnostic problems in the head and neck area. Not infrequently, significant pathology cannot be found in the anatomic site identified by the patient, and the possibility of pain referred from another site must be considered. Proper diagnosis requires a familiarity with anatomy and the common sources of referred pain. It also requires that the physician have self-confidence in his diagnostic abilities in the head and neck area to exclude significant occult causes of pain. The purpose of this chapter is to review common disorders that may result in pain referred to the ear and other sites in the head and neck region.

CAUSES AND CLINICAL IMPLICATIONS OF PRIMARY OTALGIA

Before seeking a source of referred otalgia, the clinician must rule out a primary otologic cause for pain. The more common primary causes of ear pain are infections.

Acute suppurative otitis media

This infection produces intense pain that usually resolves in 24 hours of initiation of antibiotic therapy. If this does not occur, the efficacy of the antibiotics, the possibility of other underlying systemic disorder or source for pain, or the possibility of early coalescent mastoiditis should be evaluated.

External otitis

An abscess in the external canal usually located near the meatus is easily diagnosed by point tenderness and occasionally fluctuance at the site. In diffuse external otitis, or swimmer's ear, the pain may linger for 3–5 days even after initiation of management. Worsening or persistent pain after 3–5 days should raise the question of another diagnosis such as neoplasia with superinfection or malignant external otitis.

Ramsay Hunt syndrome

Pain in the ear may precede the telltale vesicular eruption by several days. For chronic suppurative otitis media, pain is rare and uncomplicated.

Chronic otitis media

The presence of pain in chronic otitis media should alert the clinician to

135

impending neurological complications including meningeal irritation, meningitis, brain abscess or thrombophlebitis of the lateral venous sinus, or to an underlying malignancy.

Squamous cell carcinoma of the external auditory canal and mastoid is most commonly seen in the setting of chronic infection; therefore malignancy may be easily confused with simple chronic infectious process.

Petrous apicitis or Gradenigo's syndrome

The full clinical triad includes otitis media, ipsilateral sixth nerve paralysis and deep pain secondary to inflammation of the trigeminal ganglion.

Other infections such as chondritis or bullous myringitis may cause intense pain.

Neoplasia

Benign tumors of the temporal bone rarely produce pain. Occasionally acoustic neuromas may produce ipsilateral mastoid discomfort, but not tenderness. On the other hand, malignant tumors, particularly squamous cell carcinoma and adenoid cystic carcinoma, generally produce significant pain.

CAUSES OF REFERRED OTALGIA

Several cranial nerves and part of the cervical plexus contribute to the sensory innervation of the auricle (Figure 6.1), external canal and middle ear. Hence, it is not surprising that disease processes in quite distant sites may refer pain to the ear. In order to determine the cause of ear pain, the physician must develop a search strategy, such as is suggested below.

(1) A careful history should be taken to determine whether the pain is primary in the ear or is referred. The history of physiological disturbances in the head and neck, including such disorders as malocclusion, salivary gland disturbances, significant sinus disease, recurrent bleeding from the nose, pain in the oropharynx and hypopharynx, dysphagia, hoarseness or masses in the head and neck area, will give the first indication of a probable origin of referred pain.

(2) A careful ear examination will rule out a primary disorder of the ear. This should include otoscopy, manipulation of the external canal and auricle to rule out tenderness in this area, and tests of auditory

a

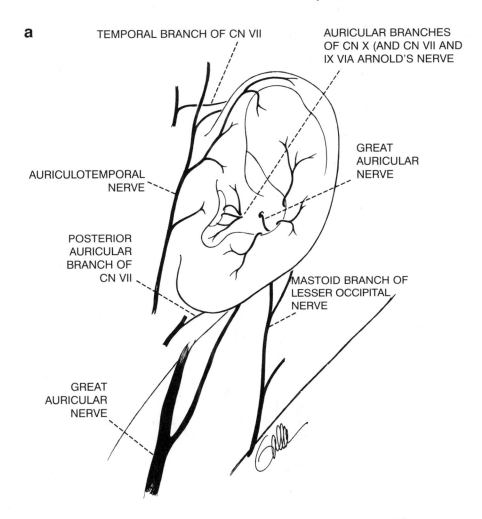

TEMPORAL BRANCH OF CN VII

AURICULAR BRANCHES OF CN X (AND CN VII AND IX VIA ARNOLD'S NERVE

AURICULOTEMPORAL NERVE

GREAT AURICULAR NERVE

POSTERIOR AURICULAR BRANCH OF CN VII

MASTOID BRANCH OF LESSER OCCIPITAL NERVE

GREAT AURICULAR NERVE

Figure 6.1 (*see also following page*) Sensory innervation of the auricle (a and b)

function. If no local dysfunction or source of referred pain is found, a computerized tomography (CT) scan of the mastoid and temporal bones will help rule out the presence of a neoplasm in the petrous bone or along the petrous ridge.

b

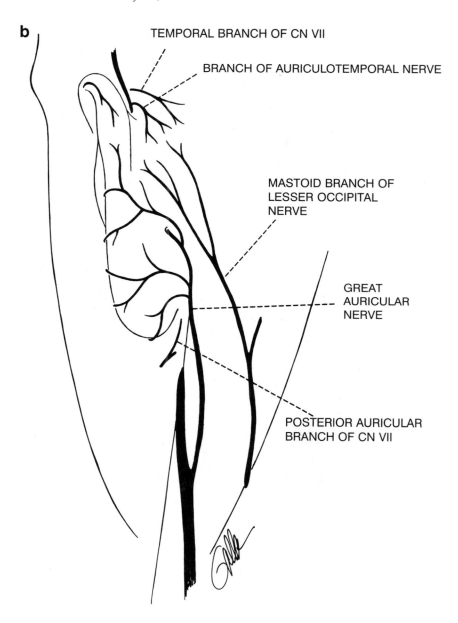

TEMPORAL BRANCH OF CN VII

BRANCH OF AURICULOTEMPORAL NERVE

MASTOID BRANCH OF
LESSER OCCIPITAL
NERVE

GREAT
AURICULAR
NERVE

POSTERIOR AURICULAR
BRANCH OF CN VII

(3) If primary otologic disease is not found, the examiner must then rule
out significant diseases in the head-and-neck area that may refer pain
to the ear.

I prefer to investigate referred pain in a systematic way, proceeding from the auricle to the most common sites of referred pain (Table 6.1).

Dental pain and the temporomandibular joint syndrome

By far the most common causes of non-otogenic otalgia are disorders of the teeth and temporomandibular joint. Malocclusion, ill-fitting dentures, caries, periapical abscesses, fractures and dislocations of the mandible, unerupted molars, bruxism and ulcerative lesions of the oropharynx may cause pain in the ipsilateral ear by way of the auriculotemporal branch of V3.

In temporomandibular joint syndrome, palpation over the joint while opening and closing the patient's mouth may reveal clicking, subluxation, lateral displacement of the mandible during opening and tenderness. Spasm of the medial pterygoid muscle, which is common in temporomandibular joint syndrome, may be manifest by tenderness at the site of attachment of this muscle on the medial surface of the mandible just anterior to its angle. X-ray results are negative except in the most advanced

Table 6.1   Sensory innervation of the ear

Cranial nerve V (auriculotemporal portion of V3) innervates the skin of the tragus, the anterior wall of the external auditory canal, a portion of the helix, the tympanic membrane, a portion of the middle ear and the tympanic plexus

Cranial nerve VII supplies cutaneous sensory innervation to the concha, a portion of the posterior canal wall and the posterior aspect of the auricle. There may be interconnections with cranial nerves IX and X

Cranial nerve IX (via tympanic or Jacobson's branch) innervates the medial aspect of the tympanic membrane and forms a major component of the tympanic plexus on the medial wall of the middle ear

Cranial nerve X, by way of its auricular branch (Arnold's nerve), mediates cutaneous sensation in a portion of the concha, the posterior aspect of the auricle and part of the posterior wall of the external auditory canal. Some anatomists believe that there are interconnections between the sensory branches of nerves VII, IX and X. A portion of the postauricular skin over the mastoid is also supplied by the auricular branch of cranial nerve X. It is probable that the cough reflex, commonly induced by manipulating the external auditory canal, is mediated by the auricular branch of cranial nerve X

Cervical nerves C2 and C3, by way of the posterior branch of the greater auricular nerve (C3), supply most of the posterior aspect of the auricle and its lateral surface. The lesser occipital nerve (C2) innervates the posterior aspect of the auricle and the adjacent skin overlying the mastoid cortex

cases, in which there is also trismus related to advanced degenerative changes in the temporomandibular joint. Examination of the dental arches may reveal abnormalities predisposing to the temporomandibular joint syndrome (e.g. malocclusion) or other sources of dental origin of referred otalgia (e.g. caries).

Salivary glands

Disorders of the salivary glands, including infection and other inflammatory and neoplastic disorders in the parotid, submandibular, sublingual and minor salivary glands, may be the source of referred pain in the ipsilateral ear via cranial nerves V, IX and X.

A careful history and an examination for masses and tenderness are usually sufficient to exclude this possibility. Sialography or other imaging is usually unnecessary unless there is some positive finding in the salivary tissues. However, adenoid cystic carcinoma of the salivary glands may produce pain as the presenting symptom before there is clinical or even radiographic evidence of a mass within the gland.

Nose and paranasal sinuses

Structural abnormalities, inflammatory disorders and neoplasms in the nose and paranasal sinuses may cause otalgia via cranial nerves V and IX. Tumors of the nose and paranasal sinuses, or acute, and occasionally chronic, sinusitis, particularly of the maxillary and sphenoid sinuses, may be the source of such pain. Most commonly, pain from the sphenoid sinus radiates to the vertex or occiput. Alternatively, the pain may radiate by way of the vidian nerve to the ear. Some authors believe that spurs of the nasal septum impinging on the middle turbinate may also cause ear pain.

A careful inquiry for suggestive symptoms, such as chronic drainage, tenderness, intermittent swelling and recurrent epistaxis, is followed by a thorough, careful anterior and posterior examination of the nose. CT scans of the sinuses are usually deferred unless there are other suggestive symptoms or findings.

Nasopharynx

Inflammatory disorders and, especially, neoplasms of the nasopharynx are common causes of pain referred to the ear via cranial nerves V and IX.

The history may include suggestive symptoms such as bleeding from the nose into the pharynx or chronic discharge. However, the most common presenting signs are ipsilateral serous otitis media and the presence of a node in the anterior or posterior cervical triangles.

Cranial nerve paresis, especially of the sixth nerve, is not uncommon. There is a much higher than average incidence of nasopharyngeal carcinoma among young adult males from mainland China.

Tumors of the nasopharynx are most commonly diagnosed by way of a mirror or transnasal nasopharyngoscopy. Some tumors of the nasopharynx spread out in a submucosal plane, and the physical findings by endoscopy may be extremely subtle or nonexistent. Therefore, if there is a high suspicion of nasopharyngeal tumor, radiography, including a lateral view of the nasopharynx, CT of the skull base to look for bony erosion and direct nasopharyngoscopy and biopsy may be indicated.

Oropharynx

Inflammatory or neoplastic disease of the oropharynx may refer pain to the ear by way of cranial nerves IX and X which form the pharyngeal plexus. In children, tonsillitis is a common cause of otalgia, even, paradoxically, when the child does not complain of throat pain. Parapharyngeal and retropharyngeal tumors or inflammation are other common sources of ear pain. Neoplasms of the lateral pharyngeal wall and the base of the tongue very commonly refer pain to the ear.

Careful examination of the oropharynx with proper light to check for asymmetry, masses and inflammatory disorders of the posterior oropharyngeal area and mirror examination of the hypopharynx and the base of the tongue are essential. Because neoplasms of the tongue base may spread submucosally and show little or no visual evidence of tumor, palpation of the tongue base and the floor of the mouth is also essential.

Laryngopharynx and esophagus

Disorders in the area of the laryngopharynx and esophagus may cause referred ipsilateral otalgia by way of cranial nerves IX and X. The most common causes are neoplasms of the epiglottis, pyriform sinus and postcricoid area. In advanced neoplastic disease, otalgia is considered a negative prognostic sign, because it suggests deep invasion.

A careful history should be taken of functional disorders of this area. A careful mirror or fiberoptic endoscopic examination is performed, particularly of the laryngeal surface of the epiglottis, pyriform sinus and postcricoid area. Appropriate X-ray studies, including fluoroscopy, barium swallow and CT of the larynx, are usually not performed, unless there is positive symptomatology, or unless the physician has a high index of suspicion of disorders in this area or is unable to accomplish a thorough examination. Even when they are performed, X-ray studies, including barium swallow, are not sufficient to rule out neoplasms of the laryngopharynx and esophagus. Relatively large tumors can be missed even by sophisticated radiographic techniques. Mirror and/or fiberoptic endoscopic examination is still essential in the diagnosis of neoplasms of the hypopharynx and larynx.

Neck

Disorders of the muscles, spine and organs of the neck may refer to the ear by way of the cervical nerves C2 and C3. Such disorders include arthritis of the spine, tumors of the thyroid gland or lymph nodes or carotidynia.

Taking a careful history of dysfunction in the area and palpation of the neck, including assessment of mobility of the spine, are usually sufficient to rule out disorders in this area.

Neuralgia as a cause of otalgia

Glossopharyngeal neuralgia (tympanic neuralgia)

Glossopharyngeal neuralgia consists of attacks of pain at one or more sites along the course of the distribution of cranial nerve IX. Typical localizations of pain include the base of the tongue, the soft palate, the tonsillar area and deep within the ear. The pain may be triggered by certain acts, such as swallowing or talking, or by temperature change in the throat.

The character of the pain is usually described as severe, intense and boring, and lasts only seconds. A few cases of syncope associated with glossopharyngeal neuralgia have also been described. Tympanic neuralgia is considered to be a subcategory of glossopharyngeal neuralgia in which pain is limited to the ear. The pain is usually felt deep within the ear and may be trigged by the stimulation of other areas innervated by the glossopharyngeal nerve, particularly in the throat. If there is a trigger point within the throat, local anesthesia of the area may prevent pain. If there is no trigger point within the throat, glossopharyngeal neuralgia is diagnosed by excluding other possible causes of pain.

If this neuralgia cannot be controlled medically, using Tegretol® (Novartis Pharmaceutical Corp., Saffern, NY, USA) or Dilantin® (Parke-Davis, Morris

Plains, NJ, USA), nerve section may be indicated. If pain is limited to the ear, transection of Jacobson's nerve by way of a transcanal tympanotomy may be curative. The glossopharyngeal nerve may also be approached through an external cervical route or an oral route through the tonsillar fossa.

Trigeminal neuralgia

A classical presentation of trigeminal neuralgia includes paroxysmal, severe, lancinating pain in the face. However, in atypical cases the pain may have trigger zones. Lesions of the middle cranial base must be excluded. Pain uncontrolled with Dilantin or Tegretol may be controlled with selective section of branches of cranial nerve V, posterior rhizotomy, intracranial decompression or radiofrequency lesioning of the ganglion.

Sphenopalatine neuralgia

Pain characteristic of sphenopalatine neuralgia is located in the lower aspect of the external ear, mastoid, occipital area, neck or shoulder. The pain is described by the patient as deep and boring and may last minutes to hours. Associated symptoms may include unilateral or bilateral lacrimation, nasal congestion and pain and tenderness in the upper teeth, face or mastoid region. A deviated nasal septum, infringing on the sphenopalatine ganglion, may act as a trigger in some cases.

Local anesthesia of the sphenopalatine ganglion may abort the pain during an attack. This may be accomplished by the use of 10% cocaine on a nasal pledget or the injection of 1% Xylocaine® by way of the greater palatine foramen. If pain is frequent or severe enough to warrant a surgical procedure, the sphenopalatine ganglion may be removed by a transantral approach.

Geniculate neuralgia

There have been a few reports of pain caused by neuralgia originating in the geniculate ganglion. The pain is characterized as deep within the ear, but it may radiate to other parts of the face. If analgesics are not successful in controlling the paroxysms of pain, relief may be achieved by sectioning the nervus intermedius portion of the facial nerve intracranially. Certainly, the diagnosis of geniculate neuralgia is one of exclusion. Some authors consider this another manifestation of tympanic neuralgia.

Eagle syndrome

An elongated styloid process or a calcified stylohyoid ligament may cause referred otalgia, in addition to difficulty with swallowing, owing to pain in the lateral aspect of the posterior oropharynx. The pain lasts seconds to minutes. The diagnosis of Eagle syndrome is confirmed by the presence of tenderness over an elongated styloid process and calcification verified by radiography.

Often the pain will regress spontaneously, but if it persists the styloid process may be removed either by an external cervical or a transoral approach.

Carotidynia

Carotidynia is usually localized to the neck and may radiate to the ear. It may be aggravated by head movement or swallowing. After other possible causes of pain have been excluded, the diagnosis of carotidynia is confirmed by reproducing or aggravating the pain by applying pressure on the carotid artery in the area of its bifurcation. The artery will feel otherwise normal. The injection of a local anesthetic should relieve the pain temporarily.

Most cases of carotidynia are self-limited and regress spontaneously within a year. To treat severe cases, the use of a short course of corticosteroids has been recommended.

Follow-up for idiopathic otalgia

If, as will occur in a great number of cases, a thorough head and neck examination and evaluation of all possibly significant symptoms has failed to lead to a reasonable, working diagnosis or a cause of otalgia, the 'test of time' may be invaluable. That is, it is not unreasonable to inform a patient that no significant disease has been found but that the symptoms should not be ignored. The patient should be re-examined in 2–3 months or sooner if the pain worsens or if new symptoms develop.

SOURCES OF REFERRED HEAD AND FACIAL PAIN

It is not the purpose of this section to review all the various causes of headache and facial pain. It is assumed that the reader is familiar with the fact that headache may be caused by inflammatory or vascular disturbances of the scalp, blood vessels of the head, muscles, meningeal structures and an increase in intracranial pressure, and that common syndromes include migraine, cluster headaches, lower-half headaches, tension headaches and cranial neuralgias.

In the evaluation of headache, it must be understood that referral of pain to the head may occur in disorders of the ear, nose, paranasal sinuses, dental structures, neck, orbit and even the heart.

Ear

Inflammatory or neoplastic diseases of the ear may refer pain to the postauricular, or mastoid, area and the temporal area of the head. Severe pain in the presence of infection of the ear may be a sign of impending serious complications. With acute or chronic active otitis media, headache may be an early sign that the disease has spread to the petrous apex, meninges or lateral venous sinus.

Nose and paranasal sinuses

Pain from inflammatory and neoplastic disorders of the nose and paranasal sinuses is usually well localized to the area of disease, but some referred pain is not unusual. For example, a patient with a disorder of the maxillary sinus will often complain of pain in his upper teeth. With ethmoid sinus disease, the pain may be localized behind the patient's eyes or deep between the eyes. With sphenoid sinus disease, the pain may be referred to the vertex or occiput.

Teeth

Disorders of the teeth and temporomandibular joint may refer pain to other areas in the trigeminal distribution or to adjacent structures, such as the ear or temporalis musculature.

Neck

Disorders of the cervical spine may refer pain to another location in the distribution of the upper cervical nerves, particularly of C2 and C3.

Orbit

Disorders within the orbit are a frequent source of headache. The most common of these is an increase in intraocular pressure. The most common problem in differential diagnosis is determining whether the pain is of frontal sinus origin or ocular origin. Other suggestive symptoms in the history, radiography of the sinuses and an ophthalmologic examination will almost always differentiate between the two.

Other sources of referred pain

Occasionally, structures distant from the head and neck may refer pain to the head area. An example of this is atypical angina pectoris, in which intense pain is felt in the throat, jaw or lower teeth.

7

Ear emergencies

Joseph B. Nadol, Jr

Auricle
  Hematoma
    Treatment
  Lacerations
  Perichondritis and chondritis
    Etiology
    Diagnosis
    Treatment
External auditory canal
  Foreign body
    Etiology
    Diagnosis and treatment
  Trauma
    Treatment
Tympanic membrane and middle ear
  Trauma
    Diagnosis
    Treatment
  Damage to the ossicular chain with or without perilymph leak
  Barotrauma
    Etiology and treatment
Inner ear trauma and temporal bone fracture
  Acoustic trauma
    Diagnosis
  Rupture of the round window or oval window
  Basilar skull fracture
    Diagnosis
  Traumatic cerebrospinal fluid otorrhea
  Sudden idiopathic hearing loss
    Diagnosis
    Treatment

Discussion of trauma and other ear emergencies is best approached from an anatomic orientation rather than from a symptom-oriented approach. Because the inner ear is not easily examined, the challenge to the primary care physician is to determine the extent of anatomic involvement in an injury. This is important, for example, in a case in which the danger from traumatic rupture of the tympanic membrane may be greatly overshadowed by that from undetected ossicular fracture, perilymph leak and injury to the inner ear. Primary infections of the external canal, middle ear and mastoid are discussed in Chapter 3.

AURICLE

Hematoma

Hematomas of the auricle are usually the result of direct trauma. The collection of blood elevates the perichondrium from the underlying auricular cartilage. This compromises the blood supply to the cartilage and, if left undrained, may result in a cauliflower ear owing to dissolution of part of the cartilaginous support of the auricle. In addition, auricular hematoma is very susceptible to superinfection, compounding the risk of loss of cartilage.

Treatment

The hematoma is evacuated using a large bore needle and sterile precautions. A pressure dressing is required to prevent reaccumulation (Figure 7.1). A conforming dressing is applied first, with the use of cotton strips impregnated with benzoin, normal saline or antibiotic ointment to fill in the interstices of the auricular cavities. A mastoid dressing is then applied using cotton, 4 × 4 surgical gauzes and preferably non-elastic rolled gauze. The ear should be re-examined and the dressing changed daily. If reaccumulation of the hematoma occurs, it may be reaspirated. If the hematoma has already organized so that needle aspiration is impossible, or if the hematoma accumulates repeatedly, incision of the overlying skin and evacuation of the hematoma cavity may be necessary. Although antibiotics are not strictly necessary, many practitioners prefer to use prophylaxis against *Staphylococcus aureus*. Some otologists believe that the use of a short, tapered course of corticosteroids will help prevent reaccumulation of a hematoma after aspiration.

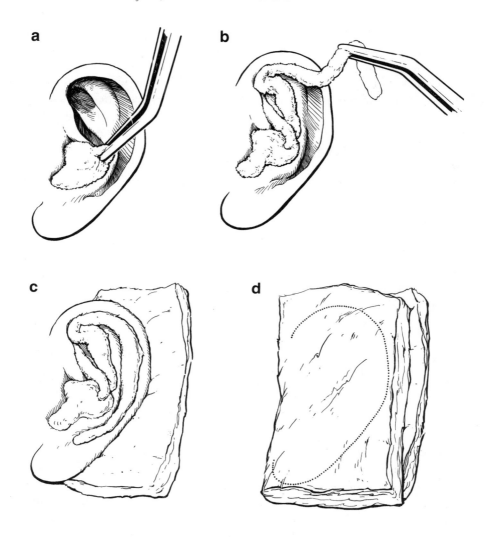

Figure 7.1 (*see also following page*) Conforming dressing for treatment of auricular hematoma (a) and (b). Cotton moistened in saline is placed in the concha and interstices of the auricular folds to prevent reaccumulation of the hematoma. This step is not necessary for the routine mastoid dressing, which begins with step (c). (c) and (d) Sterile cotton cuts are placed behind the ear and over it to provide a comfortable bed of cotton. (e) Three or four 4 × 4 surgical gauze pads are fluffed and placed over the cotton. A strip of 2-inch (5-cm) roller gauze is placed vertically over the temple, just lateral to the eye. (f) Roller gauze is wrapped around the head from the base of the occiput to the forehead. The dressing should not cover the opposite ear. (g) The dressing is tightened and moved away from the eye by tying of the vertical strip

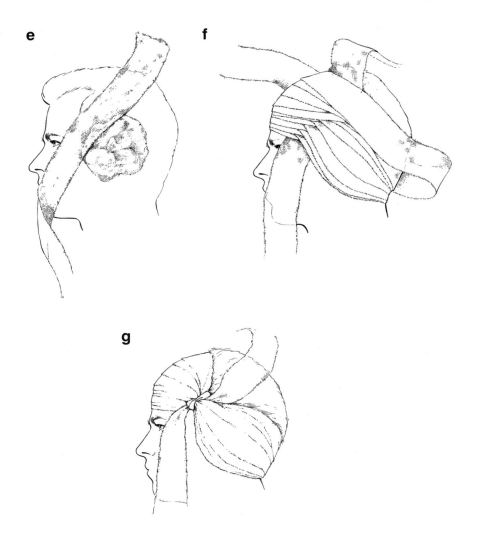

Lacerations

In the case of laceration of the auricle, standard surgical techniques for good wound repair are practiced. Macerated or clearly devitalized tissue is debrided. However, large segments of the auricle with little or no obvious vasculature may be reapproximated with hope for at least partial survival of the segment. Thus, successful reattachment of the entire auricle, or major segments of the auricle, have been reported. Macerated cartilage and cartilage without good skin coverage should be debrided. The use of tetanus toxoid prophylaxis and antibiotics follows the usual surgical indications.

Perichondritis and chondritis

Etiology

Infection of the perichondrium or auricular cartilage may occur secondary to infection of a hematoma, as a complication following surgical procedures, minor abrasions or burns of the auricular skin.

Diagnosis

Local erythema and tenderness suggest the diagnosis. The edema often thickens and distorts the normal configuration of the auricle, giving it a doughy appearance. The usual organisms involved are *Pseudomonas aeruginosa* and *S. aureus*. Perichondritis and chondritis must be distinguished from relapsing polychondritis, a disease thought to be autoimmune in etiology and which results in recurrent episodes of pain, erythema and an inflammatory response in cartilaginous structures, including the nose and auricle. On the first occurrence of relapsing polychondritis, differentiating between it and suppurative perichondritis may be difficult; the diagnosis may be based largely on the response to steroids, which usually produce a sudden and dramatic response in relapsing polychondritis. Biopsy of auricular cartilage may also be helpful in making this differentiation in difficult cases.

Treatment

The treatment of auricular perichondritis or chondritis requires the administration of parenteral antibiotics based on the results of a Gram stain and culture. If no pus is available, antibiotic coverage for *Pseudomonas* and *Staphylococcus* is selected. Aspiration of the subcutaneous tissues using a small volume of sterile saline without preservatives may provide sufficient material for culture. Parenteral treatment is continued until all signs and symptoms have resolved, usually for 2–3 weeks. If little progress is made, or if obvious abscess formation occurs, drainage, debridement of devitalized cartilage and the insertion of drains may be necessary.

EXTERNAL AUDITORY CANAL

Foreign body

Etiology

The usual clinical situation is the accidental insertion of a small object or plaything into the external canal of a child, or an insect gaining access to a patient's external auditory canal while the patient is asleep or unconscious.

Diagnosis and treatment

The most important aspect of managing a foreign body is determining the extent of the injury. This is particularly true of injuries from penetrating objects such as pencils or paper clips. To determine the extent of injury, the following two questions must be addressed. Has there been damage to the tympanic membrane and the ossicular chain? Is there any evidence of inner ear damage that might be caused by puncture of the round window, disruption of the stapediovestibular joint or fracture of the promontory? Sensorineural hearing loss, as determined by tuning fork and whisper tests or the presence of nystagmus, subjective unsteadiness or vertigo, suggests inner ear damage and may require emergency surgical intervention. During the initial evaluation, the function of the facial nerve should also be assessed.

The second most important tenet of treatment is to avoid producing further damage in abortive attempts to remove a foreign body. Removal of a foreign body requires a cooperative patient. In an adult this may require the use of a local anesthetic; in a child a general anesthetic may be necessary. Proper otologic equipment and microscopic control are essential. Living insects may be drowned in otic drops or mineral oil before removal with alligator or Hartmann's forceps. Irrigation is generally avoided, especially with organic foreign bodies that may absorb water and expand. In addition, the extent of the damage to the tympanic membrane may not be easily assessed until the foreign body is removed. If a perforation is present, irrigation may produce otitis media or labyrinthitis. Round foreign bodies may be removed with a right-angle hook, which is passed beyond the foreign body, or they may be removed with the Schuknecht foreign body aspirator. Once the foreign body is removed, careful assessment is made of the tympanic membrane. Perforations are then treated as discussed in the section Tympanic Membrane and Middle Ear (see pages 154–156).

Trauma

Abrasions commonly occur in the external canal during attempts by either a patient or a physician to clean it, because the skin of the bony external canal adheres tightly to the periosteum. Profuse bleeding may occur, which prevents proper evaluation of the tympanic membrane.

Treatment

Good light, magnification and suction with a no. 5 ear suction are used to determine the site of bleeding. The bleeding may be controlled by the application of silver nitrate to the external canal or by the use of an ear wick moistened with a few drops of epinephrine (adrenaline; 1 : 1000). Once the bleeding is controlled, the prophylactic use of otic antibiotic drops is usually recommended for 5–7 days.

Lacerations of the external canal may result from longitudinal basilar skull fractures that pass through the squamous and tympanic portions of the temporal bone. These fractures also often cause the leakage of cerebrospinal fluid (CSF). After an initial evaluation using a sterile suction tip, no immediate treatment is required other than occluding the ear with sterile cotton. Antibiotic drops or frequent manipulation are contraindicated, to avoid contamination of the CSF. The use of prophylactic antibiotics to treat traumatic CSF leaks is controversial; if used, they should be administered in doses appropriate for meningitis.

TYMPANIC MEMBRANE AND MIDDLE EAR

Trauma

Direct trauma to the tympanic membrane may occur during attempts to clean the ear with a cotton-tipped applicator or bobby pin, or it may result from debris, such as slag from welding, falling into the external canal. Indirect trauma, such as a slap to the auricle, may also result in perforation of the drum.

Diagnosis

Again, one of the most important aspects in evaluating a traumatic perforation of the eardrum is to determine the extent of injury and, in particular, whether there has been any injury to the ossicular chain or inner ear. Once the blood and debris have been removed by aspiration, the perforation is examined. Posterosuperior traumatic perforations are the most likely to result in damage to the ossicular chain. The presence of a sensorineural hearing loss, nystagmus and significant vestibular symptoms suggests the possibility of a perilymph leak, and the case should be referred to an otologist for an urgent evaluation.

Treatment

Most uncomplicated perforations of the tympanic membrane will heal spontaneously. Some authors feel that large segments of infolded tympanic membrane should be returned to their normal anatomical position and should be held in place using cigarette paper impregnated with antibiotic ointment on the lateral surface of the drum. This may be done under a local anesthetic. If the perforation occurs in a contaminated situation, such as during swimming, or if it is caused by a grossly contaminated foreign body, scrupulous cleaning of the canal and middle ear is performed, and antibiotics are often prescribed. With a clean perforation of the tympanic membrane, neither topical nor oral antibiotics are necessary. However, the patient must not allow water to enter the ear canal. On a short-term basis this can be accomplished by occluding the external meatus with commercial ear plugs or with cotton impregnated with petroleum jelly during showering or bathing. The tympanic membrane should then be re-examined by an otologist within 10 days, or sooner if drainage occurs after the first 2 days. Unlike most acute traumatic perforations, those produced by hot slag during welding accidents seldom heal and may be complicated by superinfection with profuse otorrhea. Treatment consists of removing the foreign body if it can be located and allowing resolution of the intense inflammatory response and infection, followed by delayed tympanoplasty.

Damage to the ossicular chain with or without perilymph leak

In the presence of significant injury to the ear, the initial examination should include assessment for possible ossicular damage, rupture of the round window membrane or dislocation of the stapes footplate resulting in perilymphatic leak. The ossicles may be visible if there is a perforation; if the drum is intact, a large, unexplained conductive hearing loss suggests discontinuity or fracture of a portion of the ossicular chain. Fracture or dislocation of the malleus and incus does not usually require emergency treatment.

However, ossicular injuries may be associated with the rupture of either the stapediovestibular joint or the round window, either of which constitutes an otologic emergency. The presence of vestibular signs and symptoms, including nystagmus, subjective vertigo, a positive fistula test and positional vertigo, and the presence of a high-tone sensorineural hearing loss with reduced discrimination, suggest injury to the inner ear secondary to perilymphatic leak. If there is measurable hearing, many otologists prefer to hospitalize these patients, put them at bedrest and follow the progression of their injury by daily audiograms, since many leaks will heal spontaneously. If there is no hearing at the initial evaluation, or if hearing deteriorates under such observation, urgent surgery is required to ascertain the damage precisely and to repair the leak with a fat graft. Ossicular fractures uncomplicated by perilymph leaks are usually better handled in a delayed fashion once the acute inflammatory response has resolved.

Barotrauma

Etiology and treatment

Sudden, uncompensated pressure changes may occur during rapid descent in an aircraft or during scuba diving, and may result in pain in the ear, bloody effusions in the middle ear space, rupture of the tympanic membrane or, less commonly, damage to delicate inner ear membranes or rupture of the round or oval windows.

A hemotympanum resulting from barotrauma requires little treatment. Some practitioners use decongestants to improve eustachian tube function and to achieve more rapid resolution of the effusion. Paracentesis or aspiration of the effusion is seldom necessary. Again, as with the treatment for other injuries to the ear, the examiner should include in his initial assessment the consideration of possible inner ear injury by noting auditory and vestibular signs and symptoms. An acute hemotympanum is quite painful and may require narcotic analgesics for a few days. A hemotympanum may take several weeks to resolve, and all patients should be re-examined in 2–3 weeks, both to check for resolution of the hemotympanum and to evaluate any residual hearing loss.

Rupture of the tympanic membrane by barotrauma is treated in the same way as other traumatic injuries to the eardrum.

INNER EAR TRAUMA AND TEMPORAL BONE FRACTURE

Acoustic trauma

Acoustic trauma may result from exposure to a sudden loud noise, from the cumulative effects of protracted exposure to loud noise or from a concussive injury to the skull. The usual rule of thumb is that a noise loud enough to be painful is loud enough to cause temporary or permanent injury to the inner ear. A sharp blow to the skull may produce enough mechanical energy to produce hearing loss. This is usually more severe in the ear on the side of the injury, but a bilateral hearing loss may occur in such cases.

Diagnosis

Immediately following acoustic trauma, the patient will complain of a plugged or full feeling and tinnitus in the ear. Except in extreme cases, tuning-fork and whisper tests are normal or near normal, because the hearing loss is almost always above 3000 Hz. Therefore, adequate evaluation of acoustic trauma requires behavioral audiometry with particular attention to the high frequencies. Acoustic trauma usually has two components: a temporary threshold shift and a permanent threshold shift. The temporary threshold shift is that part of the sensorineural hearing loss that resolves within 3–7 days. The permanent threshold shift connotes the permanent decrement of threshold for the high frequencies (Figure 7.2). A hearing loss that is present 3 weeks after acoustic trauma may be considered permanent. Audiometry may be performed acutely, but this is not essential, since no treatment is required. All patients, however, should be examined after 3 weeks to evaluate permanent injury.

Rupture of the round window or oval window

Rupture of the round window or oval window resulting in a perilymph leak may occur in conjunction with barotrauma, direct trauma to the temporal bone or a penetrating injury to the external canal and tympanic membrane. For diagnosis and treatment, see the previous discussion of injuries to the tympanic membrane and ossicles.

Occasionally a perilymph leak may be caused by relatively minor injury or straining such as weight-lifting. The clinical signs and symptoms include sensorineural hearing loss, unsteadiness, positive fistula sign and positive Hallpike positional testing. Absolute diagnosis is generally made by

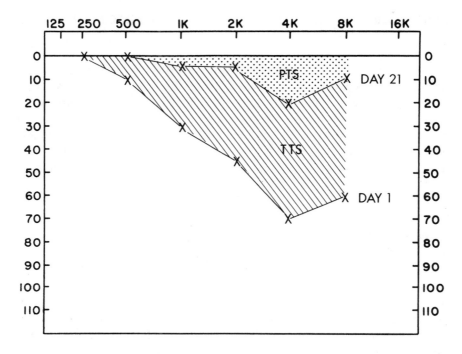

Figure 7.2 Schematic illustration of temporary (TTS) and permanent threshold shift (PTS) following acoustic trauma of the left ear. An audiogram done immediately after noise exposure demonstrates a sensorineural loss of 70 db at 4 kHz. Part of this loss may be recovered over several days, leaving only a partial high-frequency sensorineural loss at day 21

exploration of the middle ear. Repair of such leaks at the oval or round windows is accomplished using free tissue grafts, such as fat or perichondrium.

Basilar skull fracture

A blow to the head may produce a longitudinal, transverse, or mixed fracture of the temporal bone (Figure 7.3). Primary longitudinal fractures occur most often, constituting approximately 75% of all fractures involving the temporal bone. Most of these fractures pass through the squamous portion into the tympanic portion of the temporal bone, resulting in fracture or fracture-dislocation of the superior portion of the bony tympanic ring and perforation of the tympanic membrane. This will result in bleeding into the middle and external ear and perhaps CSF leak. Disruption of the ossicular chain may occur. Less commonly, the fracture may pass through the mastoid, bypassing the external canal and resulting only in bleeding into the mastoid and middle ear space without rupture of the drum.

In transverse fractures, which constitute approximately 25% of fractures of the temporal bone, the fracture line is transverse to the long axis of the petrous bone and hence across the internal auditory canal or inner ear.

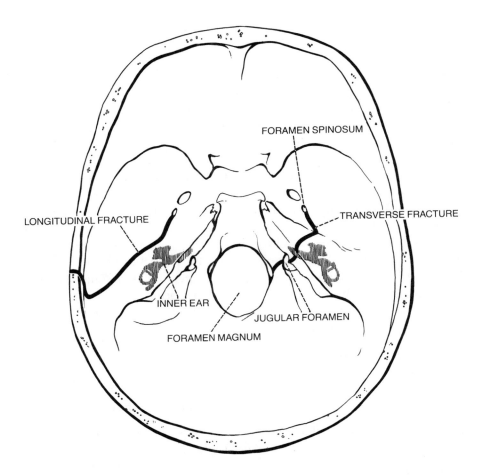

Figure 7.3 Basilar skull fracture. On the left, a longitudinal fracture passes along the axis of the petrous bone but does not enter the inner ear or internal auditory canal. On the right, there is a transverse fracture, which usually begins at the foramen magnum, extending to the jugular foramen across the internal auditory canal or inner ear, passing anteriorly to the carotid canal and foramen spinosum area. Severe injury to the inner ear and facial nerve can be expected

Therefore, in this type of fracture, significant injury to auditory, vestibular and facial nerves may occur. The tympanic membrane remains intact, and a hemotympanum is almost always present.

A mixed, or complex, fracture involves the presence of both transverse and longitudinal fractures. These often pass through the geniculate ganglion area and result in immediate or delayed facial paresis or paralysis.

Diagnosis

A longitudinal fracture-dislocation of the temporal bone is diagnosed when plain films or computerized tomography (CT) of the skull and examination of the ear canal reveal a fracture step-off, laceration of the posterosuperior canal wall, rupture of the tympanic membrane, bloody otorrhea or CSF otorrhea. However, in non-displaced fractures or transverse fractures, radiographic assessment, including tomography, may fail to reveal a fracture line. Even if X-ray films do not reveal the fracture, the presence of a hemotympanum and a history of significant skull injury are sufficient to make a diagnosis of basilar skull fracture. Retroauricular ecchymosis (Battle's sign) is considered pathognomonic of a basilar skull fracture. The initial radiographic assessment may not reveal the fracture, because of poor radiographic conditions, including time of day, cooperation of the patient and other patient care considerations. Such fractures may be more evident by tomographic evaluation at a later date, especially after some remineralization and early healing of a fracture site has occurred.

The evaluation of a patient with a suspected temporal bone fracture should include consideration of:

(1) Associated neurologic status;

(2) Possible cervical spine injuries;

(3) The extent of injury to the tympanic membrane and ossicular chain;

(4) Evidence of inner ear injury, resulting either from perforation of the round window membrane or dislocation of the stapes footplate, or from transection of the auditory nerve or fracture through the cochlea;

(5) Evidence of vestibular injury, such as subjective vertigo or nystagmus;

(6) Status of the facial nerve.

From an otologic perspective, it is very important to know whether facial nerve paralysis was immediate and complete or delayed and incomplete, for accurate assessment of the need for further treatment, including exploration or decompression of the facial nerve. Many authors feel that immediate paralysis or even a delayed paralysis in which there is electrophysiologic evidence of rapid degeneration of the nerve requires surgical exploration. This is not a universally accepted opinion, and some otologists insist that there be clear-cut evidence that surgical exploration can be expected to help, as in radiographic demonstration of a step-off in the Fallopian canal or an injury from a bullet or other missile that can be expected totally to transect the facial nerve. Exploration of the facial canal, especially its intralabyrinthine portion, is a formidable surgical procedure and may require combined middle or posterior fossa and mastoid approaches.

An isolated injury to the round window or stapedial footplate may occur without fracture through the inner ear. Diagnosis of this injury is difficult or impossible to make without surgical exploration. The decision of whether to proceed with surgical exploration is based on the individual clinical situation. Delayed treatment of trauma to the temporal bone may include repair of perforations of the drum and fracture-dislocations of the bony tympanic ring, and reconstruction of the ossicular chain.

Traumatic cerebrospinal fluid otorrhea

Fracture through the temporal bone involving the floor of the middle cranial fossa often results in profuse CSF otorrhea. The role of antibiotics in treating such cases is controversial. There is some evidence that antibiotics should be withheld until there is clear-cut evidence of infection, and the best evidence suggests that, if antibiotics are used, they should be given in doses appropriate for meningitis. In most cases, profuse CSF otorrhea due to a fracture will cease spontaneously within the first 10 days, but repair of a CSF leak is required if it is persistent. The surgical approach to repairing a persistent leak depends on the site of injury. Some leaks are best repaired by a neurosurgical approach; others are best repaired by an otologic approach.

Sudden idiopathic hearing loss

The usual presenting clinical situation in sudden idiopathic hearing loss involves a patient who suddenly hears a pop in his ear or who states that 'his hearing has been turned off'. A subjective sense of plugging and fullness also occurs. Less commonly, the hearing may be lost over several hours or days. The patient may or may not have vestibular symptoms.

Diagnosis

The diagnosis of sudden idiopathic sensorineural hearing loss is arrived at by excluding other possible causes. Most other treatable causes of sudden hearing loss can be eliminated from consideration simply by history and physical examination. These include the obvious examples of acoustic trauma to the temporal bone, the presence of obvious middle ear or mastoid infection, surgical trauma or the administration of ototoxic drugs. Other less common causes of sudden sensorineural hearing loss may require laboratory assessment. These include, for example, primary or secondary syphilis, which may cause sudden loss of auditory and vestibular function, and tumors of the cerebellopontine angle, which, rarely, may cause sudden deterioration of hearing, perhaps by hemorrhage into the tumor and compromise of the vascular supply to the inner ear.

Initial evaluation of sudden hearing loss should include a thorough history to eliminate traumatic and toxic causes and medical disorders, including blood dyscrasias and malignancies. Serology should be evaluated. A CT scan or magnetic resonance imaging (MRI) may be useful to detect the presence of a vestibular schwannoma (acoustic neuroma) and to rule out a lytic lesion in the temporal bone. Some authors believe that certain metabolic conditions, such as arteriosclerotic cardiovascular disease, diabetes mellitus, thyroid disease, renal disease or hyperlipidemia, may produce deterioration of hearing. However, because conclusive proof is wanting at this time, screening tests for these entities are of questionable importance in management. A history consistent with injury, including strain that may result from heavy lifting or from straining at stool, may suggest the possibility of a rupture of the round window membrane. In such a case, an otologist should be consulted concerning the advisability of exploring the middle ear. Once other possible causes of sudden hearing loss have been excluded by history, examination and a limited number of laboratory tests, a diagnosis of sudden idiopathic sensorineural hearing loss is made. The etiology of this disorder is unknown. A primary viral infection of the inner ear or a complex virus–host immune interaction may be the cause.

Treatment

The treatment of sudden idiopathic hearing loss is controversial. The literature abounds with various treatment protocols, including the use of anticoagulants, antihistamines, vasodilators, steroids, Hypaque® (Nycomed Amersham Imaging US, Princeton, NJ, USA), carbon dioxide rebreathing and plasma expanders. There is little or no convincing evidence that any of these treatments is effective, with the exception of steroids. In a double-blinded study, Wilson and colleagues[1] have demonstrated that certain subcategories of sudden idiopathic sensorineural hearing loss need no treatment, that others will not benefit from any treatment and that a third subgroup may be alleviated significantly by the administration of corticosteroids. Mild midfrequency or flat sensorineural hearing losses up to 30 db almost always recover spontaneously. Immediate profound losses rarely recover spontaneously and are not influenced by steroid therapy. The chance of recovery in idiopathic sudden hearing loss of moderate degree, 30–90 db, is enhanced by corticosteroid therapy. For an adult the usual dosage is 60 mg prednisone/day for 5 days, followed by a tapered course over the next 7 days.

Selected readings

Silverstein H. Trauma of the tympanic membrane and ossicles. In Nadol JB Jr, Schuknecht HF, eds. *Surgery of the Ear and Temporal Bone*. New York: Raven Press, 1993:325–8

Cheney ML. Acquired deformities of the auricle. In Nadol JB Jr, Schuknecht HF, eds. *Surgery of the Ear and Temporal Bone*. New York: Raven Press, 1993:449–70

Bibliography

1. Wilson WR, Byl FM, Laird N. The efficacy of steroids in the treatment of idiopathic sudden hearing loss. *Arch Otolaryngol* 1980;106:772–6

8

Anatomy, physiology and examination of the nose and paranasal sinuses

William R. Wilson

The nose
  Anatomy of the external nose
  Anatomy of the internal nose and paranasal sinuses
  Anatomy of the upper respiratory tract
  The neural supply of the nose
  The vasculature of the nose
The nasal examination
  Differential diagnosis
  Nasopharyngeal examination
  Sinus examination
Radiographic examination of the nose, nasopharynx and paranasal sinuses
The nasopharynx
  Anatomy
  Chronic nasal obstruction and adenoidal hypertrophy
  Carcinoma
  Cysts
  Chronic nasopharyngitis exclusive of adenoiditis
Diagnosis of palatal dysfunction
Sleep apnea syndrome
  Snoring
Olfaction
  Disorders of the sense of smell

THE NOSE

The nose is a relatively complex organ that functions as a portal for air into the respiratory system and serves to warm, humidify and cleanse the air as it passes through. It also aids in the control of infection in the airway. It is the center of olfaction (the sense of smell and fine taste). It is vital in the lower animal forms for the procurement of food and a mate.

Anatomy of the external nose

In discussing the anatomy of the external nose (Figure 8.1), the following terms are useful for the description of injuries and tumor sites. The root is where the nasal and frontal bones articulate; it is divided into the nasion and glabella. The dorsum is the ridge line from the root to the apex. The apex is the tip of the nose; the base is the triangular portion between the

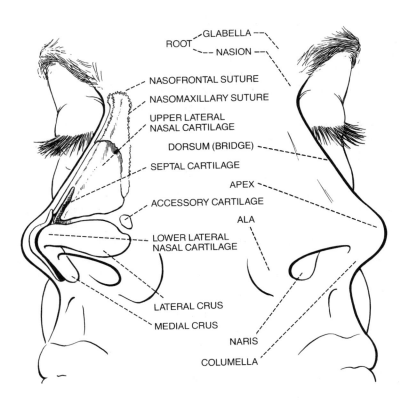

Figure 8.1   The structures of the external nose

apex and the lips; the anterior nares are divided by the columella and bounded by the alae; the columella is the membranous portion of the nasal septum; the bridge is the bony structure of the nose, the frontal portion of the maxilla plus the frontal bone; the alae are the lateral rounded eminences at the base of the nose, formed by the lower lateral cartilages. The nasal septum is made up of the septal cartilage plus the vomer and the perpendicular plate of the ethmoid.

Anatomy of the internal nose and paranasal sinuses

The lateral wall of the nose has three turbinates or conchae; however, the third turbinate is very small, located high and posterior, and cannot be seen on examination. Turbinates have a thin, bony framework but are covered with highly vascular subcutaneous tissue that is composed of a dense arterial network and venous plexuses (lakes) similar to erectile tissue. This covering is particularly evident on the inferior turbinate. The turbinates can swell by means of vascular engorgement to occlude the nose.

Beneath each turbinate lies a meatus. The inferior meatus receives drainage from the nasolacrimal duct only, at a point about one-third of the way back from the anterior margin. The middle meatus receives drainage from the nasofrontal duct and anterior ethmoid cells anteriorly, from the middle ethmoid cells and maxillary sinus ostium medially and from the posterior ethmoid cells posteriorly. Mucopurulent material can often be seen draining from these regions during acute sinus infections, thereby identifying the site of the infection.

The sphenoethmoidal recess is a long, narrow space located between the upper portion of the middle turbinate and the nasal septum. The cribriform plate forms the roof of this area, and the posterior limit is the anterior face of the sphenoid sinus. The sphenoid ostium empties into this region. More importantly, the olfactory epithelium is located here.

The nasal septum is formed by cartilage anteriorly and by bone posteriorly. It may grow irregularly or may be traumatized so that it obstructs breathing on one or both sides of the nose. If the deviation is severe enough, it will inhibit proper drainage or will obstruct sinus ostia by putting pressure on the turbinates.

The function of the paranasal sinuses is unknown. The ethmoid sinuses are a complex of 10–25 small sinuses that as a group form a roughly rectangular shape front to back. The posterior length is 4–5 cm, the height is 2.5–3 cm and the width bilaterally between the eyes is 1–1.5 cm. Some of these sinuses are present at birth; they are often involved in nasal infections and allergic disease in children. As the head enlarges, the ethmoid sinuses increase in size and complexity.

The maxillary sinuses, sometimes present at birth, remain small until the development of permanent teeth. At that time the maxillary sinuses gradually enlarge to their full size. The small ostium (2–3 mm in diameter) is located high on the medial wall of the sinus under the middle turbinate, and for these anatomical regions these sinuses drain very poorly once infected. The bony canal encasing the infraorbital nerve travels through the roof, and the roots of the second premolar and first and second molars often project into the sinus floor. Localized pain and pain in the distribution of the infraorbital nerve are common symptoms of maxillary sinus infections, owing to neural irritation, particularly on bending forward or tapping the sinus or teeth.

The sphenoid sinuses begin to develop by the sixth year. They are highly variable in size and ramifications. The ostium is located high on the anterior wall at the end of the sphenoethmoidal recess, and therefore, as with the maxillary sinuses, there is no dependent drainage from this sinus.

The frontal sinuses are the last to develop and continue to enlarge during the teenage years. Not uncommonly, the frontal sinuses may be absent or, at the other extreme, may be very large with multiple ramifications. No particular size or configuration of the frontal sinuses portends frontal sinus disease.

The nasal and sinus mucous membrane is pseudostratified columnar epithelium which is covered by a thin mucous blanket. Like the skin, the mucosa has nocioceptors: free, naked nerve endings that respond to chemicals and to changes in temperature, humidity and pressure. These receptors serve to alert and protect the lower airway following exposure to extremes of temperature or pollutants by means of the nasopulmonary reflex. They stimulate vasodilatation, mucous production and bronchial constriction.

Anatomy of the upper respiratory tract

The upper respiratory tract is an irregular, double-tubed structure, but even in normal circumstances it is not static. Eighty per cent of individuals have a cycle of congestion and decongestion involving first one side of the nose, then the other, known as the nasal cycle. In the normal nose, one passage opens up, accompanied by secretion by the serous and mucous glands, while the opposite side closes down, with increasing obstruction and decreasing secretion. There is a shift of autonomic balance, occurring every 0.5–4 hours. However, the combined or total airway resistance remains unchanged. This cycle becomes evident to most people when they try to sleep. Inspiratory air currents fan out superiorly, while expiratory currents swirl in the nose. The nasal cycle ensures that the air 'sheets' are formed in the nose and that, at some point, these sheets are no more than 1 mm in thickness; it therefore becomes more likely that inspired foreign particles can be trapped by the nasal mucous coat. Patients with cause for a reduced airway secondary to a deviated septum, or with a chronically engorged mucous membrane from perennial allergy, will complain that their nose is never completely open and that the airway shifts from side to side. In other words, they become aware of the nasal cycle because of their abnormally limited nasal space, while patients with normal nasal patency do not.

The blocked nose creates hyponasal (denasal) speech, recognizable by the substitution of other sounds for the normal nasal consonants of /m/, /n/ and /ng/. Smaller changes in resonance are noted with minor nasal swelling, as with a mild cold. Experienced rhinoplasty surgeons know that the resonances change by narrowing the alar region, not the dorsum. This phenomenon can be tested by pinching the skin of the nose at the upper portion of the cartilaginous septum.

The nose will efficiently warm cold air, no matter what the temperature of the air. Warming of the air permits humidification up to 95% before the air reaches the trachea. Experience with laryngectomized patients, however, indicates that this process is not vital. The nasal mucosa and sinus linings are composed of respiratory epithelium that is covered by a sticky, mucoid layer. This mucous blanket is produced at a rate of approximately 1 liter/day by the goblet cells and the submucosal serous–mucinous glands. The mucus serves to waterproof the nose, preventing loss of water outward and drying of the mucosa. It is a thin, sticky, clear sheet with a pH of 7 or slightly lower, and is composed of mucin, a long molecule of mucopolysaccharide that forms a sponge-like meshwork (2.5–5%); salts (1–2%); water (95%); and proteins, among which are included lysozymes and immunoglobulins. The mucus is propelled posteriorly in the nose by the nasal cilia, 10–20 cilia per cell. Mucus and particulate matter advance slowly in the anterior nose, but more rapidly in the posterior, taking 20–30 min in all to reach the nasopharynx.

The mucus serves to protect the nose from infection. The lysozymes present in the mucus cause weakening of the bacterial cell walls. Of immunoglobulins, IgA is the most prominent; there are smaller amounts of IgG. IgA is produced locally by mucosal plasma cells and is secreted as a dimer into the nasal mucus. It can inhibit viral growth and is probably a significant factor in immunity to viral infections. In the case of bacterial infection, the usefulness of IgA is unknown, because it does not bind complement and therefore will not lyse bacteria. There is some evidence that it may work in concert with lysozymes. IgG and IgM are routinely observed in the connective tissue spaces beneath the mucous membrane. Increasing amounts of IgG occur in the mucus in association with inflammatory reactions. The outpouring of this antibody represents the principal host defense once a bacterial infection has been established. IgE is present in the nasal mucus of individuals with allergies, generally in proportion to the serum IgE value. It is manufactured locally by submucosal plasma cells.

The neural supply of the nose

The first and second divisions of the fifth nerve are responsible for sensation, and hence these are the nerves responsible for referred pain patterns in the nose and sinuses.

The preganglionic fibers of the sympathetic nervous system arise from the cervical spinal cord and synapse in the middle or superior cervical ganglia with 30 or more postganglionic fibers. Fibers travel by way of the carotid plexus – the deep petrosal nerve that forms the vidian nerve – and pass through the sphenopalatine ganglion to the arterioles of the nasal mucosa. Stimulation of the sympathetic plexus produces vasoconstriction and mucinous secretion. Following sympathetic nerve injury, as occasionally occurs after a sympathectomy for Raynaud's phenomenon, there is unopposed activity of the parasympathetic nerve supply and subsequent vasodilatation, mucosal swelling, nasal obstruction and hypersecretion. The result is a nasal disorder characterized by nasal obstruction and rhinorrhea that resembles nasal allergy and is known as vasomotor rhinitis (VMR).

The path of the parasympathetic nerves is as follows: they arise in the superior salivary nucleus, form the nervus intermedius, join the facial nerve, pass to the greater superficial petrosal nerve and go through the vidian nerve and synapse in the sphenopalatine ganglion. The postsynaptic fibers are distributed to the nose. Sectioning of the vidian nerve (vidian neurectomy) results in a pale, dry, shrunken mucosa and is used as a treatment for severe cases of vasomotor rhinitis.

The vasculature of the nose

The principal arterial supply of the internal nose is through the sphenopalatine arteries, which enter through the sphenopalatine foramen at the back of the middle meatus. Here posterior lateral branches spread in dense, parallel rows over the turbinates at two levels. The deeper vessels supply venous sinuses or lakes. The superficial arterioles supply a submucosal capillary network and are responsive to changes in temperature. The ethmoid, labial and palatine arteries also contribute to the nasal blood supply.

THE NASAL EXAMINATION

Tools for an office examination are shown in Appendix 2. In a child, an examiner can view the anterior nares by pushing the nasal tip up with his thumb. The anterior septum and tip of the inferior turbinate are then in view. However, with a cooperative child or an adult, a nasal speculum is preferable. The proper technique is to place the speculum blades under the ala to the desired depth; the ala is lifted as the blades are opened down to the nasal floor, and the naris is gently spread. With a head mirror or headlight, the inferior turbinate and septum will be in immediate view. If the mucosa is swollen, a vasoconstricting nasal spray, such as oxymetazoline (Afrin®, Schering-Plough Inc., Memphis, TN, USA), is administered. The examiner re-examines the nose after a few minutes, looking for inflammation or discharge, deviations, masses and so forth.

For a more detailed examination of the nose, either straight Hopkins rod rigid nasoscopes or a flexible nasopharyngoscope may be employed after decongesting the nose and topically anesthetizing the nose with a nasal spray consisting of a 50 : 50 mixture of 1% oxymetazoline and 4% Xylocaine® (AstraZeneca Pharmaceuticals LP, Wilmington, DE, USA).

Differential diagnosis

The nasal mucosa should be pink to dull red in color. Thickened, bright red mucosa suggests an inflammatory reaction, often owing to a viral or bacterial infection. Discharge from a viral infection is mucoid, copious and gray. The bacterial infections result in yellow-tinged secretions. Old mucus, as is found in nasal stasis, develops a greenish discoloration, but this change does not necessarily mean that an inflammation is present. Allergic rhinitis may present as bright red, inflamed mucosa or with a reddish hue or bluish white mucous membrane. Allergic patients and those with vasomotor rhinitis have copious, watery, yet ropey, crystal clear secretions that will strand between the turbinate and the septum.

Any odor to the drainage, whether noted by the patient or perceived by the examiner, suggests a bacterial infection, such as a dental root abscess, chronic nasal infections or atrophic rhinitis. In general there is no odor to the drainage from acute viral rhinitis or sinusitis.

Nasopharyngeal examination

The nasopharyngeal examination is facilitated, if necessary, by the administration of tetracaine HC1 spray (Cetacaine, Cetylite Industries, Pennsauken, NJ, USA) to the soft palate and oropharyngeal wall. The patient should attempt to breathe through his nose while his tongue is depressed sufficiently to permit a small mirror to slide behind the soft palate. Many patients are unable to accomplish this, because of a sensitive gag reflex or a long palate, and a flexible or rigid nasopharyngoscope may be required to complete the examination.

Sinus examination

The sinuses are best tested clinically by gentle tapping with the examiner's third finger. Beginning laterally on the forehead, the examiner taps across the patient's brow. An infected frontal sinus will be tender locally. There will also be rather marked tenderness with pressure placed on the sinus floor by the examiner's index finger. In addition, if the maxillary sinus is infected, the first and second molars may be sensitive to gentle tapping or pressure from a wooden tongue depressor. The examiner's finger may be pressed along the alveolar ridge at the level of the dental roots to determine sensitivity secondary to a dental abscess. The ethmoid sinuses can be only very superficially visualized on nasal examination, and the sphenoid sinus is best examined radiographically. Drainage from the nasofrontal duct can be seen streaming from under the anterior end of the middle turbinate and over the inferior turbinate. Drainage from the maxillary sinus would be found more posteriorly (Figure 8.2).

RADIOGRAPHIC EXAMINATION OF THE NOSE, NASOPHARYNX AND PARANASAL SINUSES

When the source of nasal obstruction and discharge is not apparent, and sinusitis, tumor, polyps, foreign body or choanal atresia are suspected, a sinus X-ray series should be obtained. In most radiology departments this series consists of the following four basic views (Figure 8.3), which, within the limits of practicality, should be obtained in the upright position so that secretions within the sinuses will form air–fluid levels. The open-mouth

a   b   c

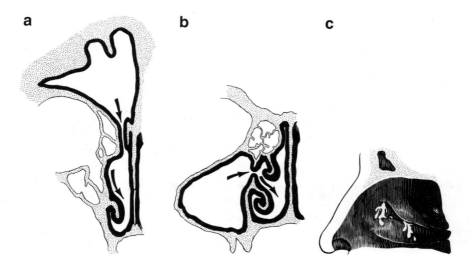

Figure 8.2 (a) Frontal sinus drainage by way of the nasofrontal duct. (b) Maxillary sinus drainage from the maxillary sinus ostium. (c) Relative location of drainage from the frontal and maxillary sinuses

upright Waters' view is the best all-purpose film, giving a particularly good view of the maxillary and sphenoid sinuses, and less satisfactory visualization of the ethmoid and frontal sinuses. The Caldwell view gives the best visualization of the frontal and ethmoid sinuses. The lateral and submental vertex views round out the series. For more complicated sinus cases or in anticipation of surgery of the sinuses, however, the computerized tomogram of the sinuses in the axial and coronal planes should be obtained. This detailed radiologic examination can demonstrate mucosal thickening and obstruction of nasal sinus ostia as well as small areas of symptomatic ethmoid sinusitis.

THE NASOPHARYNX

Anatomy

The nasopharynx (Figure 8.4) is formed superiorly by the inferior surface of the sphenoid sinus, posteriorly by the cervical vertebrae, and anteriorly by the posterior portion of the nasal septum and posterior choanae with the tips of the inferior and middle turbinates immediately adjacent to it. The lateral wall of the nasopharynx is the most complex portion. The eustachian tube orifices are located immediately posterosuperior to the soft

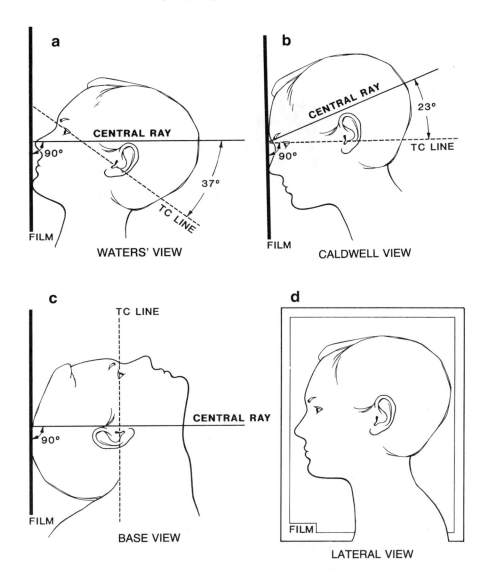

Figure 8.3 Sinus X-ray positions. (a) The Waters' view represents an inclined posteroanterior view with the tragocanthal line (TC line) forming a 37° angle with the central ray. (b) In the Caldwell view, or posteroanterior projection, the TC line is perpendicular to the plane of the film, and the central ray is directed caudally at 23°. (c) In the base, or submentovertical view, the TC line is placed parallel to the X-ray plate, and the central ray passes submentally and perpendicular to the TC line and X-ray plate. (d) In the lateral view, the sagittal plane is parallel to the X-ray plate

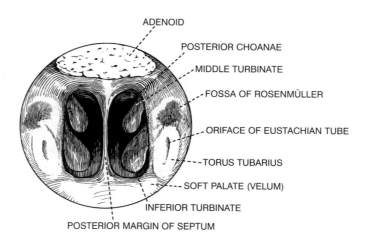

ADENOID

POSTERIOR CHOANAE

MIDDLE TURBINATE

FOSSA OF ROSENMÜLLER

ORIFACE OF EUSTACHIAN TUBE

TORUS TUBARIUS

SOFT PALATE (VELUM)

INFERIOR TURBINATE

POSTERIOR MARGIN OF SEPTUM

Figure 8.4 Mirror view of the nasopharynx, looking from the posterior end towards the anterior end

palate and immediately posterior to the inferior turbinate. The surrounding eustachian tube cartilages form a mound-like structure around the orifice itself. Immediately above the eustachian tube cartilages is a depression known as the fossa of Rosenmüller. For some reason as yet unknown, it is in this area that carcinoma of the nasopharynx will usually arise.

The nasopharynx is a relatively dirty region, and positive cultures can be obtained in this area more often than not. Therefore, the vestibule of the nose and the nasopharynx are similar in that they often harbor pathogens, while the nasal cavities are relatively free of disease-producing organisms. Therefore, when culturing the nose, care should be taken that the culture is obtained from well within the nasal cavities. In children and young adults, the pharyngeal tonsil or adenoid may be present. It is a mass of lymphoid tissue adherent to the roof of the nasopharynx. In some children, the adenoid becomes markedly enlarged and may obstruct the posterior choanae of the nose. Also, a chronically enlarged and inflamed adenoid will result in irritation and edema of the surrounding eustachian tube orifice, resulting in serous otitis media and conductive hearing loss. The primary disorders involving the nasopharynx include adenoid hypertrophy and chronic adenoiditis in children. In adults, the adenoid tissue may be enlarged in HIV-positive patients and patients with lymphoma or plasmacytoma.

Chronic nasal obstruction and adenoidal hypertrophy

When children are affected by chronic nasal obstruction and adenoidal hypertrophy, it is not possible in most cases to determine which problem is leading the other. Allergic children with chronic nasal obstruction and mucus retention and infection will develop adenoidal hypertrophy in response to the chronic nasal inflammation. The treatment for this problem is, first, medical. Therapy should be a combination of antihistamines and vasoconstrictors and a short course of antibiotics based on cultures taken from within the nasal cavity at the outset. If this course of treatment fails to resolve the problem, a surgical approach can be considered. This would include, first, an adenoidectomy to remove the obstructing lymphoidal tissue in the posterior nose and nasopharynx, and second, a deep electro-cautery of the inferior turbinate to produce scarring of its submucosal tissue and thereby achieve mucosal retraction and improvement in the airway and mucous flow. A combination of these procedures will often result in a resolution of the problem of nasal obstruction. Children with serous otitis media secondary to eustachian tube obstruction who also have a large adenoid may require an added adenoidectomy. Serous otitis, discussed earlier, is a fickle disorder that comes and goes, and is often related to the onset of a respiratory infection or allergy problems. Patients who do not respond to conservative therapy – namely, the combination of antihistamines and vasoconstrictors – should undergo myringotomy with aspiration of the middle ear fluid. If the fluid is thin and serous, most surgeons defer placement of the pressure-equalization tubes in the tympanic membrane. However, if the fluid is thick and mucinous (e.g. glue-like), a pressure-equalization tube is placed in the tympanic membrane in order to prevent the reaccumulation of mucus. If myringotomy and place-ment of pressure-equalization tubes are followed by a recurrence of middle ear fluids, an adenoidectomy is combined with the reinsertion of the pressure-equalization tubes. In most instances, this combination of procedures will result in a resolution of the problem.

Carcinoma

Carcinoma of the nasopharynx is not an uncommon disorder. It affects men and women equally and is found in patients who are approximately 20 years of age and upward with a peak incidence between 40 and 60 years of age. For some reason as yet poorly understood, the tumor is most common among the Chinese. There is a relationship between carcinoma of the nasopharynx and the Epstein–Barr (EB) virus; patients with nasopharyngeal carcinoma have been found on serodiagnostic studies to have high titers against the EB virus, which diminishes with effective therapy.

Carcinoma of the nasopharynx in general is a silent tumor causing few symptoms. In approximately half the cases, the presenting symptom is a lymph node metastasis in the neck. Nasopharyngeal carcinoma has a propensity to metastasize to the lymph nodes of the posterior cervical chain, which is palpated just anterior to the margin of the trapezius muscle. A second, common presenting symptom is the presence of unilateral serous otitis media or bacterial otitis media, and for this reason any adult with either of these should have a careful examination of the nasopharynx.

The most common nasopharyngeal tumor is lymphoepithelioma, although lymphoma makes up approximately 10% of the cases. Treatment involves administering radiation therapy to the nasopharynx and also to the regions of lymphatic drainage in the neck. Tumors in the nasopharynx can be locally resected if small and not deeply invasive, and if they fail to respond to radiation therapy. When allowed to regress, the tumor will extend through the foramen lacerum into the cavernous sinus and middle cranial fossa, eventually involving the third, fourth and sixth nerves. Less commonly, the tumor spreads into the lateral pharyngeal space and involves the tissues and nodes surrounding the carotid and jugular foramen, and there may involve the ninth, tenth and eleventh nerves. Persistent metastatic lymph nodes in the neck should be removed by block dissection of the neck.

Cysts

The cysts of the nasopharynx can arise from the bursa that lies on the undersurface of the sphenoid, and may present as a draining sinus in the adenoidal mass. These cysts are corrected by removing the adenoid and marsupializing the underlying cystic tissue. Other cysts arise from Rathke's pouch, the site of invagination of embryonic tissues into the region of the pituitary. These cysts, which may become very large, are filled with dark brown crankcase-oil-like secretions and are treated again by marsupialization.

Chronic nasopharyngitis exclusive of adenoiditis

Chronic nasopharyngitis exclusive of adenoiditis may result from a chronic bacterial or allergic condition, causing an irritated sensation above the palate, a chronic postnasal drip and recurrent sore throats. It is a common sequela of nasopharyngeal radiotherapy. Control of associated disorders such as sinusitis requires the judicious use of nasal irrigation with sterile solutions and antibiotics.

DIAGNOSIS OF PALATAL DYSFUNCTION

The palate forms a dynamic valve between the pharynx and oropharynx, preventing saliva and food from entering the nasopharynx when swallowing. In addition, the palate is vital to the production of intelligible speech, because of its role in maintaining the patency of the nasopharynx and nose. Obstruction of the nose and nasopharynx and failure of the normal amounts of air to pass through them results in hyponasal speech. The nasal sounds that require patency of the nose and nasopharynx are again represented by the letters /m/, /n/ and /ng/. These are impossible to pronounce with an obstructed nose, and the inability to make these sounds characteristically accompanies a cold. There are five pairs of muscles that are responsible for the structure of the soft palate. Included in these pairs are the tensor veli palatini, the levator veli palatini, the palatoglossus, the palatopharyngeus and the constrictor pharyngis superior, which insert into an aponeurosis in the palatine midline and are innervated from the nucleus ambiguus by way of the glossopharyngeal and vagus nerves. Improper functioning of the palate producing hypernasal speech can result either from an anatomical defect, such as a congenital cleft palate or a congenitally short palate, or from shortening of the palate by tumor surgery or sleep apnea surgery. It may also occur secondary to neuromuscular disorders, such as myasthenia gravis or amyotrophic lateral sclerosis. Excessive amounts of air escape through the nose, and the patient is unable to articulate those sounds requiring sealing of the nasopharynx. Marked hypernasal speech is unintelligible; however, slight-to-moderate hypernasal speech can be difficult to distinguish from other disorders of articulation. The distinction is made most easily by placing a small wisp of cotton just anterior to the patient's nares, and asking him to say 'school'. If the cotton is blown, a diagnosis of palatal dysfunction is made.

Repairs of the cleft palate are performed by means of a palatal pushback procedure and the use of a posterior pharyngeal flap. A palate shortened by tumor surgery may require a flap reconstruction or an obturator to occlude the defect in order to allow for intelligible speech.

SLEEP APNEA SYNDROME

Sleep apnea syndrome has been recognized as an affliction of the obese for many centuries; however, only recently with the scientific study of sleep and sleep disorders has a categorization of sleep apnea and the standardization of an approach to these patients been developed. Most cases of sleep apnea are obstructive (OSAS) and are due to a narrowed collapsible upper airway. Central sleep apnea (CSAS) is much less common and may be seen in early infancy, advanced age or in association with central nervous system disorders. Mixed sleep apnea is a combination of the two.

OSAS is most commonly found in, but not limited to, the obese. It is affected by nasal obstruction, tonsillar hypertrophy, a long palate and copious uvula, and facial variations such as micrognathia or macroglossia. The common denominator of this group is a narrowed airway or lack of muscular turgor to prevent narrowing from the negative air pressure necessary for the respiratory effort. A lack of physical exercise, the use of alcohol and sleeping medications, and in the atopic, nocturnal antihistaminics can increase symptoms.

Suspicion of the diagnosis occurs with complaints of loud snoring, daytime somnolence and poor work performance, reduced libido, depression and personality changes. Physical signs, in addition to obesity, are hypertension and cardiac disease. Often a sleeping partner will report noticing the apneic periods or excessive restlessness at night, e.g. nocturnal myoclonus.

Diagnostic evaluation is by means of a sleep study (polysomnography), during which a number of measures are made simultaneously on the sleeping patient in a sleep laboratory while under observation by a technician. These measures include a limited electroencephalogram, an electrocardiogram, an electronystagmagram (to measure rapid eye movement (REM) sleep), chest and abdominal respiratory excursions, airflow at the nose and mouth, oxyhemoglobin desaturation by pulse oximetry, as well as observed or recorded snoring and nocturnal myoclonus. Analysis of radiographic cephalometric studies are of use in a limited number of patients.

A polysomnograph report contains a number of useful parameters. Time to sleep onset or latency is usually very short in apneic patients. Apnea is defined as cessation of respiration for longer than 10 seconds, whereas hypopnea is defined as a decrease in airflow of at least 50%. The apnea-plus-hypopnea index is a measure of the number of apneas and hypopneas per hour of sleep. A normal study may have a few per hour. An oxygen desaturation below 80% is significant, and at lower levels may become dangerous.

There are five stages of sleep: one and two are considered light; three, four and five (REM) are considered deep; normal sleep is roughly divided between light and deep levels of sleep. The obstructive events and associated hypoxia occur principally in deep sleep, particularly in REM sleep, thus arousing the patient and reverting him for a time to a lighter level of sleep. A simultaneous release of catecholamines may be responsible for the progressive hypertension noted in these patients.

The most effective treatments for sleep apnea are nasal continuous positive airway pressure and tracheotomy. Uvulopalatopharyngoplasty combined with correction of nasal airway obstructions such as septal deviation or turbinate hypertrophy is successful only in roughly 50% of patients, although it is usually helpful.

Snoring

The observation that palatoplasty was very often successful in controlling snoring has led to the repopularization of the uvulectomy or uvuloplasty procedure to control snoring due principally to palatal flutter. Several office techniques have been developed, some using standard surgical methods and others employing the destructive and hemostatic advantages of the CO_2 laser. To date, the efficacy of these procedures has not been thoroughly studied; however, their popularity is testimony to the ubiquitous nature of the problem (or their apparent usefulness).

OLFACTION

In lower animals, including fish, the olfactory organs are used for the recognition of food and for procreation. In man, however, reliance on smell has been superseded by reliance on sight.

The olfactory region is a small, yellow-brown area made up of the superior turbinate and the nasal septum opposite from it. The epithelium is made up of 10–20 million bipolar olfactory cells, each an olfactory rod extending into the mucous blanket. From each rod extend fine cilia known as olfactory hairs. These are thought to be the sensors. The central process of each olfactory cell joins with the neighboring processes to form bundles, which, as they become larger, are sheathed in myelin and pass on a dural sheath through the cribriform plate to the olfactory bulb. Following synapse there, connections are complex and run to the hypothalamus and brain stem.

At present there is no adequate explanation of the transducing mechanism that determines the quality and quantity of an odor. In order to be smelled, a substance must not only be volatile, but also be soluble in water and lipids. The fine discrimination tasks of taste, such as distinguishing veal from lamb, are mediated by a combination of taste and smell.

Disorders of the sense of smell

The first complaint is reduction or absence of the sense of smell (hyposmia, anosmia) and taste (ageusia, hypogeusia). This may be caused by:

(1) Congenital anosmia, resulting from birth trauma or, rarely, agenesis of the olfactory bulb; at times, it can be associated with hypogonadism;

(2) Injury, such as cribriform fracture, frontal lobe laceration or hemorrhage injury, contrecoup or complication of intranasal or intracranial surgery;

(3) Nasal obstruction, caused by mucosal swelling from upper respiratory infection (viral or bacterial), allergy (the most common cause), nasal polyps, chronic ethmoiditis or neoplasia in the region of the cribriform plate;

(4) Mucosal injury, from atrophic rhinitis, or such as a chemical injury or viral injury after influenza;

(5) Intracranial lesions, caused by a meningeal neoplasm in the frontal lobe or resulting from intracranial surgery;

(6) Hysteria.

The second complaint is enhancement (hyperosmia) or perversion of the sense of smell or taste (parosmia, dysgeusia). Normal smells become putrid and food smells rotten. The patient finds it difficult to eat or cook. This disorder may result from idiopathic, viral or drug-related causes, or from a vitamin deficiency or trauma. It may also occur because of olfactory hallucination (in schizophrenic and obsessional patients) or from an injury to the uncus of the temporal lobe.

Evaluation of olfactory disorders is as follows:

(1) History: fracture, infection, allergies and chemical exposure.

(2) Careful examination of the nose for obstruction, infection or atrophy.

(3) Cranial nerve examination, including funduscopy.

(4) Testing of olfactory sense with vials of coffee grounds, lemon extract and ammonia (each side of the nose is tested separately).

(5) Computed tomography scan of sinuses with sections through the cribriform plate.

(6) Allergy testing.

(7) Therapeutic trials.
    (a) Prednisone
    (b) Vitamin A.

9

Nasal and sinus congestion and infection

William R. Wilson

Nasal infections
  Nasal furunculosis
  Recurrent nasal vestibulitis
  Viral rhinitis
Unilateral nasal obstruction
  Choanal atresia
  Meningoencephalocele
  Foreign bodies
  Trauma
Bilateral nasal obstruction
  Allergic rhinitis
  Vasomotor rhinitis
  Rhinitis medicamentosa
  Polypoid rhinosinusitis
Sinus headache, pain and drainage
  Acute sinusitis
    Acute frontal sinusitis
    Acute sphenoid sinusitis
    Acute maxillary sinusitis
    Acute ethmoiditis
  Chronic sinusitis
    Chronic frontal sinusitis
    Chronic sphenoid sinusitis
    Chronic maxillary sinusitis
    Chronic ethmoiditis
  Sinusitis in HIV-positive patients
  Sinus surgery
    Caldwell–Luc procedure

Ethmoidectomy
Osteoplastic frontal sinus obliteration
Functional endoscopic sinus surgery
Unusual causes of nasal obstruction and drainage
Tuberculosis
Sarcoidosis
Rhinosporidiosis
Rhinoscleroma
Syphilis
Wegener's granulomatosis
Midline granuloma
Mucormycosis
Aspergillosis

NASAL INFECTIONS

Nasal furunculosis

Nasal furunculosis is a minor *Staphylococcus aureus* infection involving the follicles of the vibrissae of the nares. Redness, swelling and pain are usually limited to the inner surface of the vestibule, and any drainage occurs spontaneously into the vestibule. However, prompt antibiotic treatment plus incision and drainage are required if the infection becomes more than superficial. The reason for special concern is that infections involving this portion of the nose may seed the cavernous sinus by way of the facial veins, occasionally leading to a cavernous sinus thrombosis. In general, patients with severe nasal furunculosis may require several days of intravenous antibiotic therapy.

Recurrent nasal vestibulitis

A chronically irritated nasal vestibule may be the result of recurrent staphylococcal infections. Patients should be evaluated for rhinologic or sinus infections, although often these are not present. A patient can control vestibulitis by keeping his hands away from his nose and face, by washing his hands and face twice daily with hexachlorophene soap and by applying bacitracin ointment to the nasal vestibule twice daily with a sterile cotton applicator. Patients with a mustache may have to remove it to control vestibulitis.

Viral rhinitis

Viruses are spread by droplet dissemination or by fomite transfer from a patient's hands to his nose. There are a host of viruses responsible for occurrences of the common cold: rhinovirus will cause about one-third, parainfluenza types 1–4 and influenza A and B are responsible for 15–20%, and respiratory syncytial virus, adenovirus, enterovirus and all others combined are each responsible for 5% or less.

During the first 24 hours of a viral cold, there is a significant increase in the IgA level of nasal mucus, owing to the release of stored specific and non-specific IgA into nasal secretions. During the secretory phase of viral rhinitis (days 2 to 5), there is necrosis and shedding of epithelial cells, accompanied by marked transudation of serum albumin and IgG. At this point, the nose is most inflamed and obstructed, and bacterial rhinitis and sinusitis may occur secondary to stasis of mucus. The normal flora of the anterior of the nose and nasopharynx include many pathogens that live symbiotically but that, under altered conditions of anatomy and physiology, can become pathogenic to the host. These include *S. aureus, Hemophilus influenzae, Streptococcus pneumoniae* and β-streptococcus. In general, although the nasal vestibule and the nasopharynx will often culture positively for potential pathogens regardless of the state of the patient's health, the intervening mucosal surfaces should be pathogen-free. For this reason, when culturing the nose, it is best to place the tip of the cotton-tipped applicator along the lower surface of the middle turbinate, because this is an area bathed by drainage from the sinuses as well as the nose. Care should be taken to avoid touching the vestibular surfaces during this procedure.

Cultures are taken when the mucus becomes thickened and creamy or tinged with yellow. In small children this is an indication of bacterial rhinoethmoiditis and should be treated with appropriate antibiotics, although some physicians would choose not to use antibiotics for these symptoms. In an adult, these symptoms will be accompanied by complaints of nasal discomfort, namely obstruction, copious rhinorrhea and headache or facial pain; the indications for antibiotics are more apparent. Antibiotic treatment for 5–7 days is sufficient to resolve rhinitis. However, sinusitis requires a longer course of treatment.

The treatment for viral rhinitis often includes a mild analgesic for the accompanying achy malaise as well as an antihistamine–vasoconstrictor combination for the nasal symptoms. Most antihistamines have an atropine-like drying effect; the vasoconstrictor reduces congestion by reducing vascular engorgement. Further relief of congestion is obtained from the temporary use of vasoconstricting nasal sprays. Excessive rhinorrhea can be controlled with ipratropium bromide spray (Atrovent®, Boehringer Ingelheim Pharmaceuticals, Ridgefield, CA, USA).

Our preference of medication for viral rhinitis includes acetaminophen 325 mg to 650 mg every 4 hours as circumstances may require, and chlorpheniramine (Chlor-Trimeton®, Schering-Plough Inc., Kenilworth, NJ, USA) 4 mg to 8 mg every 4 hours for 3 days, in addition to steam inhalations through a hot towel. There are many similar medications that will accomplish the same therapeutic goals. When bacterial infections are present, an antibiotic is added to the regimen.

UNILATERAL NASAL OBSTRUCTION

Unilateral nasal obstruction may present as a continuous discharge from or as an irritation around one naris of the nose. This symptom requires a thorough evaluation. The diagnostic possibilities include the following congenital anomalies.

Choanal atresia

Undetected unilateral choanal atresia is an unusual anomaly that can result from bony or membranous obstruction of the posterior nose. The diagnosis can be made readily in the office by attempting to pass a soft catheter through the nose or by instilling a small amount of methylene blue in the nostril being examined. Failure of the dye to appear in the pharynx strongly suggests the presence of choanal atresia. Axial and coronal computerized tomography (CT) scans must be obtained to confirm the diagnosis. A small amount of radiopaque dye in the nose will help outline the structures during that procedure. Treatment is surgical correction.

Meningoencephalocele

Meningoencephalocele may present extranasally or intranasally and, when intranasal, it will at times present as a mass involving the septum or as a pedunculated structure resembling a polyp. CT scans will demonstrate a bony defect in the floor of the anterior or middle cranial fossa. Biopsy should not be considered. Patients should be referred for neurosurgical and otolaryngologic evaluation.

Foreign bodies

A foreign body in the nose may be one of an endless variety of inanimate objects. By far the most common objects are parts of toys, such as wheels, beads and buttons. Pebbles, bits of cotton, beans, peas and nuts may also be found. Persistent unilateral fetid mucopurulent discharge should arouse clinical suspicion. To prevent aspiration of the dislodged object, a co-operative child should be placed in a supine position with his head down. The nose should be carefully anesthetized topically before forceps or a wire loop are introduced. Other methods, such as passing a Foley or Fogarty catheter beyond the object, inflating the catheter slightly and withdrawing it, are occasionally useful. The use of a general anesthetic may be required in uncooperative children or a retarded adult. It is prudent when removing one foreign body to make a quick check for others.

Trauma

Nasal obstruction may result from a traumatic dislocation of the caudal cartilage of the nasal septum or from a septal hematoma (Figure 9.1).

BILATERAL NASAL OBSTRUCTION

Allergic rhinitis

Allergic rhinitis is very common and affects at least 10% of the population to some degree. It takes two forms: seasonal and perennial. Seasonal allergy may be recognized as hay fever and is associated with inflamed conjunctival membranes as well as nasal and, in some patients, bronchial symptoms. In the Northeast USA, patients who are sensitive to tree pollen will begin to notice symptoms beginning in late March or early April. Grass-sensitive patients will be symptomatic from mid-May to the end of June. July and the first 2 weeks of August is a good, relatively allergy-free period for most of these patients. Ragweed and other summer weeds pollinate from mid-August until the first frost, usually early in October. Pollens and their seasons, of course, vary from region to region.

The first treatment program for seasonal allergy involves the antihistamines. These medications can be used alone or in combination in a

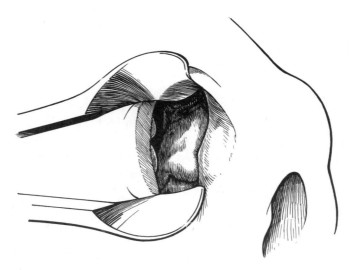

Figure 9.1 Nasal speculum examination. One of the most common findings is a deviated nasal septum, which may obstruct breathing. It may also become a source of bleeding, owing to trauma or excessive drying from the air stream

standard-release or sustained-release form. The patient should be made aware that these medications prevent the effects of histamine release by competing with histamine for binding sites and that, therefore, they should be taken in a regular, prophylactic manner. The side-effect of drowsiness common with the older antihistamines often abates after several days of use. The standard dosage form may be too strong for women or for persons with low body weight; therefore, the dose should be titrated by breaking the pills or by using the liquid form. Newer antihistamines (H-1 blockers) do not cause significant drowsiness, have the convenience of dosing once or twice a day, and are equally efficacious; therefore, they have become the drugs of choice for allergic rhinitis (Table 9.1). An especially effective therapeutic combination is to use an H-1 blocker in the morning and diphenhydramine (Benadryl®, Warner-Lambert, Morris Plains, NJ, USA, or Sominex®, Smith Kline Beecham, Philadelphia, PA, USA) at bedtime to improve sleep.

Vasoconstrictors can be used in combination or separately. Because of the relatively long symptom period of seasonal allergy, vasoconstricting nasal sprays should be avoided. The rebound phenomenon may develop

Table 9.1   Recommended antihistamines

	Remarks
Fexofenadine (Allegra®, Aventis Pharmaceuticals, Parsippany, NJ, USA), 60 mg twice a day	Use with caution in liver disease. Contraindicated for patients taking keto conazole, macrolide antibiotics, or in heart conditions leading to Q-T prolongation. Use with caution with tricyclic antidepressants and monoamine oxidase inhibitors.
Fexofenadine 60 mg + pseudoephedrine HCl 120 mg (Seldane D), tablet twice a day	In addition to precautions for fexofenadine, should not be used in patients with severe hypertension.
Loratadine (Claritin®, Schering-Plough Inc., Memphis, TN, USA), 10 mg every day (with food)	Use with caution with liver disease.
Diphenhydramine (Benadryl®), 25 or 50 mg three times a day or q.i.d.	Sedation, sleepiness. Avoid alcohol use. Thickened secretions. Useful as a night-time antihistamine, as promotes sleep.
Chlorpheniramine, 4 mg every 4–6 h, 12 mg long-acting form two or three times a day	Effective, the standard by which the efficacy of other antihistamines is measured. May cause drowsiness and thickened mucus.

or be made worse in these patients, owing to rhinitis medicamentosa, by the use of these sprays. On the other hand, topical steroid nasal sprays are often very helpful.

Patients who are so uncomfortable that they are unable to function normally despite these measures can be given corticosteroids for the duration of their allergy season if the allergy season is short – a few weeks to a month – and if there are no medical contraindications. For nasal allergy, 20 mg of prednisone on alternate mornings is usually very effective and has minimum suppressive effects on the adrenal–pituitary axis. Prednisone should be withdrawn gradually as the end of the season approaches. An alternative is a slowly absorbed steroid such as Depo-Medrol® (Pharmacia & Upjohn, Peapack, NJ, USA) 40 mg administered subcutaneously.

Skin testing or antigen-specific serum IgE levels (PRIST test) should be undertaken in order to determine sensitivities. By combining the results of these tests with an allergic history, the physician and patient can better understand the etiologic basis of the patient's symptoms and develop an appropriate plan of allergen avoidance and therapy. When allergic rhinitis becomes sufficiently troublesome, many physicians attempt allergic hyposensitization. This form of therapy is successful in providing partial or complete relief to approximately 80% of allergic patients. There are a variety of materials and techniques employed. In general, injections should be begun soon after the allergic season and should be gradually increased to the highest tolerable dose prior to the next allergic season.

The largest amounts of antigen, as measured by protein nitrogen units, can be administered with alum-precipitated extracts of pollens, because these are absorbed more slowly by the patient. The host responds by producing antigen-specific IgG that serves as a blocking antibody by combining with the antigen in the respiratory tissues, thus preventing the combination of the antigen with IgE bound to the surface of mast cells.

Perennial nasal allergy is also very common, and patients suffering from it complain of year-round nasal stuffiness, particularly at night when they try to sleep, although there may be exacerbations during pollen seasons. Sleep is often fitful, and patients awaken early in the morning with a blocked nose and begin to sneeze immediately upon arising. There is some gradual, but not complete, improvement during the day. Thick postnasal drip accompanies this disorder. Other common symptoms are intermittent loss of smell and taste, frontal headaches, facial pain, a dry throat and cough. Common allergies include house dust, house-dust mites, molds, feathers and animal danders. The role of food allergy in allergic rhinosinusitis is controversial and poorly understood. When these patients are questioned closely, many describe an increased incidence of symptoms following the social use of alcohol and exposure to cigarette smoke, perfumes and exhaust and paint fumes. In general, it is this group of perennial allergy patients who develop polypoid degeneration of the mucous membrane of the nose and paranasal sinuses (nasal polyps).

An evaluation of these patients should include full skin testing, testing for serum IgE level and CT sinus films. The films should include axial and coronal cuts through the sinuses for better assessment of mucosal thickening and sinus ostia obstruction.

Skin testing in these patients usually demonstrates a diffuse sensitivity to many antigens, but principally to those from house dust and pets. Based on this information, the patient should be instructed on how to eliminate sources of irritation from his environment. If there is little or no polypoid degeneration of the mucosa of the nose and paranasal sinuses, hyposensitization may be tried. Allergy injections will not reverse polypoid degeneration. Most patients with perennial nasal allergy have suffered for many years and have tried almost every form of antihistamine and vasoconstrictor. Although these medications are beneficial to some patients, many patients are not helped, because thickened secretions become thicker and the mucosa becomes refractory. Topical medications, such as cromolyn sodium (Nasal Crom®, Pharmacia & Upjohn) and beclomethasone (Beconase®, Glaxo Welcome Research, Triangle Park, NC, USA and Vancenase®, Schering Corp., Kenilworth, NJ, USA) are of some value. Patients with perennial allergy are difficult to help medically.

Vasomotor rhinitis

Symptomatically, vasomotor rhinitis seems identical to nasal allergy. Although it is approximately ten times less common than allergy, these are not mutually exclusive and at times are seen in conjunction. In pure vasomotor rhinitis, skin tests are negative and there is no elevation of IgE level. Unlike allergy, this condition is not improved by a short clinical course of cortisone, such as prednisone 20 mg orally every morning for 5 days. A course of treatment such as this is useful when doubt exists as to how much nasal symptomatology is due to allergy, and how much is due to vasomotor rhinitis or structural dysfunction, such as a deviated septum. The allergic symptoms will clear, leaving residual symptoms secondary to other nasal disorders.

In general, vasomotor rhinitis is poorly controlled by medications, although an antihistamine–vasoconstrictor combination should be tried. In our experience, ipratropium bromide (Atrovent®) works well. If obstruction persists despite therapy, one of a number of surgical treatments becomes necessary. In patients bothered primarily by obstruction, cryosurgical treatments of the inferior and middle turbinates (cryoturbinectomy), electro- or laser cautery plus surgical trimming of the inferior turbinate are useful. For profuse rhinorrhea, sectioning of the parasympathetic nervous supply to the nose may be necessary (vidian neurectomy). This therapy is reserved for the most severe cases; there is often a recurrence of the disorder several years later.

Rhinitis medicamentosa

Rhinitis medicamentosa is a common disorder associated with the chronic use of vasoconstricting nasal sprays. The mucosa becomes red and swollen, and the nose becomes completely obstructed with engorged turbinates because of irritation from the continual use of nasal spray and the recurring rebound phenomenon. Initially, the use of nose spray gives the patient relief, but in time the periods of improvement become shorter and shorter. Treatment consists of complete abstinence from nose spray for 2 weeks or more.

Corticosteroids, such as prednisone 20 mg every other morning for 2 weeks, are helpful in reducing some of the inflammation associated with this disorder, and they will help the patient do without the spray. If the obstruction fails to clear and there is no underlying nasal disorder, a procedure that reduces the size of the inferior turbinates such as electrocautery and trimming of the turbinates or cryoturbinectomy is required, to establish a satisfactory airway.

Polypoid rhinosinusitis

Both allergic and non-allergic patients may develop hyperplastic, boggy, thickened mucosa of the ethmoid, maxillary and, less frequently, the other sinuses. The causative factor is unknown. The majority of allergic patients never develop polyps, but there may be increased polyp formation in the presence of viral or bacterial infections. Also, there is a relationship between aspirin sensitivity, nasal polyps and bronchial asthma (aspirin triad syndrome). Patients with this condition should be advised to avoid tartrazine (US FD & C yellow no. 5) and indomethacin as well. Polyps should be removed as often as is necessary to maintain a satisfactory airway and to prevent obstruction and interruption of mucous flow and infection from stasis. Repeated or chronic infection compounds the problem by leading to increased inflammation and polyp formation. Polypectomy is a short office procedure and, for some patients with complaints only of nasal blockage secondary to polyps, this minor procedure is sufficient. When polypoid sinus disease becomes complicated by constant sinus headache pain or chronic infection, sinus surgery may often be required.

The surgery for polypoid rhinosinusitis should be based on a CT scan study which includes axial and coronal views of the paranasal sinuses. These films should be reviewed with the patient at an office visit, as with some explanation they are not difficult for patients to understand. The patients are given a demonstration of extent and location of their polyps and the relationship to their symptoms. In addition, the operative procedures can be explained with the films thus providing a visual explanation of what the proposed surgery will achieve as well as a demonstration of risk of complications involving the orbit and anterior skull base.

In general, surgery for polypoid rhinosinusitis includes bilateral ethmoidectomy and removal of polyps from the sphenoid or maxillary sinuses as well. These procedures may be combined with septoplasty, if a deviated septum is obstructing either the airway or access to the ethmoids, and trimming of the inferior one-third of the inferior turbinates if turbinate hypertrophy is part of the pathological complex. Local monitored or general anesthesia are commonly employed, and most often these patients do not require hospital admission. Most often these procedures are performed with endoscopes and, at times, with computer guidance, which will become the norm in the future. This technique eliminates the need for incisions external to the nose.

SINUS HEADACHE, PAIN AND DRAINAGE

Acute sinusitis

All forms of paranasal sinusitis are usually precipitated by nasal congestion from a viral, upper respiratory tract infection or nasal allergy, or both. Although occasionally acute sinusitis is a purely viral infection, much more commonly it is the result of a bacterial acute superinfection. Whether it occurs in the frontal, maxillary or ethmoid sinuses, the most frequent causative pathogens are *S. pneumoniae*, *H. influenzae*, *S. aureus*, *Moraxella catarrhalis*, β-streptococcus and occasionally anaerobes (anaerobes are frequently found in chronic sinusitis).

For patients with the clinical symptoms of sinusitis, a sinus X-ray study should be performed to establish the diagnosis. As a minimum, the views should include an upright, open-mouth Waters' view (so that air–fluid levels will be seen), a Caldwell view, a submental vertex view and a lateral view. Transillumination is too inexact a technique to use for diagnosis, but it is helpful in assessing the progress of therapy. Cultures are also helpful, but only if pus is cultured as it streams from a sinus ostium or, in the case of maxillary sinusitis, by antral puncture; otherwise, contamination from nasal flora makes the results open to question. Therapy should not await the culture report. Antibiotic selection is based upon the known frequency of occurrence of the pathogens and regional bacterial sensitivities, but it may be adjusted on the basis of clinical progress and the culture report. The spectrum of appropriate antibiotics necessary to provide coverage for the bacteria primarily responsible for acute sinusitis is in slow, constant evolution. In the past, ampicillin was an excellent choice; however, the emergence of resistant *H. influenzae* in a significant percentage of infections requires a change to drugs that give coverage for this and other β-lactamase-producing bacteria. Treatment for non-hospital acquired sinusitis does not need to include coverage for methicillin-resistant *S. aureus*, however. On a cost basis, trimethoprim–sulfamethoxazole is the most reasonable, but the list of effective antibiotics includes amoxicillin–clavulanate, certain cephalosporins, semisynthetic macrolide and quinolone antibiotics (Table 9.2). Along with the antibiotic, a long-acting, vasoconstricting nasal spray, such as oxymetazoline hydrochloride (Afrin®, Schering-Plough Inc.), should be prescribed. The most effective way to use these sprays is to spray the nose once, wait 5 min for the nose to clear, then spray again so that the second spray can reach the swollen sinus ostia. Following this, the patient should breathe through a very hot, wet towel for several minutes. The warm, moist air helps to liquefy the secretions. A patient with maxillary sinusitis should be instructed to lie across his bed and hang his head over the other side, with the affected sinus uppermost to promote drainage. This routine should be followed for 5 min three times a day for 3–4 days after the initiation of therapy. Antihistamines are not recommended in the treatment of acute sinusitis, because they tend to thicken, rather than to liquefy, the purulent material trapped within the sinus. Guaifenesin (Duratuss®, UCB Pharma Inc., Smyrna, GA, USA) will act to liquify secretions and, in combination with phenylpropanolamine (Duratuss G®, Pharma Inc.), will simultaneously vasoconstrict the nose and improve drainage. Analgesics are used according as circumstances may require.

Acute sinusitis may resolve slowly because of a narrowed nasofrontal duct or because of the lack of dependent drainage from the maxillary sinuses. A follow-up X-ray study consisting of the Caldwell view and an

Table 9.2 Some recommended antibiotics for sinusitis. Hypersensitivity to any of the listed medications is a contraindication to use. Medications for pregnant patients should be cleared with the obstetrician

	Sensitivities	Remarks
Amoxicillin (Amoxil®, Smith Kline Beecham Pharmaceuticals), adult dose 250–500 mg three times a day	(Gram⁺) *Staphylococcus aureus*, *Streptococcus pneumoniae*, *Streptococcus pyogenes*. (Gram⁻) *Haemophilus influenzae*, *Moraxella catarrhalis*	While amoxicillin is cost effective, there is a good proportion of *H. influenzae* and *M. catarrhalis* that produce β-lactamase. May have a cross-reaction with cephalosporins and other penicillins
Amoxicillin–clavulanate (Augmentin®, Smith Kline Beecham Pharmaceuticals), adult dose 250–500 mg three times a day	(Gram⁺) *Staphylococcus aureus*, *Streptococcus pneumoniae*, *Streptococcus pyogenes*. (Gram⁻) *Haemophilus influenzae*, *Moraxella catarrhalis*	Effective for β-lactamase-producing bacteria. May have cross-reaction with cephalosporins and other penicillins. Antibiotic-associated colitis, sometimes from *Clostridium difficile*
Azithromycin (Zithromax®, Pfizer Laboratories, New York, NY, USA), adult dose 250 mg once a day for 5 days	(Gram⁺) *Staphylococcus aureus*, *Streptococcus pneumoniae*, *Streptococcus pyogenes*. (Gram⁻) *Haemophilus influenzae*, *Moraxella catarrhalis*	Contraindicated with pregnancy, liver disease, or with terfenadine
Cefixime (Suprax®, Lederle Pharmaceuticals, Pearl River, NY, USA), adult dose 200 mg twice a day	(Gram⁺) *Streptococcus pneumoniae*, *Streptococcus pyogenes*. (Gram⁻) *Haemophilus influenzae*, *Moraxella catarrhalis*	Cross-reactions with cephalosporins, penicillins and β-lactam antibiotics
Cefuroxime axetil (Ceftin®, Glaxo Welcome), adult dose 250 mg twice a day	(Gram⁺) *Staphylococcus aureus*, *Streptococcus pneumoniae*, *Streptococcus pyogenes*. (Gram⁻) *Haemophilus influenzae*, *Moraxella catarrhalis*	Cross-reaction with cephalosporins, penicillins. May occasionally lead to pseudomembranous colitis
Clarithromycin (Biaxin®, Abbott Laboratories, Abbott Park, IL, USA), adult dose 500 mg twice a day	(Gram⁺) *Staphylococcus aureus*, *Streptococcus pneumoniae*, *Streptococcus pyogenes*. (Gram⁻) *Haemophilus influenzae*, *Moraxella catarrhalis*	Contraindicated in pregnancy, liver disease, and with terfenadine
Trimethoprim–sulfamethoxazole (Bactrim DS®, Roche Pharmaceuticals, Nutley, NJ, USA), adult dose one tablet twice a day	(Gram⁺) *Streptococcus pneumoniae*. (Gram⁻) *Haemophilus influenzae*	Severe reactions can occur such as Stevens–Johnson syndrome, toxic epidermal necrolysis, fulminant toxic epidermal necrolysis, agranulocytosis, aplastic anemia

upright Water's view should be obtained after 2–3 weeks of antibiotic therapy to ensure complete resolution of the infection. These are important films for the following reasons. First, acute sinusitis often resolves slowly, and the films may show only partial resolution of the infection. At this point the decision to continue antibiotic therapy for another 2 weeks should be made. Failure to treat an acute sinus infection adequately may result in troublesome chronic sinusitis. Second, this X-ray film occasionally reveals an underlying mechanism for the infection that is obscured by the inflammation and the secretions on the original films. Acute sinusitis that fails to clear after 3–4 weeks of treatment should be re-evaluated for further medical and surgical treatment by means of a CT scan and cultures. There are special diagnostic and therapeutic considerations that pertain to each sinus.

Acute frontal sinusitis

Acute frontal sinusitis causes pain in the forehead immediately over the sinus. This pain is intensified by bending forward or by tapping with a finger over the sinus. In general, the diagnosis of acute frontal sinusitis is simple to make; the difficulty lies in determining how much of a risk the infection represents to the patient. An infection of a frontal sinus that is not draining through the nasofrontal duct may potentially induce bacterial phlebitis of the diploic veins of the posterior wall of the sinus; therefore, it may spread centrally and result in an epidural, subdural or brain abscess. In other words, because the frontal sinuses, and sphenoid sinuses as well, are contiguous with the cranial vault and can become completely obstructed, when infected they represent a greater hazard to patients than infected maxillary and ethmoid sinuses. Also, improperly treated acute frontal sinusitis may become chronic sinusitis, a more difficult problem to treat.

If a patient with frontal sinusitis is febrile or has intense pain associated with edema of the overlying skin and tissues of the upper lid, he should be placed on intravenous antibiotics and topical vasoconstrictors. When rapid improvement fails to occur within 24 hours, surgical drainage by means of a trephine procedure is recommended. This procedure, performed with the patient under a local or general anesthetic, requires a 2-cm incision along the inferior medial edge of the eyebrow. The floor of the sinus is exposed (in the roof of the orbit), and a 5–7-mm opening is made in the bone. The contents are cultured for aerobes and anaerobes and aspirated, and a small catheter to be used for irrigation with an antibiotic solution is sutured in place for several days. The wound heals without significant scarring.

A common cause of acute frontal sinusitis is from water being forced into the sinus during diving into fresh water. These patients are often hospitalized because of the difficulty encountered with antibiotic therapy for an enteric bacterial infection from swimming water.

Acute sphenoid sinusitis

Acute sphenoid sinusitis occurs in otherwise healthy adults in conjunction with pansinusitis. In general, because the sphenoid sinuses will clear as the other sinuses clear, there is no cause for particular concern. However, acute sphenoid sinusitis can present as an isolated and potentially lethal infection in immunosuppressed, diabetic or elderly debilitated patients. The early signs are few and, therefore, the physician must have a high index of suspicion. Symptoms include fever, headache referred to the vertex of the skull and some purulent nasopharyngeal secretions. If the symptoms do not resolve rapidly upon institution of antibiotic therapy, the sphenoid sinus should be opened, cultured and drained with an endoscopic sphenoidotomy. If acute sphenoid sinusitis is not quickly recognized and treated, there is risk of central spread of infection either by direct extension through phlebitic veins or by the development of osteomyelitis of the sphenoid bone, particularly if the sphenoid sinus is well pneumatized. Because the lateral sinus wall is contiguous with the superior orbital fissure and the cavernous sinus, the infection may spread to these areas. The superior orbital fissure syndrome consists of panophthalmoplegia involving the third, fourth and sixth cranial nerves. In addition, the first division of the fifth and sympathetic nerves may also be involved. Cavernous sinus thrombosis is associated with spiking fever, exophthalmos and edema of the orbit and lids, decreased vision, papilledema and panophthalmoplegia.

Acute maxillary sinusitis

Acute maxillary sinusitis causes tenderness over the sinus that is also felt in the teeth that are contiguous with the sinus. These include the ipsilateral second premolar and the three molars. In some patients the tooth roots protrude into the antrum and are covered by only a thin layer of bone. The teeth may be sensitive to hot and cold liquids. Also, achy pain is referred to the orbital, zygomatic and temporal regions. Unilateral, isolated maxillary sinusitis requires increased diagnostic attention because it can arise secondary to carcinoma of the maxillary sinus or to a dental root abscess. X-ray films of the sinus should be carefully examined for any bone destruction indicative of a tumor. A survey X-ray film of the teeth that includes the roots should be obtained as well.

Patients in whom acute maxillary sinusitis does not resolve may require antral irrigation. This procedure is performed in the doctor's office. The lining of the nose is anesthetized, and a trocar needle is placed in the inferior meatus and pushed into the antrum. Warm sterile saline is then used to irrigate the sinus. Persistent infections will require surgical exploration, such as creating a nasal–antral window by means of endoscopic surgery or performing a Caldwell–Luc procedure (see Chronic maxillary sinusitis).

Acute ethmoiditis

Viral ethmoiditis accompanies many severe upper respiratory infections. It can produce frontal or orbital headache and a reduced sense of smell and taste. There are no additional symptoms associated with a bacterial infection, other than an observable change in the nasal secretions from a mucoid consistency to a yellow–gray purulence. Acute ethmoiditis is the only form of sinusitis that occurs in young children, because the other sinuses are yet to develop.

The ethmoid sinuses are separated from the orbital contents by a very thin plate of bone, the lamina papyracea. As a result, ethmoid sinusitis is occasionally complicated by orbital cellulitis. Patients with this complication are immediately hospitalized for intravenous antibiotic therapy and CT scans. If the infection fails to resolve rapidly (in 24–48 hours), the ethmoid sinus and orbit are explored and drained as a combined ophthalmology–otolaryngology procedure. Orbital cellulitis must be differentiated from cavernous sinus thrombosis.

Chronic sinusitis

Chronic frontal sinusitis

Chronic frontal sinusitis takes several forms. It may result from improperly treated acute frontal sinusitis, allergic polypoid sinus disease or obstruction of the nasofrontal duct secondary to scarring or fracture of the sinus wall. The sinus membrane is thickened, and infected secretions are retained. Patients may complain of a steady headache, associated with dull, localized tenderness and intermittent, purulent nasal and postnasal drainage. The sinus X-ray films of these patients demonstrate opacification of the sinus and sclerosis of the bony sinus margins.

Chronic frontal sinusitis may take the form of a mucocele, an expanding mucosal cyst filled with mucinous secretion. When infected, this cyst becomes a pyocele. Mucoceles slowly erode the walls of the sinus, and can reach the dura or expand into the orbit. Physical symptoms include headache and, at times, a soft mass protruding below the medial aspect of the brow or into the upper lid. Because the expanding cysts cause rarefaction of the bony walls of the sinus, radiologic determination of chronic sinusitis prior to CT scans was difficult to make.

The treatment for chronic frontal sinusitis is endoscopic widening of the nasofrontal duct in conjunction with an anterior ethmoidectomy. In the case of mucocele or failure of endoscopic surgery, obliteration of the sinus with osteoplastic frontal sinus obliteration is the best choice.

Chronic sphenoid sinusitis

Chronic sphenoid sinusitis occurs as an isolated infection in the chronically ill and the elderly. Physical findings are scant, except for a headache deep to the eyes and to the vertex and occiput of the skull in conjunction with complaints of intermittent purulent nasopharyngeal drainage. CT scans will demonstrate thickened mucosa, sometimes an air–fluid level and some-times complete opacification plus sclerosis of the surrounding bone. Cases that are refractory to medical care require surgical drainage by means of endoscopically removing the anterior wall of the sinus.

Chronic maxillary sinusitis

Chronic maxillary sinusitis presents with a generalized facial ache in the region of the sinus, in addition to intermittent ipsilateral mucopurulent discharge. In the absence of a dental root abscess, carcinoma, or very thick allergic or hyperplastic sinus mucosa, the condition may respond to a series of antral wash procedures along with a 3–4-week course of treatment with a properly selected antibiotic based upon the antral cultures. Otherwise, a Caldwell–Luc procedure to remove the diseased sinus membrane and to establish improved drainage through a window between the sinus and the nose is often curative.

Chronic ethmoiditis

Chronic ethmoiditis is seen most commonly as a complication of polypoid allergic sinusitis or polypoid hyperplastic sinusitis in which mucus and bacteria become entrapped. Patients suffer recurrent or continuous mucopurulent nasal discharge. Blockage of the upper portions of the nose produces midface headache and a diminished or absent sense of smell or taste. CT scans demonstrate a dissolution of the bony ethmoid septa and replacement by soft tissue. Satisfactory medical treatment of infections is often difficult; therefore, consideration must be given to ethmoid sinus surgery. With the advent of CT scanning, radiologic changes in the ethmoid sinuses have been a relatively common finding.

Sinusitis in HIV-positive patients

Those patients infected with the HIV-1 virus are broken into three groups based on symptoms. First, are the asymptomatic HIV$^{(+)}$ individuals. Second, are the early symptomatic patients with AIDS-related complex who may be experiencing weight loss, unexplained temperature elevations, weakness, oropharyngeal candidiasis or diarrhea. Third, are patients in the final stage of AIDS, with the characteristic frequent infections. Sinusitis, often in association with pulmonary infections and/or otitis media, has been reported in 20–70% of the AIDS population, depending on whether the diagnosis is made on a clinical basis or by CT scanning or magnetic resonance imaging (MRI). The most severe sinusitis is seen in conjunction with the greater levels of immunosuppression, namely CD4$^{(+)}$ counts below 200/mm^3 and alterations in humoral immunity secondary to B lymphocyte dysfunction. In general, IgE levels increase with advancing AIDS.

Almost all patients have more than one sinus involved; the frequency of involvement is maxillary and ethmoid commonly, sphenoid and frontal sinusitis occurs with advancing, therapeutically unresponsive disease. Approximately half the patients have asymptomatic sinusitis; the remainder experience occult fever, nasal congestion, discharge and headache most commonly. As many AIDS patients have had previous hospitalizations or have received antibiotics over a period of time, bacterial pathogens include a wider and more resistant spectrum than is found in a community population, in addition to sinus infections due to HIV-1, respiratory and herpes virus, as well as opportunistic fungal infections, especially *Aspergillus*.

When sinusitis is demonstrated, treatment begins with vigorous medical management. Most patients exhibit a partial response to antibiotics; however, incomplete resolution of the sinusitis is the rule, as measured by CT or MRI scans. Surgery is reserved for those patients with severe sinusitis that worsens or fails to improve on therapy.

Sinus surgery

Asymptomatic chronic sinusitis does not require surgery, except in special circumstances where there may be a question of osteomyelitis or the possibility of tumor. Ordinarily surgery should be proposed only to correct specific symptoms, and these include chronic nasal obstruction, chronic headache or facial pain, or chronic purulent drainage or recurring infections. Sinuses opacified on CT scan by polypoid mucosal linings in an otherwise asymptomatic patient do not automatically require surgery. A surgeon cannot improve an asymptomatic patient. In other words, sinus surgery is as much art as science, as overzealous surgery can result in symptoms worse than the original. For example, excessive tissue removal (especially turbinal) deprives the nose of protection from dry air as well as the moisturizing and cleansing effects of mucus-covered ciliated surfaces, thereby leading to chronic rhinitis sicca. Large areas where scar rather than respiratory epithelium has relined an ethmoid cavity or maxillary sinus, even following well-performed ethmoid or maxillary sinus surgery, will result in mucus stasis (crusting), bacterial growth and odor. Alternatively, the formation of an excessively large nasal–antral window will make the maxillary sinus a catchbasin for static mucus, creating chronic maxillary sinusitis.

Caldwell–Luc procedure

The Caldwell–Luc procedure is the most common surgical procedure used in the treatment of chronic maxillary sinusitis. In this operation, a 2-cm incision is made at the buccogingival junction above the canine and premolar teeth. The tissues of the cheek are then elevated, and an opening of 1 cm in diameter is made in the anterior bony wall with a drill. A smaller opening can be made if endoscopes are to be used. After culture of the contents of the sinus, the diseased membrane lining is removed, and an enlarged opening is made between the middle meatus and the sinus (a nasal–antral window) to provide improved drainage. The incision heals rapidly, but an occasional oral antral fistula may require secondary closure. Rarely, patients can be left with temporary or permanent numbness of the cheek in the area of distribution of the inferior orbital nerve. More commonly, there may be some numbness of the one or two teeth that are adjacent to the area of bone removal.

Ethmoidectomy

Ethmoidectomy can be performed through the nose (intranasal

ethmoidectomy) or by way of a 1.5–2-cm vertical incision placed halfway between the medial canthus of the eye and the dorsum of the nose (external ethmoidectomy). The external ethmoidectomy provides better exposure than the intranasal procedure, and as a rule a more thorough exenteration of the sinus cells can be achieved by this method. It is the method of choice when a mucocele or tumor is present. Wounds from ethmoidectomy heal well with little scarring. Ethmoidectomy can be bloody, because the only method of controlling bleeding is by tamponade and electric cautery; therefore, transfusions are occasionally required. Gauze packing is usually left in the sinuses for several days postoperatively. Complications, though rare, may be of a serious nature, and may include cerebrospinal fluid leak, epiphora, ophthalmoplegia and blindness. The usual hospital stay is 1 day following surgery, followed by a 1–2-week convalescent period at home.

The external ethmoidectomy provides an approach to the sphenoid sinus for sphenoidotomy and hypophysectomy. A sphenoidotomy includes removal of the anterior wall of the sphenoid and exenteration of the contents of the sinus. The complications and hospital stay are the same as for ethmoidectomy. Intranasal endoscopic and external ethmoidectomy can be combined with the Caldwell–Luc procedure and others when necessary.

Osteoplastic frontal sinus obliteration

Osteoplastic frontal sinus obliteration has been the procedure of choice for chronic frontal sinusitis. The incision can be hidden in the scalp or hair or, less satisfactorily, it can be placed above the eyebrows. The anterior bony wall of the sinus is elevated as a flap based on the periosteum inferiorly. The infected lining of the sinus is completely removed, and the sinus is obliterated with subcutaneous abdominal fat. This is an effective and relatively complication-free procedure with a high success rate. The patient is hospitalized for approximately 4–5 days, followed by several weeks of convalescence.

More recently, endoscopic frontal sinus procedures have been tried, reserving fat obliteration of the frontal sinus for failures.

Functional endoscopic sinus surgery

In nasal and sinus surgery there are a myriad of small and large unexpected good and bad effects of seemingly minor alterations of the anatomy which, in this region, have a profound effect upon the delicate balance of nasal health and disease. It is for these reasons that functional endoscopic sinus surgery was developed and has rapidly gained wide acceptance, as it permits close inspection of infected tissues, enabling the removal of disease in a manner that preserves or improves nasal physiology over the diseased state.

Endoscopic sinus surgery employs solid glass rod nasal telescopes with a light source and optional chip television camera, which provide a direct magnified view of the small sinonasal surgical field, a view that, if need be, may be redirected by means of 30° and 70° prisms, allowing the surgeon an improved view in the maxillary sinuses or nasofrontal duct region. The surgery requires a three-dimensional understanding of the anatomy in general and, using the patient's sinus CT scans as a guide in the operating room, a detailed understanding of the patient's anatomy and disease in particular, in order to produce the desired effect, namely marked improvement or total relief of the patient's sinus complaints.

With the advent of CT scanning of the paranasal sinuses, it was recognized that patient complaints of headache, upper nose congestion and recurring sinusitis, which until this time had been unexplained, were due frequently to anterior ethmoiditis and an associated condition known as osteomeatal complex disease. The infected ethmoid causes swelling, which results in obstruction of the natural ostium of the maxillary sinus. Limited surgery, using endoscopic techniques, results in a restoration of the normal function of this area and, in a high percentage of cases, relief of symptoms. The uses of endoscopic surgery have increased exponentially so that practically every sinus procedure has an endoscopic surgical equivalent.

The technical details of this surgery are beyond the scope of this book; however, the surgery accomplishes the following:

(1) For the ethmoid sinuses, partial or complete (depending on the disease) intranasal ethmoidectomy with or without preservation of the middle turbinate;

(2) For the maxillary sinus, clearing of the obstruction of the normal ostium, removing infected debris and preserving the ciliated epithelium to provide a normally functioning sinus;

(3) For the frontal sinuses, an anterior ethmoidectomy as well as a wide opening (and at times connecting) of the nasofrontal ducts to provide ample dependent drainage and relief of symptoms secondary to pressure and retained infection;

(4) For the sphenoid sinus, enlarging of the natural ostium almost to the point of removing the entire anterior wall.

UNUSUAL CAUSES OF NASAL OBSTRUCTION AND DRAINAGE

Tuberculosis

There had been a decrease in the incidence of tuberculosis in the USA until 1985; however, since that time, a resurgence has occurred secondary to increased homelessness and the developing HIV[(+)] population, as well as crowded conditions in prisons and shelters. Resistant tuberculosis (to at least one drug) has gradually spread through these groups. Superficial mucosal infections may result from the spread of infectious pulmonary aerosolized bacteria. Even so, tuberculous rhinitis and otitis are very unusual infections, even among HIV[(+)] and immunosuppressed patients. In the nose, tuberculosis presents as beefy red edema, an ulceration, or a granulomatous growth or polyp. Diagnosis is made by biopsy, smears, cultures and purified protein derivative. In general, isoniazed 300 mg daily combined with rifampicin 600 mg for 9 months is sufficient therapy in drug-sensitive infections.

Sarcoidosis

Sarcoidosis, a multisymptom disorder of undetermined etiology, occasionally presents as, or includes, nasal congestion and rhinitis. The condition is not considered serious in the absence of hilar adenopathy, pulmonary infiltrations, or ocular or skin lesions. The otolaryngology referral is commonly made by chest physicians or ophthalmologists, and usually patients are female more commonly than male, in the 20–40-year age range and, for unknown reasons, Blacks and Scandinavians predominate.

The nasal manifestations are principally those of obstruction secondary to low-grade inflammation with characteristic yellowish 1–3-mm nodules of the turbinal or septal mucosa. Inflammation may be followed by intense fibrosis. Other ear, nose and throat manifestations of sarcoidosis include cervical lymphadenopathy and parotid enlargement, which, when associated with keratoconjunctivitis, represents Heerfordt's syndrome.

Diagnosis is made by biopsy. In its milder form, the disease may have a self-limited course. Corticosteroids provide some relief of symptoms. Surgery can be counter-productive due to intense scarring.

Rhinosporidiosis

A condition found primarily in India, rhinosporidiosis is manifested by a chronic painless, purplish, pedunculated nasal mass, which, on pathological examination, contains minute cysts appearing as white submucosal spots containing the pathogen *Rhinosporidium seeberi*. Treatment is surgical excision.

Rhinoscleroma

This is a chronic infection involving the mucosa of the upper respiratory system that is found in economically depressed areas of Africa, the Americas, southern Asia and Eastern Europe. The disease, secondary to *Klebsiella rhinoscleromatis*, leads to atrophic rhinitis due to destruction of mucosa and replacement by scar. In advanced cases, the nose can become obstructed by granulations turned to scar. Diagnosis is based on characteristic histopathologic findings of foamy-appearing histiocytes called Mikulicz cells. Treatment is by a 2-month course of trimethoprim–sulfamethoxazole, streptomycin and tetracycline, which may require repeating. Scarring is corrected by surgery.

Syphilis

Primary syphilis may rarely present as a chancre on the nasal epithelium–mucosa junction. Diagnosis requires a dark-field microscopic examination because serological, reagin and specific treponemal tests are negative for the first 8–12 weeks. Syphilis can be an occupational hazard to medical personnel.

Secondary syphilis can present as gray, mucinous patches on the nasal mucous membranes as well as on the oral mucosa. The lesions are highly infectious. Rhinitis, nicknamed 'the snuffles' in infants, is classically seen in early congenital syphilis and is characterized by mucosal inflammation and bloody, mucopurulent discharge.

Congenital syphilis in the adult is analogous to tertiary syphilis and, if unrecognized, it can lead to nasal saddle deformities from luetic chondritis and osteitis.

Late syphilis presents as a gummatous reaction of the bony nasal septum and foul-smelling drainage. Patients often develop septal perforations. Intramuscular penicillin remains the principal therapy for syphilis as *Treponema pallidum* has remained sensitive to this antibiotic.

Wegener's granulomatosis

Wegener's granulomatosis is an uncommon disease characterized by focal necrotizing vasculitis that most commonly affects the upper respiratory tract initially, followed by the lower respiratory tract, skin, joints and kidneys. Patients may present with a secondarily infected and painful ulceration of the nose or a granular draining otitis media – both of which are unresponsive to antibiotic therapy. Nasal or otic, as well as pulmonary and renal, biopsies are often necessary to confirm the diagnosis. Prednisone is useful in controlling symptoms; however, cytotoxic drugs, primarily cyclophosphamide, have produced remissions and revolutionized the treatment of this previously lethal disorder.

Midline granuloma

Midline granuloma is very rare. It presents in a manner similar to Wegener's granulomatosis but tends to remain localized. The underlying disorder is an atypical lymphoid and reticulum cell proliferation in granulation tissue, identified by deep biopsy. The disease process, characterized by a rapidly growing ulcerating mass, results in destruction of the internal structures of the nose. Treatment is high-dose (4000–6000 cGy) radiation therapy when the disease is localized.

Mucormycosis

Mucormycosis is an opportunistic fungal infection caused by *Rhizopus* in patients with diabetic ketoacidosis or blood dyscrasias, or patients who are immunosuppressed or require long-term treatment with high doses of steroids and antibiotics. Patients complain of nasal pain and have a serosanguineous nasal discharge. Examination of the nose reveals a black, necrotic turbinate. Biopsy and smear for *Mucor* are diagnostic. The treatment of mucormycosis is prompt debridement and immediate initiation of amphotericin B. The prognosis is grave.

Aspergillosis

Aspergillus has several presentations in the nose and sinuses. In non-immunosuppressed patients who typically have been on antibiotic therapy for chronic sinusitis, it may form a collection or fungus ball, usually in the maxillary sinus. The organism does not invade the sinus mucosa, and treatment consists of removal of the fungus from the sinus, generally by the Caldwell–Luc operation.

In atopic patients, the fungus can create an allergic reaction resulting in an edematous mucosa and sequestered, inspissated gray–green gum-thick mucus involving single or multiple sinuses. Again, the disease is not invasive, therefore a thorough surgical removal of the infective debris and a course of prednisone will control the disorder.

The third form is similar to mucormycosis in that the organism invades the mucosa and especially the blood vessel walls of immunocompromised patients, resulting in progressive necrosis of the sinonasal structures and inexorable progression intracranially. Vigorous surgical debridement and aggressive therapy with amphotericin B may be life-saving.

10

Nasal and facial emergencies

William R. Wilson

Epistaxis
  Anterior septal bleeding
  Rare disorders
  Arterial epistaxis
Treatment for persistent nasal bleeding
  Nasal tampons
  Nasal balloons
  Anterior and posterior nasal packs
  Surgical options
  Treatment of rare disorders associated with epistaxis
Nasal fractures: office or emergency room repair
  Examination
  Treatment
Septal drainage procedures
  Septal hematoma
  Septal abscess
Repair of soft tissue lacerations of the head and neck
  Evaluation
  Preparation of the wound for closure
  Repair of facial lacerations
  Repair of mucosal lacerations
  Repair of through-and-through lacerations of the lip

EPISTAXIS

Anterior septal bleeding

Anterior septal bleeding from the Kiesselbach plexus (Figure 10.1), primarily venous, is by far the most common variety of nosebleed. Almost without exception, it is the type of nosebleed seen in children, and it is the most common site of bleeding in adults. Often there is a history of trauma or hay fever, and most commonly there are repeated episodes of bleeding. In adults, the possibility of clotting disorders should be ruled out, especially secondary to regular aspirin use, and familial histories of epistaxis should be sought.

Examination demonstrates venous bleeding from one side of the nasal septum. A check should be made for septal spurs and deviations, ulcerations, septal perforations, granulomas, foreign bodies and tumors. There is a great deal of folklore regarding the treatment of epistaxis. Patients, and in the case of children their parents, should be questioned about treatment methods, because many old tricks or misconceptions, such as lying down, merely serve to prolong the bleeding. Taking the time to teach patients the principles of treatment for minor epistaxis will help them have fewer bleeding episodes.

The patient should sit up and lean forward to reduce venous pressure in the head and to prevent the swallowing of blood. A small piece of cotton

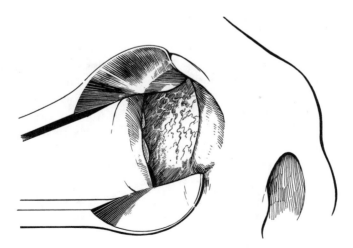

Figure 10.1 Speculum examination. The venous plexus located on the anterior nasal septum is the most frequent source of epistaxis, particularly in children

soaked with a vasoconstricting nose drop such as phenylephrine hydro-chloride (Neo-Synephrine®, Bayer Corp., Morristown, NJ, USA) or oxymetazoline hydrochloride (Afrin®, Schering Plough Inc., Memphis, TN, USA) is placed in the vestibule of the nose and pressed against the bleeding site for 10–15 min. This will stop almost all venous bleeding of this type. The patient should be given precautions to prevent retraumatizing the area: children's nails should be trimmed; humidity is helpful in dry weather or homes; and a lubricant, such as bacitracin ointment or petroleum jelly, helps promote healing.

If these remedies fail, the mucous membrane can be anesthetized using cotton soaked with 4% cocaine or 4% lidocaine (Xylocaine®, AstraZeneca Pharmaceuticals LP, Wilmington, DE, USA) for 5 min. A silver nitrate stick can be applied to the membrane over the bleeding site and to any vessels that appear prominent.

Occasionally, a small artery in the septal mucous membrane either will fail to stop bleeding or will rebleed a short time later. These episodes can usually be controlled by anesthetizing and recauterizing the area, and by placing a small amount of oxidized regenerated cellulose (Surgicel®, Ethicon, Somerville, NJ, USA) against the bleeder or a small packing of petrolatum gauze strip in the nasal vestibule for 24 hours.

Problems that may require an otolaryngologic consultation include chronic nasal ulcerations due to bony septal spurs or septal deviations that become dried and easily traumatized by the flow of air through the nose. Correction may require a submucous resection or septoplasty in order to remove the spurs and correct the deflection.

Patients with clotting disorders or liver or renal disease require especially careful treatment so that the mucous membrane does not suffer further abrasions. These cases are best handled with soft cotton tamponades wetted with long-acting nasal vasoconstricting drops, such as oxymetazoline hydrochloride 0.5% (Afrin nasal solution), humidity and copious lubricants. Packing should be avoided at all costs; but, if excessive blood loss necessitates, it can be accomplished with a piece of Surgicel, which does not require removal.

Rare disorders

Bleeding secondary to granulomas is uncommon, but if it is seen, the patient should be referred for biopsy and further management. Osler–Weber–Rendu disease, or familial hereditary telangiectasia, presents with frequent epistaxis, up to several times daily in extremely severe cases.

If local measures do not control the bleeding, a surgical procedure involving skin grafting of the nasal septum (septal dermoplasty) can be used. Long-standing nasal foreign bodies can cause epistaxis. They are usually impacted and often require removal by a nasal surgeon with the patient under a general anesthetic.

Arterial epistaxis

Arterial epistaxis is a less common variety of epistaxis, involving primarily middle-aged or elderly adults. The patient's history may include hypertension, nasal trauma or surgery. When arterial epistaxis presents in young males, examination for a vascular tumor is required in order to rule out juvenile nasopharyngeal angiofibroma. This can be easily accomplished with sinus X-rays.

Examination for arterial epistaxis requires a headmirror or surgical headlight and nasal suction. The most common finding is unilateral brisk arterial epistaxis from a branch of the sphenopalatine artery on the posterolateral wall of the nose, either below or above the inferior turbinate. Less commonly, the bleeding is from an ethmoid artery; if this is the case, bleeding is seen from the superior aspect of the nose, above the level of the middle turbinate.

Treatment of arterial epistaxis involves the following steps:

(1) The patient must be seated and leaning forward slightly so that the blood runs from his nose. This permits an assessment of the bleeding and helps prevent nausea in the patient from ingested blood.

(2) A vasoconstrictor such as phenylephrine hydrochloride (Neo-Synephrine) or oxymetazoline hydrochloride (Afrin) must be sprayed into the nose.

(3) Using bayonet forceps, the nose is packed gently with long cotton pledgets soaked in 4% cocaine or 4% lidocaine (Xylocaine solution) in order to induce anesthesia and to tamponade the bleeding temporarily, for 10–30 min. A hematocrit is obtained.

(4) Upon removal of the pledgets, the bleeding site is electrocauterized, and a small piece of Surgicel is placed over the area.

Once the bleeding is controlled, the patient is given the following instructions to help prevent recurrence.

(1) Do not blow your nose forcibly.

(2) If you must sneeze, expel the sneeze through your open mouth.

(3) Avoid strenuous exercise and stooping.

(4) Sleep with two or three pillows to elevate your head at night.

(5) Avoid hot drinks, alcohol (a nasal vasodilator) and smoking.

(6) Do not take aspirin or medications that contain aspirin.

(7) Use a laxative if constipated.

(8) It is advisable to use a long-lasting vasoconstricting nasal spray, such as oxymetazoline (Afrin) three times a day for several days.

TREATMENT FOR PERSISTENT NASAL BLEEDING

If bleeding persists or recurs, the nose must be packed or tamponaded. There are several varieties of tampons and balloons available commercially.

Nasal tampons

Nasal tampons, made of compressed Merocel® (Xomed Surgical Products, Jacksonville, FL, USA) sponges, are sometimes useful in the treatment of epistaxis. The sponge swells with hydration and acts as a tamponade. They come with or without a silicone-cannula airway through the packing. Tampons are most effective when the bleeding is in a relatively confined space, such as under the inferior turbinate, where they can be wedged into position. These sponges must be anchored anteriorly to prevent slippage into the pharynx. If the tampon is placed in the posterior portion of the nose, the patient should be hospitalized for observation. Tampons should be removed after 5 days. They may be regularly soaked with vasoconstricting nasal sprays, antibiotic solutions (1 ml of bacitracin solution 1 : 1000), and thrombin. All patients treated with tampons should receive antibiotic coverage.

Nasal balloons

In general, a nasal balloon is placed more easily, and without as much discomfort for the patient, than nasal packing. Unfortunately, balloons are not always as successful as packing in controlling bleeding, because they cannot conform as well to the nasal interstices. Balloons often cause mucosal ulcerations from pressure necrosis, and they have a tendency to leak and, occasionally, burst. Balloons, and to a lesser degree packing, can result in intranasal scarring and partial nasal obstruction. This becomes apparent several weeks after their removal.

Before a balloon or pack is put in place, the patient's nose must be well anesthetized with a topical anesthetic. Premedication with morphine sulfate intramuscularly or Demerol® (Sanofi-Synthelabo, New York, NY, USA) intramuscularly is recommended. In general, the balloons leak less when inflated with normal saline than when inflated with air. The balloons must be carefully secured anteriorly in order to prevent their displacement into the lower airway.

It is our practice to hospitalize patients with balloons or posterior nasal packing. Arterial hypoxemia and hypercapnia are frequent sequelae of posterior nasal packs, and arterial oxygen saturation should be monitored in some patients. Obstructed airways can occur secondary to a slipped packing or balloon, swelling of the palate or relaxation of the tongue secondary to exhaustion and pain medication. Nurses must be aware of these potential airway problems. A rubber nasopharyngeal airway placed in the opposite side of the nose can be of benefit. Patients must be placed on antibiotics, such as penicillin, clindamycin or cephalexin, in order to prevent sinusitis. In addition, good mouth care should be maintained with lemon and glycerine swabs and oral irrigations with half-strength hydrogen peroxide four times a day.

The packing or balloon is removed after 5 days. Ferrous sulfate, 300 mg orally every day, helps to replenish lost hemoglobin. In general, our patients are transfused only if they are symptomatic from blood loss or if the stabilized hematocrit is below 25%.

Anterior and posterior nasal packs

With the advent of improved sponge and balloon packings, the gauze packings are rarely used but are included in the event that they are required.

A method of cinching an anterior packing tightly into the nose has been described, which accomplishes a tight packing that does not slip into the nasopharynx (M. Joseph and M. Strome, personal communication; Figure 10.2). This modified anterior pack eliminates the need to place a packing into the posterior choana through the mouth and is more comfortable, and probably as effective, as standard anteroposterior packing for the patient. When a nasal balloon or tampon is not available or has not been effective, an anterior or posterior nasal pack can be put in place. The patient must

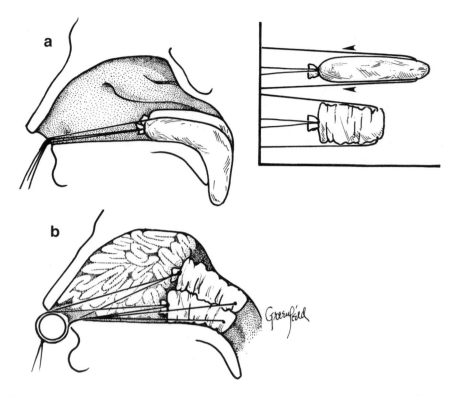

Figure 10.2 An alternative method of placing an anterior nasal pack. (a) Two finger cots are prepared by placing a second heavy silk suture, which is cut approximately 12 in (30 cm) long, through the distal end (tip). After the patient has been premedicated and the nose has been anesthetized with topical anesthetics, such as 4% cocaine solution on wrung-out cotton sponges, the finger cots are placed partway through the posterior choana. (b) The anterior nose is then packed with 0.5-in (1 cm) petrolatum (Vaseline®) gauze in a layered fashion, so that the silk sutures do not come in contact with mucosa or skin. When completed, the sutures through the tip of the finger cot are pulled tight, and all sutures are tied over a gauze in the naris. This maneuver creates a pressure packing at the posterior end of the turbinates, the region where the sphenopalatine artery enters the nose

be well medicated beforehand, and the nose and palate must be anesthetized (Figure 10.3).

The packing is prepared by folding a 4 × 4 gauze to a size estimated to be slightly larger than the posterior choanae. It is secured with two heavy silk sutures. The four ends of the sutures are left about 1 ft (30 cm) in length. Bacitracin ointment is worked into the pack to act as a lubricant and to inhibit infection.

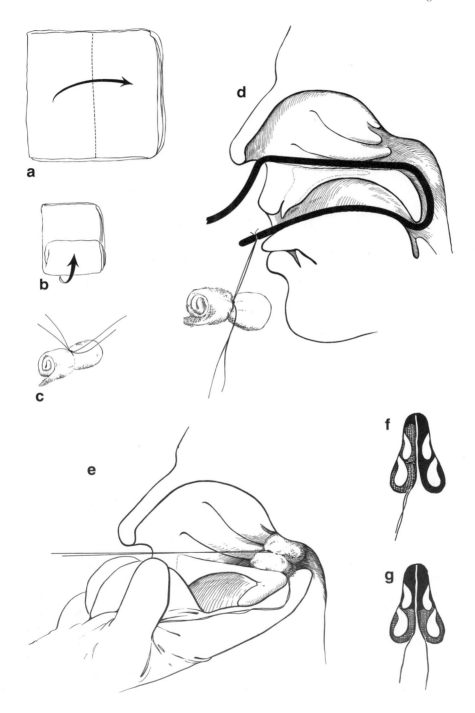

h

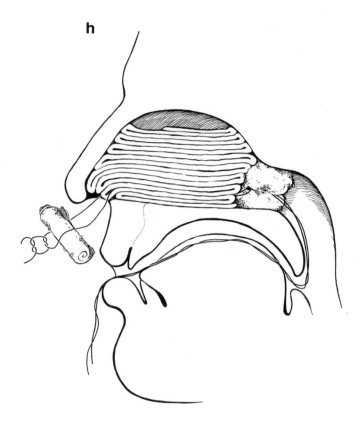

Figure 10.3 (*see also previous page*) Anterior–posterior nasal pack (a), (b) and (c). A 4 × 4-in (10 × 10 cm) gauze sponge is folded in half, trimmed, rolled and tied with heavy silk sutures so that there are four 12-in (30-cm) suture ends. The packing is coated with an antibiotic ointment, such as bacitracin. (d) Following topical anesthetization of the nose and premedication with parenteral analgesics, a rubber catheter is passed through the bleeding nostril and brought out through the mouth. Two sutures are tied to the catheter. (e) The catheter is carefully withdrawn from the nose, and the pack is guided and pressed into the posterior choana with an index finger or Kelly clamp. (f) The proper position of the posterior nasal pack. (g) A frequent error, demonstrated here, is to place one suture on either side of the septum. This does not allow the pack to be drawn tightly against the posterior bleeding site. (h) One-half-inch (1 cm) petrolatum gauze is packed by layers into the nose, inferiorly to superiorly, against the posterior pack. Care is taken to surround the sutures completely with the layering gauze, so that neither the nasal mucosa nor the nasal ala can be cut by them. The sutures are pulled tight and tied over a soft, rolled gauze at the nares

A soft rubber catheter is inserted through the side of the nose that is bleeding, until the end is seen in the oropharynx; it is then grasped with a Kelly clamp and brought out through the mouth. Two ends of the sutures are secured to the catheter, which is now withdrawn from the nose as the pack is placed into the mouth and around the soft palate, and is cinched into the posterior choana. The physician can use his fingers or a Kelly clamp to facilitate placement of the pack in the choana.

With the posterior pack held tightly in place by the silk sutures, petrolatum gauze packing 0.5 in (1 cm) wide and approximately 3 ft (1 m) in length is packed in the nose. This packing should be placed tightly and should completely surround the silk sutures to keep them from coming in contact with, and cutting, the mucous membrane. More than one of the petrolatum gauze packings may be required. Once the nose is packed, the posterior pack is secured into position by tying the ends of the suture over a rolled 1 × 1-in (2 × 2 cm) gauze placed at the anterior nares. The other suture is brought out through the mouth and taped to the cheek. Its purpose is to facilitate removal of the pack. The patient is hospitalized with the same medications and precautions as for those patients treated with nasal balloons.

Surgical options

If the bleeding persists, the patient should be advised about further treatment. Referral to an otolaryngologist should be made at this point. The surgical options are listed below in relative order of popularity, and depend in part on the facilities available:

(1) Endoscopic examination of nose and identification of bleeding site and cautery with direct visualization in the operating room, using sinus surgery instruments.

(2) Transantral ligation of the internal maxillary artery and ligation of the anterior and posterior ethmoidal arteries is almost uniformly successful and leaves only a small scar adjacent to the medial canthus of the eye and in the buccogingival sulcus. The risks are slight when this procedure is performed by an experienced surgeon, but they include possible eye injury and occasional numbness in the area of the infraorbital nerve, in the ipsilateral hard palate or in adjacent teeth.

(3) Selective internal maxillary arteriography and embolization is an elegant method available in large medical centers. A skilled head-and-neck

arteriographer is required. The success rate is approximately the same as that of arterial ligation.

Treatment of rare disorders associated with epistaxis

Juvenile nasopharyngeal angiofibroma is a benign vascular tumor unique to postpubescent adolescent males (13–21 years of age) that most often presents with a very brisk epistaxis. Once the bleeding is controlled, the diagnosis is made by X-ray studies of the paranasal sinuses. Biopsies are not to be performed, because of the risk of excessive hemorrhage. Removal should be attempted following arteriography and embolization of the feeding vessels.

Intracranial aneurysms secondary to trauma or infection occur spontaneously. They have been known to rupture into the sphenoid sinus or, from a pulsating mass, into the nasopharynx. The hemorrhage is massive and usually fatal.

NASAL FRACTURES: OFFICE OR EMERGENCY ROOM REPAIR

Patients with a history of nasal injury, some epistaxis and a question of nasal fracture are frequently seen in emergency areas. Palpation of the nasal bridge, an intranasal examination and an X-ray evaluation constitute a complete examination. Severely injured noses involving comminuted bone fractures and cartilage breaks or tears will require referral to an ear, nose and throat surgeon.

Examination

(1) If there is little or no swelling, it is particularly useful to palpate the nasal bones and orbital rims in order to identify small fractures. It should be ascertained whether the paired upper and lower lateral cartilages are torn.

(2) The nasal septum is inspected both externally and with a nasal speculum for evidence of fracture, dislocation or hematoma formation. The correction of internal deformities must accompany the correction of external deformities. Failure to drain a septal hematoma will result in gradual resorption of the septal cartilage and a saddle deformity of the nose. In addition, a septal hematoma may lead to a septal abscess and subsequent meningitis. Septal hematomas can occur gradually and, therefore, patients should be told to return in 24 hours if nasal breathing becomes obstructed.

(3) The patient is asked to lean forward in order to identify any cerebrospinal fluid (CSF) leakage. A brief check should be made for the presence or absence of the sense of smell.

(4) X-ray views for nasal fractures should include the lateral projection, Waters' view, hyperextended Waters' view and superinferior tangential view. For the superinferior tangential view, a bite-wing film is placed between the tongue and palate, providing an excellent view of the nasal bones (Figures 10.4 and 10.5). Care must be taken not to overinterpret the X-ray films, because the nasal suture lines as well as the impression made by the angular vessels in the nasal bones can be misinterpreted as fractures.

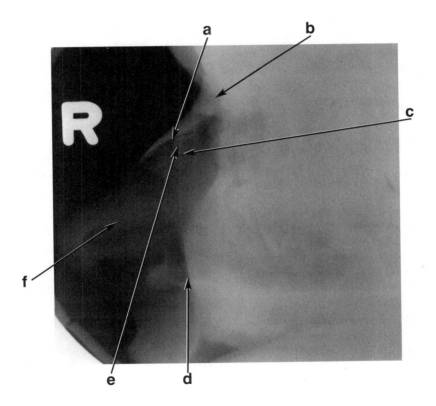

Figure 10.4 Lateral view of the nasal bones reveals (a) normal nasal bones; (b) nasofrontal suture; (c) nasomaxillary suture; (d) nasal spine; (e) normal grooves for vessels and nerves; and (f) cartilaginous structures of the nose

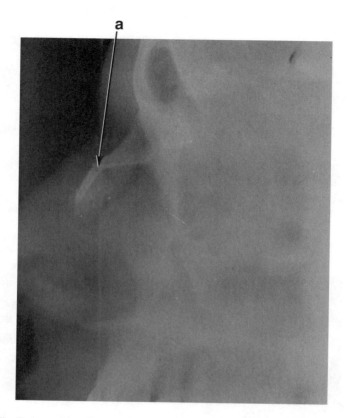

Figure 10.5 Patient with a fracture in the midnasal bones. The lateral view shows a linear fracture (a) with slight anterior buckling of the nasal bones

(5) Injuries in the region of the nasal bones and the nasal process of the frontal bone may lead to a fracture through the cribriform or ethmoid bones. Patients with such injuries should be asked whether they have noted a small amount of clear drainage after their injury. The drainage is most commonly unilateral and may be intermittent, coming in short, rapid gushes, or may present as a steady flow. The CSF is perfectly clear, has a slightly salty taste, and, unlike nasal mucus, contains protein (15–40 mg/dl) and glucose (50–80 mg/dl). A clue to CSF leak is the formation of a characteristic 'bull's-eye' when the fluid is mixed with blood and dried on a white sheet. Clear fluid can be differentiated from watery nasal secretions by means of a positive glucose test using a commercial dipstick designed for testing urinary sugar. Situations in

which CSF leakage is possible (for example, when there is a fracture through the cribriform area) should be evaluated with a computerized tomography (CT) scan. Further evaluation might require injection of markers, such as fluorescein or [I^{131}] albumin, by way of a lumbar puncture.

In general, CSF leakage should be treated by keeping the patient at bed rest with his head elevated at all times, with placement of a lumbar drain for several days and by maintaining prophylactic antibiotic coverage until the leak seals spontaneously. Leaks that do not stop require repair. In general, intranasal repair techniques work well for small defects. Large tears may require an intracranial approach.

Treatment

(1) Non-displaced nasal fractures require no treatment. However, patients should be warned to return for treatment promptly if they experience increasing nasal obstruction, unusual pain or swelling or clear drainage through the nose.

(2) Simple nasal fractures involving depressed fractures of the nasal bones or septal fractures and dislocations can be reduced in a properly equipped emergency area. Nasal fractures in adults can be reduced at any time up to 10 days. It is not uncommon to defer reduction in adults if nasal swelling at the time of the initial visit is severe enough to obscure the adequacy of reduction. In children, reduction should not be delayed more than a few days, if at all.

(3) For reduction of a nasal fracture, the patient is premedicated with Demerol or morphine. Intranasal anesthesia is achieved by packing the nose with cotton strips soaked with 4% cocaine or an appropriate substitute. An external field block is obtained by injecting 2% lidocaine with epinephrine (adrenaline) 1 : 100 000 subcutaneously with a no. 27 needle introduced at the root of the nose.

Additional injections can be made at the lateral margins of the nose and at the base of the columella if necessary.

Upon removal of the anesthetic packing, a blunt nasal elevator wrapped with moistened cotton to decrease intranasal trauma is introduced into the nose under the nasal fracture and lifted until the deformity can no longer be felt. Some reduced fractures require stabilization with an intranasal iodiform gauze-strip packing for several days.

Fractures involving the septum or a fracture of both nasal bones may require the use of Asch forceps or Walsham forceps to achieve proper reduction. If, after a week, when the swelling has decreased, it is apparent that the reduction is less than satisfactory, the fracture can be corrected further by a nasal surgeon. The technique of treatment varies with the surgical problem and the surgeon's preferences; resetting, packing, internal or external splints and reduction by means of septorhinoplasty are among the options.

Immediate referral should be made for torn cartilages and for a comminuted fracture involving either intranasal or external laceration or the nearby bony structures, such as the ethmoid, the ascending processes of the maxilla or the nasal process of the frontal bone (nasal–frontal–ethmoid complex). These patients usually require an open reduction and external nasal splinting to prevent a root-depression deformity. Every effort should be made to achieve the best possible functional and esthetic results initially because, in general, it is more difficult to achieve excellent results with chronically twisted or distorted noses.

SEPTAL DRAINAGE PROCEDURES

Septal hematoma

A septal hematoma should be treated as soon as it is identified. The septal mucosa is cocainized and 1-cm incisions are made on the right and left sides. In order to avoid the risk of septal perforation, the incisions are placed so that they are not apposed to one another (Figure 10.6). Following culture of the accumulated blood, the remaining blood is aspirated from both sides of the nose using a Frazier suction. The status of the septal cartilage can be assessed at this time. A small Penrose drain or piece of 1-in (2-cm) wide iodiform gauze is placed in each drainage site to prevent reaccumulation of the hematoma. Finger-cot packings are placed bilaterally to reapproximate the mucosal flaps. Patients with a septal hematoma should be placed on antibiotics for several days until the danger of infection is past. Patients must be warned of the possibility of saddle deformity, even if the hematoma has been treated expeditiously.

Septal abscess

A septal abscess almost always evolves from an unrecognized septal hematoma 2–14 days following nasal trauma. Patients present with nasal pain and

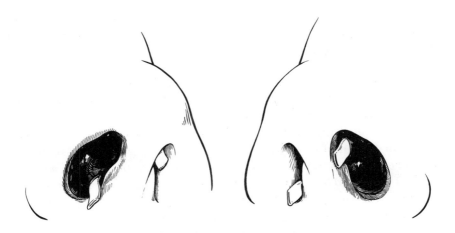

Figure 10.6 Placement of submucosal Penrose drains for septal hematoma or septal abscess

swelling, elevated temperature, headache and, occasionally, meningitis. Bacterial cultures most often grow a variety of nasal pathogens, including *Hemophilus influenzae*, *Staphylococcus aureus*, and *Streptococcus pneumoniae*. Therefore, following culture, the antibiotics of choice for treatment are synthetic penicillins, such as nafcillin. The drainage procedure is identical to that described for a septal hematoma. Parenteral antibiotics are maintained for approximately 10 days. At times, the caudal cartilage is destroyed, and a marked saddle deformity occurs. These are best repaired by augmentation rhinoplasty, using autogenous cartilaginous or bony implants 6 months or more after the infection.

REPAIR OF SOFT TISSUE LACERATIONS OF THE HEAD AND NECK

Although they have had little formal training in surgery, many primary care physicians, such as family care practitioners, pediatricians and internists, master and understand the techniques of laceration suturing and wound repair and are capable of superior closures of minor wounds in the head and neck. The difference between fair and superior results is often a matter of attention to detail prior to and during the surgery, as well as of appropriate follow-up care.

A minor surgery room or emergency room must have good lighting, co-operative help, appropriate supplies and instruments suitable for the work that is to be done. If a physician is frequently called upon to do suturing, a small investment in a few plastic surgery instruments for his own set will ensure the availability of the proper tools. Skill will be enhanced and confidence will grow as case volume increases. Familiarity with instruments will further increase surgical skill. For instance, it is very difficult to close a facial laceration while trying to hold a 6-0 suture in a long, serrated jaw needle holder designed for abdominal surgery.

This list of instruments is included only as a guide for selection. Two fine skin hooks are useful (a single and a double). These are the simplest of instruments and most atraumatic to skin. It is also important to have a fine-toothed forceps. These are used primarily to grasp subcutaneous tissue to avoid crushing margins of the epidermis. Four very fine, curved mosquito hemostats should be enough. For trimming tissues, a no. 15 or no. 11 Bard Parker surgical blade is the most useful. A few pairs of scissors are helpful. The set should include good quality, blunt, curved scissors (very delicate Metzenbaum type), curved, sharp iris scissors and straight, sharp iris scissors. A good marking pen with a fine point is a frequently omitted instrument that can be used for planning alignment, margin refinement or even a simple flap. A comfortable fine-tipped needle holder that can readily grasp 5-0 and 6-0 suture material during tying is a vital and useful instrument. Finally, binocular loops (2 power is sufficient) are useful. Delicate margins and sutures become much easier to handle with this simple optical aid.

Evaluation

When evaluating a head-and-neck laceration, the physician must consider the possibility of injury to underlying neural, vascular, ductal, cartilaginous, bony or mucosally lined structures. The wound must be examined thoroughly to its depths and must be cleansed by gentle irrigation with sterile saline. A local anesthetic, 1% Xylocaine with epinephrine as medically appropriate, can be used to achieve anesthesia with relatively little discomfort for the patient if it is administered to the subcutaneous tissues through the skin dehiscence. The wound can then be thoroughly cleansed with a dilute soapy solution, such as Hibiclens® (Astrazeneca Pharmaceuticals LP, Wilmington, DE, USA), dried, draped and re-examined for severed neural and ductal structures and foreign bodies. Impacted debris must be meticulously removed to prevent traumatic tattoo. Photographs should be taken to document the injury, and a tetanus booster should be administered.

Preparation of the wound for closure

Ragged lacerations require débridement of obviously non-viable subcutaneous tissue. Cutaneous margins must be judiciously trimmed with a scalpel so that they appose well. Wounds should be closed along skin-tension lines whenever possible, a technique that is more easily achieved with older patients, who have lax, mobile skin and readily apparent skin creases. The degree of tension on the closure determines the amount of undermining required; wounds running across lines of skin tension may require greater undermining and increased attention to the subcutaneous and dermal closure. Ideally, the wound should close with little or no tension. Loss of skin may require the use of a local flap or grafting for coverage.

Repair of facial lacerations

The choice of suture material and suture techniques for repairing facial lacerations varies, depending on the wound and the preference of the surgeon. The following is a description of one method that we use with success for facial wounds (Figures 10.7 and 10.8).

After the wound is prepared for closure, the subcutaneous tissues are judiciously approximated with a few absorbable sutures (mild chromic or Vicryl®, Ethicon) on a curved needle (the use of a non-cutting one is possible) in order to eliminate any dead space. The dermis is approximated with 5-0 mild-chromic sutures or 5-0 Vicryl sutures, which are placed to evert the edges slightly. This row of sutures usually provides strength to the closure. Physicians should practice placing all the stitches at precisely the same depth (or at compensating levels) in order to learn to appose the skin with the edges everted perfectly. In most cases, after the subcutaneous closure is completed, the wound should appear closed.

The skin sutures ensure that the wound margins remain in perfect alignment despite the swelling and movement that will occur over the next few days. A fine 5-0 or 6-0 monofilament suture, such as nylon on a cutting needle, may be used with a simple stitch, a running subcuticular stitch or a running locking stitch.

We also sometimes use a 6-0 mild-chromic suture. The advantages of this 6-0 mild-chromic closure, used only in areas of little mobility, low concentration of sebaceous glands and little tension, are that the sutures usually weaken in 4–5 days, thus reducing the chance that noticeable stitch marks will form. In addition, the necessity for stitch removal is eliminated, which saves office time and is of great benefit when dealing with children. Most importantly, the results from using this technique are excellent. The

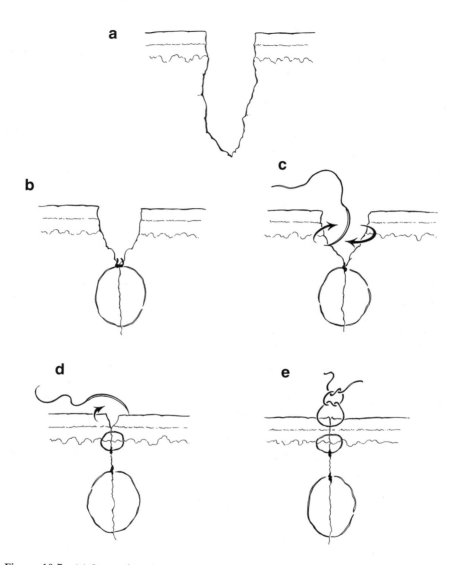

Figure 10.7 (a) Laceration through the skin and subcutaneous layer. (b) Closure of the subcutaneous fat layer with a few large, simple stitches of chromic gut tied just tightly enough to approximate but not strangulate. (c) A subcuticular stitch with the knot buried closes the dermal layer and places the knot at the deepest portion of the suture tract. (d) A small cutting needle with a 6-0 suture may be used for the skin surface layer. The needle must enter the skin 2–3 mm from the wound margin at an obtuse angle in order to evert the edges slightly. (e) The skin stitches are shallow and should be placed 2–3 mm apart. Sutures should just approximate the edges with as little tension as possible to allow for swelling. Square knots are preferred

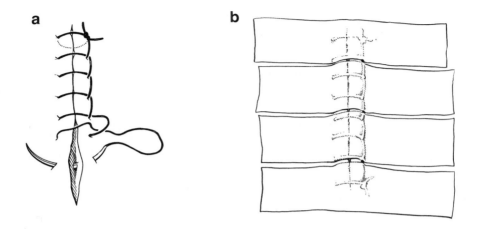

Figure 10.8 (a) Each stitch or every second or third stitch must be locked. Locked stitches should not be used when drainage is expected (e.g. if there are contused surfaces or if there is a diffuse surface and wound-edge bleeding). (b) The wound is then covered, and tension released, with a Steri-strip®, and the wound is kept dry. A return appointment is given after 4–5 days. Antibiotics appropriate to the medical circumstances are used

physician must remain aware that occasionally patients have a sensitivity to gut suture.

A tension-releasing, moderate-pressure antibiotic dressing that is appropriate to the area is the last (but a crucial) part of the closure, because it protects and supports the wound and absorbs drainage. Components of the dressing from inward out are antibiotic ointment, Xero-form® (Sherwood Medical, St. Louis, MO, USA) gauze, an absorbent gauze layer and supportive adhesive materials such as Steri-strip® (3M Healthcare, St. Paul, MN, USA).

Repair of mucosal lacerations

Mucosal wounds are often closed with gut suture. Silk sutures are also used; they provide longer lasting alignment strength, but require removal. A tapered needle should be used rather than a cutting one, because the latter will cause mucosal tears. The mucosal margins should be joined loosely. Knots must be square, and at least three to four throws of the knot are used in the mouth, because the movement of the surfaces and moisture tend to untie the sutures. Any laceration that passes through the vermilion border must be perfectly joined at that border (mucocutaneous junction) by the initial stitches of the repair. Mucosal surfaces heal rapidly, usually without complication and with little or no scarring.

Repair of through-and-through lacerations of the lip

In the repair of a through-and-through laceration of the lip, the principles of repair for the skin and subcutaneous tissue are identical to those described earlier (see Figure 10.7); however, the mucosal layer of the lip should be approximated by means of a deep layer closure and a loosely closed surface layer. This technique provides for intraoral drainage and prevents abscess formation from contamination by oral flora that might disrupt the skin closure.

11

Anatomy of the neck, examination of the head and neck and evaluation of neck masses

Gregory W. Randolph

Anatomic considerations
   Triangles of the neck
      Anterior triangles of the neck
      Posterior triangles of the neck
   Contents of the cervical triangles
   Skeletal landmarks of the neck
   Lymph nodes of the head and neck
      Occipital nodes
      Retroauricular (mastoid) nodes
      Preauricular nodes
      Parotid nodes
      Facial nodes
      Submandibular nodes
      Submental nodes
      Retropharyngeal nodes
      Superficial cervical nodes
      Deep cervical chains: anterior and posterior
      Central cervical nodes
Techniques for physical examination
Diagnostic strategy for the evaluation of a neck mass
   Lymphadenopathy
   Lymphadenitis
      Infectious lymphadenitis
      Human immunodeficiency virus
      Cat scratch disease
      Toxoplasmosis

        Mycobacteria

        Actinomyces

        Rare forms of infectious lymphadenitis

        Non-infectious inflammatory lymphadenitis

Fine needle aspiration

Lateral neck masses

   Branchial cleft cyst

   Laryngocele

   Deep neck abscess

   Cystic hygroma and hemangioma

   Teratoma and dermoid

Midline neck masses

   Thyroglossal duct cyst

   Thymic cysts

   Plunging ranulas

Masses associated with normal structures of the neck

   Masses associated with the skin

   Masses derived from neural tissue

   Tumors associated with blood vessels or related structures

   Masses within the thyroid gland

   Lesions within the esophagus

   Tumors arising from cartilaginous structures

   Head and neck nodal metastasis

   Head and neck lymphoma

The differential diagnosis of a neck mass involves all classes of disease processes including metastatic disease from practically any part of the body, a variety of neoplasms and cysts of normal organs and structures of the neck, and neurogenic and vascular disorders. Therefore, the examiner must follow a strategy that is designed to reduce diagnostic possibilities to a minimum and allow intelligent selection of further diagnostic procedures such as blood testing, imaging, fine needle aspiration or open biopsy. Assessing a neck mass requires a working knowledge of both the regional anatomy of the neck and the disorders likely to occur in the specific area of the neck in which the mass is found. Although all of the disorders listed in this chapter occur in the neck, the physician can usually reduce the number of diagnostic possibilities to one or a few, based on the location and other characteristics of the mass.

ANATOMIC CONSIDERATIONS

The exact position of a mass within the neck often provides key diagnostic clues. A thorough understanding of regional neck anatomy is, therefore, essential. For the purposes of evaluating a neck mass, the neck is best understood by division into triangles. In addition, there are a few landmarks that will help the examiner remember the relative position of relevant structures of the neck.

Triangles of the neck

The neck can be divided into anterior and posterior triangles. These are further subdivided into four anterior subtriangles, and two posterior subtriangles (Figure 11.1).

Anterior triangles of the neck

The anterior triangle is delineated by the body of the mandible superiorly, the midline of the neck anteriorly and the sternocleidomastoid muscle posteriorly. It is subdivided into submandibular (digastric), carotid, submental (suprahyoid) and muscular triangles. The submandibular (digastric) triangle is bounded superiorly by the body of the mandible, anteriorly by the belly of the digastric muscle and posteriorly by the posterior belly of the digastric muscle. The carotid triangle is bounded superiorly by the posterior belly of the digastric muscle, anteriorly by the superior belly of the omohyoid and posteriorly by the sternocleidomastoid muscle. The

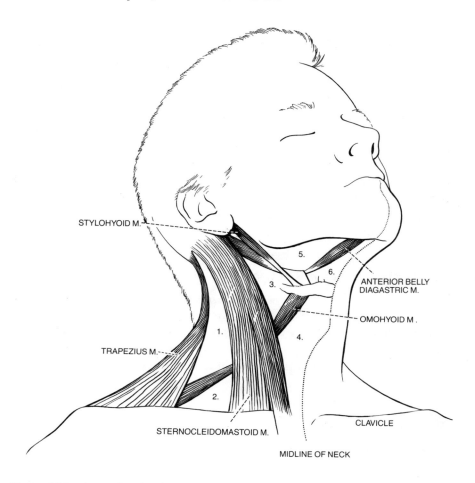

Figure 11.1 Anatomic triangles of the neck: 1) occipital; 2) subclavian; 3) carotid; 4) muscular; 5) submandibular; 6) submental

submental (suprahyoid) triangle is bounded anteriorly by the midline of the neck, posteriorly by the anterior belly of the digastric and inferiorly by the body of the hyoid. The muscular triangle (also called central compartment) is bounded anteriorly by the midline of the neck, posteriorly by the anterior border of the omohyoid muscle and posteroinferiorly by the sternocleidomastoid muscle.

Posterior triangles of the neck

The posterior triangle of the neck is bounded anteriorly by the sternoclei-domastoid muscle, posteriorly by the trapezius muscle and inferiorly by the body of the clavicle. It is further subdivided into the occipital and sub-clavian (omoclavicular) triangles. The occipital triangle is bounded anteriorly by the sternocleidomastoid muscle, posteriorly by the trapezius muscle and inferiorly by the posterior belly of the omohyoid muscle; the subclavian (omoclavicular) triangle is bounded superiorly by the posterior belly of the omohyoid muscle, anteriorly by the sternocleidomastoid muscle and inferiorly by the body of the clavicle.

Contents of the cervical triangles

The most significant anatomic structures located in the triangles are listed in Table 11.1, and are illustrated in Figure 11.2.

Skeletal landmarks of the neck

The greater cornu of the hyoid bone is in close proximity to several impor-tant structures of the neck, including the carotid bifurcation, the internal jugular vein, the vagus nerve, the hypoglossal nerve, the superior thyroid artery and the superior laryngeal nerve.

The transverse process of the first cervical vertebra (atlas) is located one finger breadth anterior and inferior to the mastoid process. The internal jugular vein and the lower cranial nerves (nerves IX, X, XI and XII) are located just anterior to this bony process.

The transverse process of the sixth cervical vertebra (carotid tubercle) is located at the level of the arch of the cricoid cartilage and approximately at the anterior border of the sternocleidomastoid muscle. Just anterior to this bony prominence is the common carotid artery, which can be compres-sed against the carotid tubercle to control hemorrhage. Also, the vertebral artery enters its vertebral foramen at this level.

Several important cartilaginous landmarks are easily recognized in the midline neck. The thyroid cartilage's upper midline notch ('Adam's apple') is present in both males and females, but is more developed and easily palpable in thin males. The cricoid cartilage's anterior ring can be easily felt in the midline directly below the thyroid cartilage's lower edge. This anterior ring of the cricoid cartilage is a key landmark for thyroid gland examination. The thyroid's isthmus rests one finger breadth below the cricoid's anterior arch, on the upper cervical trachea (see Chapter 17).

Table 11.1   The contents of triangles in the neck

A. Anterior triangles
    1. Submandibular (digastric) triangle
        a. Glands and organs
            (1) Submandibular gland
        b. Vasculature
            (1) Anterior facial artery and vein
        c. Nerves
            (1) Hypoglossal nerve
        d. Muscles
            (1) Mylohyoid muscle
            (2) Hyoglossus muscle
        e. Lymph nodes
            (1) Submandibular node
    2. Carotid triangle
        a. Glands and organs
            (1) Carotid body
        b. Vasculature
            (1) Internal and external carotid artery
            (2) Superior thyroid artery
            (3) Internal jugular vein
        c. Nerves
            (1) Vagus nerve
            (2) Hypoglossal nerve
            (3) Accessory nerve
            (4) Superior laryngeal nerve
        d. Muscles
            (1) Thyrohyoid muscle
            (2) Inferior constrictor muscle
        e. Skeleton
            (1) Greater cornu of hyoid bone
            (2) Ala of thyroid cartilage
        f. Lymph nodes
            (1) Superficial cervical node
            (2) Deep cervical nodes
    3. Submental triangle
        a. Muscles
            (1) Mylohyoid muscle
        b. Lymph nodes
            (1) Submental node
    4. Muscular triangle
        a. Glands and organs
            (1) Larynx and trachea
            (2) Thyroid gland

continued on following page

Table 11.1   *continued*

  b. Vasculature
     (1) Common carotid artery
     (2) Inferior thyroid artery
     (3) Internal jugular vein
  c. Nerves
     (1) Vagus nerve
     (2) Cervical sympathetic chain
     (3) Descendens hypoglossi
     (4) Recurrent laryngeal nerve
  d. Muscles
     (1) Sternohyoid muscle
     (2) Sternothyroid muscle
  e. Skeleton
     (1) Thyroid cartilage
     (2) Cricoid cartilage
     (3) Tracheal rings
     (4) Transverse process of sixth cervical vertebra (carotid tubercle)
  f. Lymph nodes
     (1) Superficial and deep cervical nodes
B. Posterior triangles
  1. Occipital triangle
     a. Nerves
        (1) Greater occipital nerve
        (2) C3 and C4
        (3) Accessory nerve
        (4) Brachial plexus
     b. Muscles
        (1) Levator scapulae
        (2) Splenius capitis
        (3) Scalenus anterior, scalenus medius and scalenus posterior
     c. Lymph nodes
        (1) Occipital node
        (2) Accessory node
        (3) Superficial cervical node
        (4) Transverse cervical node
  2. Subclavian triangle
     a. Vasculature
        (1) Subclavian artery and vein
        (2) Thyrocervical trunk
     b. Nerves
        (1) Phrenic nerve
     c. Muscles
        (1) Scalenus medius and scalenus anterior
     d. Lymph nodes
        (1) Transverse cervical node
        (2) Superficial cervical node

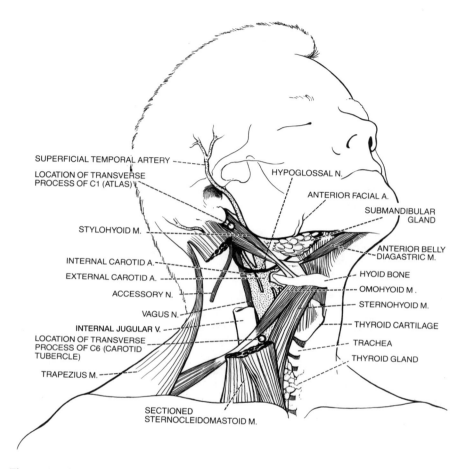

SUPERFICIAL TEMPORAL ARTERY
LOCATION OF TRANSVERSE PROCESS OF C1 (ATLAS)
HYPOGLOSSAL N.
ANTERIOR FACIAL A.
SUBMANDIBULAR GLAND
STYLOHYOID M.
ANTERIOR BELLY DIAGASTRIC M.
INTERNAL CAROTID A.
EXTERNAL CAROTID A.
HYOID BONE
ACCESSORY N.
OMOHYOID M.
STERNOHYOID M.
VAGUS N.
INTERNAL JUGULAR V.
THYROID CARTILAGE
LOCATION OF TRANSVERSE PROCESS OF C6 (CAROTID TUBERCLE)
TRACHEA
THYROID GLAND
TRAPEZIUS M.
SECTIONED STERNOCLEIDOMASTOID M.

Figure 11.2   Functional anatomy of the neck

Lymph nodes of the head and neck

Lymph nodes of the head and neck are grouped anatomically. The main groupings in the neck include the anterior or jugular chain and the posterior or accessory chain. Other important groupings in the head and neck include the occipital, retroauricular (mastoid), preauricular, parotid (extra- and intraglandular), facial, submandibular, submental and central neck nodes (Figure 11.3). The anterior cervical chain, or jugular nodes, run along the jugular vein roughly corresponding to the path of the sternocleidomastoid muscle in the neck, and are divided into the superior jugular digastric nodes, midjugular nodes and inferior jugular nodes. The posterior

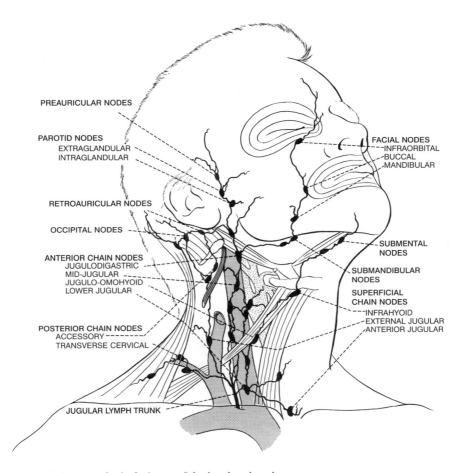

Figure 11.3 Lymphatic drainage of the head and neck

chain nodes include superiorly the accessory nodes (associated with the 11th cranial nerve) and inferiorly the transverse cervical nodes. The posterior chain runs along the front edge of the trapezius muscle, roughly approximating the course of the spinal accessory nerve.

Nodal regions of the neck can also be divided into discrete numbered regions. In this system, region 1 encompasses the submandibular and submental nodes, region 2 the jugulodigastric nodes, region 3 the midjugular nodes, region 4 the lower jugular nodes, region 5 the posterior chain nodes and region 6 the central compartment nodes. Various types of cervical lymphadenectomy (i.e. neck dissection) are classified in part according to which of these numbered regions is surgically encompassed. Head and neck malignancies from specific regions have common patterns of metastasis to specific nodal regions. For example, nasopharynx and scalp malignancies typically involve region 5, while oral cavity malignancies often initially metastasize to regions 1 and 2. Laryngeal, hypopharyngeal and thyroid malignancies typically metastasize to regions 3 and 4. While 90% of neoplastic cervical nodes represent the metastasis of a head and neck primary, 10% represent nodal metastasis from a distant site, including chest, abdomen and pelvic viscera. Such lung, gastrointestinal and genitourinary malignancies often metastasize to the supraclavicular fossa and low jugular regions. Adenopathy present in the left supraclavicular fossa is especially suspicious for metastasis from an abdominal primary. Metastatic spread from head and neck malignancies is not always completely predictable. For example, an anterior tongue primary may skip, in certain circumstances, regions 1 and 2, and metastasize to a lower jugular region 4 node.

Occipital nodes

Occipital nodes are located near the anterior attachment of the trapezius muscle to the skull. They receive afferent lymphatics from the posterior lateral scalp and drain to the posterior cervical chain.

Retroauricular (mastoid) nodes

The retroauricular (mastoid) nodes are located at the insertion of the sternocleidomastoid muscle to the mastoid bone. They receive afferent lymphatics from the posterior, temporal and parietal areas and drain into the posterior cervical chain.

Preauricular nodes

The preauricular nodes are located just anterior to the tragus of the auricle and receive afferent lymphatics from the pinna and temporal regions of the scalp. They drain to the anterior cervical chain nodes.

Parotid nodes

The parotid nodes are divided into two groups: the extraglandular and intraglandular nodes. The extraglandular nodes are located deep (medial) to the parotid fascia near the preauricular nodes, which lie more superficially. The intraglandular nodes are deep within the parotid gland, near the junction of the superficial and deep lobes. The parotid nodes receive afferent lymphatics from the anterior temporal scalp, external auditory canal, eyelids and the root of the nose, and drain into the deep cervical chain.

Facial nodes

The facial nodes are divided into the infraorbital, buccal and supramandibular nodes. The infraorbital nodes overlie the orbicularis oculi. The buccal node is in a subcutaneous plane near the junction of the buccinator and orbicularis oris muscles. The supramandibular nodes lie lateral to the mandible, near the anterior facial artery. The anterior facial artery arises from the neck and extends over the anterior mandibular body. The facial nodes receive afferent lymphatics from the eyelids, conjunctiva, nasal skin and mucosa, and cheek. These nodes, in turn, drain to the submandibular nodes.

Submandibular nodes

The submandibular nodes are located under the body of the mandible in close proximity to the submandibular gland. They are further subdivided into preglandular, retroglandular and intracapsular nodes. These nodes receive afferent lymphatics from the cheek, nose, upper and lower lips, anterior nasal mucosa, gums, teeth, soft and hard palates, anterior aspect of the tongue, submandibular and sublingual glands and the floor of the mouth. They drain, in turn, to the jugular chain. These nodes are best palpated through bimanual examination of the floor of the mouth, in the submandibular gland region.

Submental nodes

The submental nodes lie between the paired anterior bellies of the digastric muscle and receive afferent lymphatics from the lip, floor of the mouth, buccal mucosa, the incisor region of the gingiva and the anterior tongue. The submental nodes drain, in turn, to the submandibular nodes and then to the ipsilateral anterior cervical chain. Occasionally, they will drain to the contralateral jugular chain.

Retropharyngeal nodes

These nodes are situated behind the pharynx and hypopharynx in the retropharyngeal space. They are especially prominent in children, and receive afferent lymphatics from the nasopharynx and pharynx. These nodes are not assessable during the routine head and neck examination.

Superficial cervical nodes

The superficial cervical nodes are located along the course of the external and anterior jugular veins. They receive afferent lymphatics from the ear, parotid and face, and drain to the jugular chain.

Deep cervical chains: anterior and posterior

These nodal chains represent the main lymphatic groupings in the neck. The anterior cervical, or jugular, chain lies anterior to the internal jugular vein high in the neck, and posterior to the vein lower in the neck. This anterior cervical chain parallels the course of the carotid sheath through the neck and is partially covered by the sternocleidomastoid muscle. This chain includes superiorly the jugulodigastric nodal group at the level of the posterior belly of the digastric muscle; the midjugular nodes including both carotid nodes at the carotid bifurcation and jugulo-omohyoid nodes at the level of the crossing of the omohyoid muscle and internal jugular vein; and supraclavicular or inferior jugular nodal group just superior to the level of the clavicle. The posterior cervical chain consists superiorly of nodes following the course of the accessory nerve roughly along the anterior edge of the trapezius muscle. These nodes receive afferent lymphatics from the posterior aspect of the scalp, nasopharynx and mastoid regions. Inferiorly, the posterior cervical chain includes the transverse cervical nodes, which are closely associated with the course of the transverse cervical artery and vein. These nodes receive afferent lymphatics from the spinal accessory chain, the pectoral region, part of the arm and the lower cervical viscera; they drain, in turn, to the inferior jugular group.

Central cervical nodes

The central cervical nodes lie between the two carotid sheaths below the level of the hyoid bone. The deep central cervical nodes consist of prelaryngeal (delphian), pretracheal nodes and paratracheal nodes, which run along the course of the recurrent laryngeal nerve. They receive afferent lymphatics from the thyroid gland and infraglottic larynx and drain into the mid- and lower jugular chain. These deep central cervical nodes around the thyroid also communicate to anterior mediastinal nodes. Inferiorly on the right, the main jugular lymphatic channel empties into the right lymphatic duct and, on the left, into the thoracic duct.

TECHNIQUES FOR PHYSICAL EXAMINATION

During examination, the physician should mentally divide the patient's neck into triangles by delineating the sternocleidomastoid and trapezius muscles (Figure 11.1). The neck is then examined in a rostral to caudal direction in a systematic fashion with reference to cervical triangles and cartilaginous and bony landmarks. There are several maneuvers the physician can perform that will ensure a thorough examination of this area:

(1) The submental and submandibular triangles should be examined bimanually with one of the physician's forefingers in the anterior and lateral floor of the mouth. Masses in these regions can be pushed up under the mandible during the external neck examination. Bimanual examination, therefore, is mandatory.

(2) In the central neck, the hyoid bone and thyroid and cricoid cartilages as well as the tracheal rings should be delineated and checked for displacement and mobility. The thyroid gland examination can be assisted by asking the patient to swallow during palpation of the gland (see Chapter 17).

(3) The structures deep to the sternocleidomastoid muscle should be palpated by displacing the muscle both anteriorly and posteriorly.

(4) The patient's neck should be placed in a neutral or slightly flexed position to allow relaxation of cervical musculature and to allow the physician's fingers to probe deep within the triangles of the neck. The patient's natural tendency during the neck examination is to extend the head back, which tenses the neck musculature, making the examination more difficult.

During the neck examination, the neck should not be medially compressed, as any underlying cervical mass will be pushed away from the examining finger. Instead, the skin overlying the presumptive mass should be pulled or dragged over the deeper underlying structures in order to sense the quality of that underlying tissue. It is the 'jump' of the examining hand when it encounters and then slides over a mass that allows detection of the underlying mass. The physical examination of the neck should be performed systematically. One method includes three discrete passes through the neck, each pass starting superiorly. The examiner begins by assessing bilaterally the parotid glands, moving inferiorly to the mastoid and then down the posterior chain. In this way, the parotid gland is included in the neck examination. Lesions in the tail of the parotid gland can mimic high jugular nodes. The second sweep through the neck includes starting superiorly in the submandibular gland region (including the bimanual examination) and submental region, and then extending downwards along the anterior cervical chain to the clavicle. The third pass through the neck centers on the central compartment, running superiorly from the hyoid down the thyroid and cricoid cartilages, and concluding with the thyroid examination.

DIAGNOSTIC STRATEGY FOR THE EVALUATION OF A NECK MASS

When a mass is discovered, its characteristics are evaluated and recorded.

(1) *Location in a cervical triangle and proximity to known major structures* Does the mass feel attached to known structures, such as the thyroid gland or carotid artery?

(2) *Consistency* Is the mass soft, fluctuant, easily mobile, well-encapsulated and smooth, or is it firm, poorly mobile and fixed to surrounding structures? Does it pulsate? Is there a bruit? Does it appear to be superficial or attached to the skin, or is it within deeper regions of the neck? Are there overlying skin changes? Is it tender or non-tender? Does it elevate with deglutition?

(3) *Concomitant pathology* Is there any other evidence of significant disease in the head and neck? To answer this question the physician must thoroughly examine the patient's scalp, face, external ear, tympanic membrane, parotid or pharynx, nose, nasopharynx, laryngopharynx and tongue.

(4) *Growth of the lesion* What is its rate? Has the lesion been stably present for 4 months, slowly developed over a period of months or developed rapidly over a period of days?

(5) *Patient setting* Age figures prominently in the evaluation of a neck mass. It can be useful in the evaluation of a neck mass to divide patients into three age groups: less than 20, between 20 and 40, and over 40 years. While there are always exceptions, each of the above age groups has a discrete differential diagnosis. In patients less than 20 years of age, neck lesions are most often benign, and include infectious and inflammatory

adenitis, sialadenitis, branchial cleft cysts, thyroglossal duct cysts, dermoids, hemangiomas and lymphangiomas (including cystic hygromas). Rarely, neck lesions in patients less than 20 years of age will represent malignancy. Most common malignancies occurring in this age group include lymphoma, rhabdomyosarcoma, thyroid carcinoma and neuroblastoma. In patients more than 40 years of age, a discrete, persistent neck mass will often represent neoplasia, usually of epithelial origin. Common malignancies in this age group include squamous cell carcinoma, thyroid carcinoma, salivary gland carcinoma and lymphoma. In patients between 20 and 40 years of age, the differential diagnosis is broad. Malignancies that tend to occur in this age group include thyroid carcinoma and lymphoma. Also, AIDS-related lymphadenopathy may manifest in this age group. Aside from patient age, there are many factors that guide our evaluation in patients with neck lesions. A history of smoking and alcohol use increases the risk of squamous cell carcinoma. The history of past exposure to low-dose ionizing radiation increases the risk of both salivary gland and thyroid neoplasia. Fever, night sweats and weight loss may indicated lymphoma. The identification of HIV risk factors may result in the inclusion of AIDS-associated lymphadenopathy or AIDS-related lymphoma in the differential diagnosis. In a patient with cervical adenopathy, it is important also to appreciate whether this cervical adenopathy is part of a generalized lymphadenopathy, or is restricted to the head and neck.

Once the initial evaluation is complete, a working differential diagnosis is constructed (see Table 11.2 for a complete differential diagnosis of a neck mass).

Lymphadenopathy

Lymphadenopathy may consist of either inflammatory or neoplastic disorders. In both, knowledge of the afferent supply of the involved lymph node is critical for further evaluation. In the presence of acute infectious disease such as pharyngitis, tonsillitis, dental or skin infection, or upper respiratory tract infection, no further diagnostic maneuvers may be necessary to formulate a diagnosis for the cause of the lymph node enlargement. Acute inflammatory nodes are usually tender, mobile and doughy.

A frequent diagnostic problem involves the identification of a probable lymph node and the inability to determine whether the node represents a chronic infectious or inflammatory disorder such as toxoplasmosis or

Table 11.2 Differential diagnosis of neck masses

A. Lymphadenopathy
    1. Infectious disorders
        a. Routine bacterial and viral adenitis
        b. Suppurative adenitis/neck abscess
        c. Mononucleosis
        d. Salivary gland infection
        e. Cat scratch fever
        f. Actinomycosis
        g. Atypical tuberculosis
        h. Toxoplasmosis
        i. AIDS
        j. Luetic adenitis
        k. Lyme disease
        l. Tularemia
        m. Rat bite
        n. Leprosy
        o. Bubonic plague
    2. Inflammatory disorders
        a. Sarcoid
        b. Systemic lupus erythematosus
        c. Kawasaki disease
        d. Kikucki disease
        e. Castleman's disease
        f. Rossi–Dorfman disease
        g. Combined variable immunodeficiency
        h. Histiocytosis X
    3. Neoplastic disorders
        a. Primary lymphoma
        b. Metastatic tumors
            (1) Head and neck primary 90%
            (2) Distant primary 10% (lung, gastrointestinal, genitourinary, melanoma)
    4. Metabolic
        a. Amyloidosis
        b. Dilantin pseudolymphoma
B. Congenital or developmental cysts and masses
    1. Branchial cleft cyst
    2. Thyroglossal duct cyst
    3. Lymphangioma/cystic hygroma
    4. Hemangioma
    5. Laryngocele
    6. Ranula
    7. Teratoma

continued on following page

Table 11.2   *continued*

   8. Dermoid
   9. Thymic cyst
C. Neoplasia or other enlargement of structure or organ contained in the neck
   1. Skin/connective tissue
      a. Sebaceous cyst
      b. Lipoma
      c. Fibroma
      d. Fibrosarcoma
      e. Liposarcoma
   2. Muscle
      a. Torticollis
      b. Rhabdomyosarcoma
   3. Nerve
      a. Neurofibroma
      b. Schwannoma
      c. Neuroblastoma
      d. Paraganglioma
   4. Blood vessel
      a. Aneurysm
      b. Carotid body tumor
      c. Hemangiopericytoma
      d. Glomus jugulare
   5. Thyroid/parathyroid
   6. Esophagus
   7. Larynx
      a. Chondroma
      b. Laryngocele
   8. Salivary gland
      a. Neoplasia
      b. Salivary cysts

sarcoidosis, or a primary or metastatic neoplastic process. All nodes should be considered neoplastic until proven otherwise, and several steps should be undertaken before an open biopsy of the neck is considered. Although it would seem that biopsy of the node would save time in the diagnostic work-up, there is evidence that premature open biopsy of a neoplastic node later identified as having metastasized from a head and neck primary tumor may result in a poorer prognosis than if the primary node and metastasis had been treated in an orderly fashion. Proper evaluation of a node requires a careful history of associated symptoms, including the identification of dysphagia, hemoptysis, hematemesis, hoarseness or a sensation of a mass in the mouth or throat. A history of drinking and smoking should be obtained. A thorough head and neck examination, including mirror or fiberoptic examination of the larynx, is also performed.

There are differences of opinion as to how many additional diagnostic steps should be undertaken in the absence of evidence of a primary tumor in the head and neck prior to biopsy. Certainly any suggestive symptoms should be thoroughly investigated by any available means, including the use of serologic testing and radiographic imaging. If a patient complains of dysphagia, a barium swallow can be considered; however, a barium swallow or a head and neck computerized tomography (CT) scan are not substitutes for a thorough examination of the oropharynx and hypopharynx. CT scanning of the neck may be useful in certain circumstances to identify the full extent of a palpable neck lesion and appreciate its relationship to adjacent structures including, importantly, the carotid artery. CT scanning may also prove useful in the identification of subclinical, yet radiographically suspicious coexistent adenopathy. A chest X-ray may indicate primary lung disease, involvement of mediastinal nodes or other metastasis to pulmonary parenchyma. If indicated, CT scanning or magnetic resonance imaging (MRI) will provide additional information concerning tumors of the nasopharynx and skull base. Sinus malignancies infrequently metastasize to cervical nodal beds, unless extensive. Sialography is not usually performed unless there is a suggestive clinical history or findings. Any suggestive thoracic or abdominal symptoms should be elicited and appropriately evaluated.

Depending on the systemic findings, the history of the node enlargement and exposure of the patient, certain skin tests or serologic tests may be helpful in arriving at a diagnosis. These include tests for tuberculosis, AIDS, syphilis, sarcoidosis, toxoplasmosis, mononucleosis, Lyme disease, tularemia, systemic lupus erythematosus (SLE) and cat scratch disease.

Lymphadenitis

Acute cervical adenitis occurs commonly in the pediatric population, but may also occur in the adult, where it is usually associated with a viral upper respiratory tract infection or pharyngotonsillitis. When associated with infectious pharyngitis, upper jugular nodes are typically involved. For this reason, upper jugular nodes are also referred to as the 'tonsillar nodes'. Infectious adenitis associated with mononucleosis may preferentially affect the upper posterior cervical chain. Other common causes of acute cervical adenitis include insect bites and dental and facial skin infections. It should be noted that all patients with enlarged cervical nodes and fever may not have infectious adenitis. Patients with lymphomatous cervical nodal involvement may present with fever, night sweats and weight loss. Dermatopathic lymphadenitis is associated with chronic overlying skin conditions such as acne or eczema.

Common pathogens associated with acute cervical adenitis include viral agents, streptococcus group A and staphylococcus. Treatment relates in part to the underlying primary infection (e.g. pharyngotonsillitis, dental abscess, etc.) as well as to the intensity of the nodal infection. Significantly infected nodes may suppurate and lead to neck abscess. Patients with neck abscesses usually have significant systemic signs of toxicity, including fever, and may even demonstrate signs of impending respiratory obstruction. The patient with a neck abscess will typically exhibit some head tilt or deviation of the neck. The mass will be exquisitely tender and often show overlying skin changes of erythema and warmth.

Adults may often present with chronic cervical lymphadenopathy. Such adenopathy may have initially developed during an acute infectious episode (e.g. pharyngotonsillitis) but never completely resolved. These nodes, while palpable, are usually small (less than 1 cm), non-tender, mobile and often in the jugulodigastric region or posterior cervical chain. If such adults are young, and do not give a worrisome history of alcohol use, significant smoking, low-dose radiation exposure or HIV risk factors, and if their examination fails to reveal any suggestion of primary neoplasia, they may be offered a course of antibiotics in an attempt to shrink the nodes prior to any further evaluation. Appropriate serology and fine needle aspiration are reserved for patients whose nodal pathology persists after this empiric course of antibiotics.

Infectious lymphadenitis

Infectious lymphadenitis is most commonly viral. Common viral agents include those associated with common upper respiratory tract infections, such as Epstein–Barr virus, cytomegalovirus (CMV), rubella and others.

Human immunodeficiency virus

One of the common initial manifestations of HIV disease can be cervical adenopathy. Such lymphadenopathy may be due to the HIV virus itself, or it may be from a number of other infectious agents including CMV, tuberculosis, atypical tuberculosis (including *Mycobacterium avium intracel-*

lulare), histoplasmosis, toxoplasmosis and cat scratch disease. If the cervical nodes are relatively small, symmetrically distributed and, most importantly, stable over time, they can be aspirated with a fine needle and, if negative, followed without open biopsy. Open biopsy in such circumstances usually reveals nodes affected by follicular hyperplasia. Because HIV patients are at risk for Kaposi's sarcoma, which can metastasize to cervical nodes, and non-Hodgkin's lymphoma, lymph nodes that are large, asymmetric, rapidly growing, or in patients with marked constitutional symptoms without an alternative explanation, should be offered fine needle aspiration and, in appropriate circumstances, open biopsy. HIV disease can also lead to salivary gland disease (see Chapter 16). If salivary gland pathology extends to the tail of the parotid, this can be misinterpreted as cervical adenopathy. In patients with HIV disease, lymphoid changes, both benign and malignant, can occur in extranodal lymphatic tissue of Waldeyer's ring.

Cat scratch disease

Cat scratch disease is a common cause of lymphadenopathy. Most patients will note an exposure to a cat, if not an actual documented scratch. Cat scratch disease is caused by two intracellular pleomorphic Gram-negative, non-acid-fast bacilli recently named *Bartonella henselae* and *Bartonella quintana*. Identification is made by serology and the polymerase chain reaction (PCR). The bacilli stain with Warthin–Starry silver stain. Patients classically develop a small (2–5 mm) vesicular eruption at the site of the cutaneous scratch, which may or may not be noticed. The scratch is typically inflicted by a kitten. Within 2 weeks of inoculation, regional nodes become involved. Patients may develop malaise, fever, headache and anorexia, along with the subacute regional adenopathy. Lymphadenopathy usually lasts 2–3 months. Treatment is supportive, as the disease is usually self-limiting, unless the nodes suppurate, which occurs in about one-third of patients. Lymph nodes affected by cat scratch disease that are excised show relatively non-specific lymphoid hyperplasia and scattered granulomata. Cat scratch disease can occur in a Parinaud's (oculoglandular) form involving conjunctivitis, fever and regional (parotid) adenopathy.

Toxoplasmosis

Toxoplasma gondii infection occurs after exposure to infected feces (usually feline) or infectious meat (usually lamb or pork). Infection occurs in a variety of tissues. Patients may present with fever, malaise, night sweats and asymptomatic cervical adenopathy. Nodes may fluctuate in size over a period of months. The diagnosis is by acute and convalescent serologic testing of IgM and IgG. Nodal histology shows subcapsular and trabecular monocytoid cells. No treatment is usually required, unless the patient is significantly symptomatic or immunocompromised. Pyrimethamine plus trisulfapyrimidines have been used.

Mycobacteria

Tuberculous involvement of cervical nodes, especially common in children, is termed scrofula and is more common with atypical agents (usually *Mycobacteria scrofulaceum* or *M. avium-intracellulare*) than with true tuberculosis. With atypical tubercular cervical nodal involvement, the chest X-ray is usually negative and the purified protein derivative (PPD) skin test is usually negative or weakly positive (> 0, but < 10 mm of induration). Atypical tuberculous adenitis may result from oral ingestion of non-pasteurized milk. The painlessly enlarged nodes characteristically suppurate and involve the skin. Nodes affected by atypical tuberculosis are treated surgically. Standard treatment involves the excision of involved nodes and skin. Recent work suggests that conservative incisional nodal curettage may be equally effective. Such treatment may allow skin preservation and avoidance of facial nerve injury when skin of the upper neck and lower face is involved. Antibiotics may be offered postoperatively, depending on susceptibility, but surgery alone is usually sufficient for atypical nodal infections. Affected nodes show characteristic caseating granulomata. Antibiotics are the mainstay of treatment for true mycobacterial tuberculosis nodal involvement, with surgery added if nodes suppurate. Fine needle aspiration can be useful diagnostically in such cases, allowing initiation of medical treatment.

Actinomyces

Actinomyces is a slow-growing, branching, filamentous, Gram-positive anaerobic bacterium present in periodontal pockets adjacent to carious teeth and in tonsillar crypts. Usually, trauma leads to opportunistic infection of adjacent tissue. *Actinomyces* infection may present as a suppurative adenitis with prominent skin involvement (with notable purplish discoloration) and a predilection for fistula formation. Characteristic yellow particulate sulfa granules can be seen in the discharge from the fistula tract. Culture of the discharge needs to be processed for anaerobic organisms. Treatment involves surgical debridement and intravenous penicillin for 6 weeks, followed by a prolonged course of oral penicillin. *Nocardia* is an anaerobic member of the Actinomycetales which can manifest as cervical adenitis without the tendency of *Actinomyces* for fistula formation. Treatment of *Nocardia* infection involves surgical debridement and sulfonamides.

Rare forms of infectious lymphadenitis

Tularemia   Tularemia results from exposure to infected deer and rabbit ticks bearing *Francisella tularensis*, a Gram-negative pleomorphic rod. Patients may present with an impressive ulcerative cervical adenopathy that can be misinterpreted as neoplasia. Tularemia can occur in a Parinaud's variant with conjunctivitis and ipsilateral parotid nodal involvement. Diagnosis is through serologic titers. Histology of tularemic nodes shows necrotizing granulomata. Treatment is with streptomycin or gentamycin.

Syphilis   Lymphadenopathy may accompany the primary or secondary stage of syphilis. Three weeks after initial exposure, the primary stage of syphilis is characterized by the chancre and regional nodal involvement. Nodal involvement can be cervical if the chancre is oral. The secondary stage of syphilis is characterized by macular papular mucocutaneous lesions which are associated with generalized adenopathy. Diagnosis is made by serology including the Venereal Disease Research Laboratory (VDRL), rapid plasma reagin (RPR) and fluorescent treponemal antibody absorption (FTA-ABS) tests (see Chapter 12).

Lyme disease   Lyme disease is transmitted by deer ticks bearing the spirochete *Borrelia burgdorferi*. Lyme disease is a complex, multisystem disease affecting skin, joints, heart and nervous systems. Patients initially present with malaise, fever, regional or generalized adenopathy and a characteristic annular rash called erythema chronicum migrans. In the second stage of Lyme disease, which occurs weeks to months after initial presentation, patients may present with aseptic meningitis, cranial nerve palsies and cardiac arrhythmias. In the third stage of Lyme disease, which may occur months to years after initial presentation, patients may develop chronic neurologic and joint findings. Overall, about 20% of patients with Lyme disease develop adenopathy. Treatment includes tetracycline or other antibiotics including doxycycline, penicillin or amoxicillin.

Many less common forms of infectious adenitis exist. *Yersinia pestis*, the agent of bubonic plague, is transmitted by rat bite and occurs rarely in the

USA. A painful suppurative adenitis (bubo) results, with pulmonary symptoms predominating in the fulminant clinical course. *Mycobacterium leprae* results in the multiple manifestations of leprosy, typically including skin, nasal and oral mucosa, and lymphadenopathy. Pasteurellosis (*Pasteurella multocida, Pasteurella haemolytica, Pasteurella pneumotropica, Pasteurella ureae*) is associated with exposure to or bite from a variety of animals and can give a mononucleosis-like picture, with fever and cervical adenitis. Contracted through exposure to cattle and other ungulate products, brucellosis can be diagnosed by serologic testing. Brucellosis typically manifests as a recurring high spiking fever, headache, fatigue and arthralgia. Seventy per cent of patients develop cervical and inguinal adenopathy. Exposure to a variety of domestic and wild animals including rats can result in leptospirosis (Weil's disease). Leptospirosis is characterized by multiple systemic symptoms, including headache, fever, muscle aches and generalized lymphadenopathy. The bite of a rat or other rodent (*Streptobacillus moniliformis* and *Spirillum minus*) can result in fever, headache, arthralgias and regional adenopathy. Anthrax, contracted through exposure to infected sheep or goats, results in an ulcerative skin lesion with regional adenopathy. Non-diphtheria *Corynebacterium* infection can also result from exposure to infected sheep, and manifests as a granulomatous lymphadenitis. Glanders and melioidosis (*Pseudomonas pseudomallei, Pseudomonas mallei*) results from exposure to infected horses, and can present as a regional adenopathy. African trypanosomiasis (*Trypanosoma brucei*) and rickettsial infections (scrub typhus and rickettsial pox) may present with regional lymphadenopathy. *Paracoccidioides brasiliensis* infection is a systemic mycosis seen primarily in South America as a progressive respiratory disease. It may lead to mucosal granular lesions involving the nasal cavities, oral cavity and larynx, and with associated cervical adenopathy. Sporotrichosis may develop in patients working with plants and soil and exposed to the fungus *Sporothrix schenckii*. Typically, a thorn bush prick leads to a chancreform ulcer and an indolent regional adenopathy. Oculoglandular presentations (conjunctival inflammation with reactive regional adenitis, typically periparotid) are associated with infectious agents including *F. tularensis* (tularemia), *Listeria monocytogenes* (listeria) and *Chlamydia trachomatis* (lymphogranuloma venereum).

Non-infectious inflammatory lymphadenitis

A number of inflammatory disorders can result in lymphadenopathy in the head and neck.

Sarcoid   This is a systemic granulomatous disease of unknown etiology, typically associated with hilar adenopathy seen on chest X-ray and increased angiotensin converting enzyme (ACE) levels and erythrocyte sedimentation rate. Sarcoid may involve lung, skin, liver, kidney and spleen. In the head and neck, sarcoid may result in lacrimal and salivary gland enlargement, intranasal mucosal nodules and cervical adenopathy.

Systemic lupus erythematosus   This can present in the head and neck with cervical adenopathy (see Chapter 13). Histologically, lymph nodes show prominent foci of necrosis.

Kikucki disease   This is regarded as an idiopathic post-viral hyperimmune reaction. It was initially described in Asian populations, but has now been reported in the USA and Europe. Patients present with a tender cervical adenopathy associated with fever, night sweats and fatigue. Histologically these nodes show a necrotizing histiocytic lymphadenitis, somewhat similar to nodes in SLE. No diagnostic serology is available. Diagnosis is suggested by clinical features and node biopsy. No specific treatment is recommended. The clinical course is benign and self-limiting, usually resolving within 2–6 months.

Rossi–Dorfman disease   This is a rare, benign inflammatory disease characterized by painless bulky cervical adenopathy. It is usually associated with a low-grade fever, leukocytosis and a polyclonal hypergammaglobulinemia. Histologically, involved nodes show sinusoidal histiocytic infiltration. Rossi–Dorfman disease has also been called sinus histiocytosis with massive lymphadenopathy. The disease is self-limiting and no treatment is usually recommended. Extranodal Rossi–Dorfman lesions have been described in the nasal septum skin, sinus and salivary gland.

Castleman's disease   This is an idiopathic benign lymphoproliferative disease characterized by lymphadenopathy. Castleman's disease has also been called giant lymph node hyperplasia and angiolymphomatous lymphoid hyperplasia. Two histologic types exist: a more common hyaline vascular type and a plasma cell type. Castleman's disease can affect mediastinal nodes and less frequently cervical nodes. The disorder has been associated with human herpes virus 8, a variety of skin disorder (lichen planus, pemphigus vulgaris), neurologic diseases (myasthenia gravis), HIV disease, nephrotic syndrome and amyloidosis. When presenting clinically with localized adenopathy, surgical excision is recommended. When presenting with multicentric disease, surgery and chemotherapy (including steroids) are employed. Multicentric disease is associated with malignant lymphoma, Kaposi's sarcoma and other carcinomas.

Kawasaki's disease   This usually presents in the pediatric age group with fever, conjunctivitis, characteristic mucosal changes (strawberry tongue) and a desquamating rash affecting palms and soles. A non-suppurative cervical adenopathy is associated (see Chapter 12).

Histiocytosis X   This may present in three discrete forms: a localized eosinophilic granuloma; a chronic disseminated form (Hand–Schüller–Christian disease); or an acute, lethal systemic form (Letterer–Siwe disease). Disseminated forms may be associated with adenopathy. Whipple's disease (intestinal lipodystrophy) is a multisystem disease presenting with malabsorption, weight loss, anemia, skin and joint changes and adenopathy. Anticonvulsant medicine can result in nodal and gingival hyperplasia.

FINE NEEDLE ASPIRATION

Fine needle aspiration amounts to a microscopic biopsy and has revolutionized the work-up of the neck mass. Advances in cytopathology have facilitated the widespread acceptance of this technique. Fine needle aspiration allows preoperative diagnosis; this is helpful in counseling the patient preoperatively and in generating an appropriate surgical plan. For example, if an enlarged node shows squamous cell carcinoma, the physician can counsel the patient regarding panendoscopy or search for the mucosal primary and possible neck dissection, rather than open biopsy alone. Alternatively, if a large node is preoperatively aspirated and shows papillary carcinoma of the thyroid, appropriate surgical therapy encompassing the thyroid can be planned.

Fine needle aspiration can be performed in an office chair after the overlying skin is cleaned with alcohol. Patients with poor hygiene should have overlying skin cleaned with surgical soap then alcohol. An anesthetic can be administered, but this can produce an area of regional focal swelling in the skin over the underlying mass, which can lead to subsequent difficulty in palpation of the mass. Anesthesia is infrequently needed. It should be explained to the patient that the fine needle aspiration procedure is equivalent in terms of discomfort and complexity to phlebotomy, except that a smaller-gauge needle is used for fine needle aspiration. Usually, a 22- or 25-gauge needle is used and is attached to a small syringe, usually 6 ml.

A good deal of time is spent palpating the lesion prior to needle aspiration. The palpable lesion needs to be stabilized on adjacent neck structures, or by being tented relative to overlying skin. Once the lesion is appropriately stabilized between the examining fingers, the needle is placed through the skin into the mass. Usually the puncture of the skin is the only painful part of the procedure. While the needle is in the mass, approximately 1 cm of suction is applied to the syringe and the needle is oscillated in and out along the initial path of entry. The needle is not angulated widely, as this can disrupt tissue within the mass, causing bleeding within the lesion; and it is unnecessary for obtaining appropriate biopsy material. The needle is simply moved in and out of the mass along the axis of initial entry, usually about 15 to 20 times. The suction on the syringe is then released and the needle is withdrawn and pressure is placed over the region through the gauze for several minutes. Suction is applied only when the needle is in the mass, and not during entry or needle removal, so as to prevent skin contamination of the aspirate. Significant pain, ecchymosis or bleeding within the lesion is unusual. The aspirated material is typically confined to the shaft of the needle, with little material in the needle hub or syringe itself. Only if a vessel is encountered will blood be seen in the syringe. Usually this implies that blood contamination of the aspirate has occurred and that repeat aspiration will be required for diagnostic material. Usually a repeat aspiration is performed in a different position in the mass or from a slightly different orientation. If cystic fluid is encountered, this material should be smeared and the remainder placed into cytology fixative. This material can be spun down at a later time, and the pellet smeared. Repeat aspiration should then be performed to sample the collapsed cyst wall. While the patient puts pressure on the region that has been aspirated with a gauze, the specimen should be smeared. The needle is taken off the syringe. The syringe plunger is pulled back and the needle is reattached to the syringe; the contents of the needle shaft are expelled onto a labeled glass slide, which is smeared as one would smear a peripheral blood sample. The slide is then quickly placed into alcohol fixative to prevent air drying, which can occur rapidly. Several slides may be made from one needle aspiration pass by repetitively expelling the contents of the needle. The needle should then be rinsed with cytology fixative solution so as to collect any residual material contained within the needle hub or shaft. The cytology fluid can be spun down by the cytopathologist later and the pellet collected can be smeared or imbedded into paraffin for cell block analysis. Usually, three to six separate needle passes are made. Capillary sampling is a fine needle aspiration technique in which a bare needle without a syringe is used. This emphasizes the fact that, during fine needle aspiration, cytologic material is gathered up within the shaft of the needle. Capillary sampling is not appropriate if the lesion is known to be cystic. Even in cases in which surgical excision of the cervical lesion is anticipated, fine needle aspiration allows for preoperative diagnosis. This not only allows for the creation of an appropriate surgical plan, but also facilitates preoperative patient counselling.

Fine needle aspiration material can be put into single cell suspension and can be evaluated by the technique of flow cytometry. Flow cytometry analysis adds to cytologic interpretation and allows analysis of cell-surface antigen markers, cell-cycle kinetics and nuclear DNA content. During flow cytometric analysis, lymphocytes are analyzed in an effort to detect loss of normal B-cell surface-antigen heterogeneity. Flow cytometry is especially useful in the detection of clonal κ and λ light-chain expression seen in B-cell lymphoma. Reactive lymph nodes fail to demonstrate such clonality. There are no cell-surface markers of T-cell clonality, so other immunophenotypic characteristics are analyzed. Flow cytometry is not helpful in identifying the heterogeneous lymphoid populations that characterize Hodgkin's lymphoma, but fortunately the presence of Reed–Sternberg cells may be detected on routine cytological preparations in such circumstances.

Studies show that fine needle aspiration sensitivity and specificity in young patients with lymphadenitis is 93% and 95%, respectively. Tracking of malignancy to the skin with fine needle aspiration of malignant nodes is extraordinarily infrequent, unlike with larger gauge needles, such as the Vim–Silverman needle.

LATERAL NECK MASSES

Branchial cleft cyst

Branchial cleft cysts are most commonly located just anterior to the sternocleidomastoid muscle in the carotid triangle. A cystic mass with or without an external sinus tract is present. The diagnosis is more obvious in the presence of an external fistulous tract and a history of intermittent discharge. Branchial cleft cysts may become symptomatic at any age, but most are diagnosed in the first two decades of life. Often, branchial cleft cysts present with acute enlargement at the time of an upper respiratory tract infection. These lateral neck cysts are basically remnants of the gill apparatus. They represent the cystic remnants of fully developed branchial cleft arch tracts. Such lesions, as noted above, may to a varying extent have residual identifiable proximal or distal sinus tract remnants. Surgical excision is recommended for all such anomalies. Surgical excision should include both the cyst and any associated tract. Branchial cleft cysts may arise from first, second or third branchial cleft remnants. Associated branchial cleft tracts have known relationships to the adjacent cranial nerves. First branchial cleft anomalies (type I) represent duplications of the external auditory canal and extend from the external auditory canal to the preauricular skin. The tract may run between divisions of the facial nerve. First branchial cleft anomalies (type II) extend from the external auditory canal to the submandibular gland triangle. The tracts from such lesions may also have a variable relationship with the facial nerve. Second branchial cleft anomalies represent the most common branchial cleft anomaly, and extend from the tonsillar fossa to the skin at the medial edge of the sternocleido-mastoid muscle. The cystic component of the anomaly is typically adjacent to the carotid sheath. The proximal tract extends from the cyst superiorly between the internal and external carotid artery, lateral to the hypoglossal and glossopharyngeal nerves into the tonsil fossa. Third branchial anomalies are rare, and extend from the internal opening at the pyriform sinus to the external opening at the skin of the medial aspect of the sternocleidomastoid muscle. The cyst lies adjacent to the carotid sheath. The proximal tract extends superiorly lateral to the hypoglossal nerve but medial to the glossopharyngeal nerve to extend to the pyriform sinus.

Laryngocele

The laryngocele is an air-filled dilatation of the saccule, a small anterior diverticulum in the laryngeal ventricle (the lateral indentation between the true vocal cord below and the false vocal cord above). Initially, the laryn-gocele extends under the false vocal cord, resulting in the development of a submucosal mass lesion in the false cord and aryepiglottic fold. At this stage, the lesion is termed an internal laryngocele. As the internal laryngocele expands further, it extends up to and over the upper edge of the thyroid cartilage and extends through the thyrohyoid membrane into the soft tissues of the neck as an external laryngocele. Laryngoceles may become filled with mucoid fluid and may become infected. Internal laryngoceles can be endoscopically marsupialized. External laryngoceles are excised through an external approach.

Deep neck abscess

A deep neck abscess may present as a lateral neck mass. The history usually suggests an acute course and patients usually demonstrate systemic signs of toxicity. Pharyngeal or dental sources are common. On physical examination the masses are typically exquisitely tender and the overlying skin is often erythematous.

Cystic hygroma and hemangioma

Cystic hygromas, a form of lymphangioma, are almost always seen by the second year of life, although a few may be first diagnosed in adult life. They are thin walled, multiloculated cystic masses that infiltrate surrounding tissues. Their borders are typically indistinct and they fail to follow normal tissue planes, making their excision difficult. Clinically, they are diffuse, soft, doughy, irregular masses. They may represent significant cosmetic issues, or may compromise the airway, depending on their location and size. Because spontaneous regression occurs in some pediatric patients, surgery is postponed unless the airway is compromised.

Superficial cutaneous hemangiomas are easily diagnosed by their appearance. They are usually seen as bluish masses affecting the skin or mucosa. Patients with known cutaneous lesions are at increased risk for other lesions, including subglottic hemangiomas. Deeper hemangiomas may be more difficult to diagnose and may be associated with the parotid gland or neck musculature. In three-quarters of patients this condition is present at birth; in nearly 90% of these, it is diagnosed in the first year of life. There is a female preponderance. Larger hemangiomas, especially cavernous hemangiomas, may have a palpable thrill. Although hemangiomas may grow initially, they have a high rate of spontaneous regression within the first two years of life. Therefore, expectant observation is usually practiced. Deeper invasive lesions, or lesions affecting vision or interfering with upper aerodigestive tract function, may require surgery.

Teratoma and dermoid

Teratomas are cystic or solid, discrete soft tissue masses. True teratomas contain tissue from all three germ layers. If they are large, tracheal or esophageal obstruction may occur. When complete organ or body parts are formed, they are termed epignathi. Dermoid lesions are cystic or solid lesions that usually occur as firm midline submental lesions. Dermoids contain epidermal and mesodermal remnants.

MIDLINE NECK MASSES

Thyroglossal duct cyst

The thyroglossal duct cyst is a remnant of the tract of descent of the thyroid gland into the neck from the tongue base (see Chapter 17). It is, therefore, almost always found in the midline. Thyroglossal duct cysts may be found at any age, but most are found in the first or second decades of life. A thyroglossal duct cyst must be differentiated from dermoid cysts, lymphadenopathy and cutaneous lesions such as lipomas or sebaceous cysts. It may be located above or below the hyoid bone and moves with it. Surgery is almost always required, not only because of cosmetic considerations, but also because of the high incidence of recurrent infection, including abscess formation.

Thymic cysts

Thymic cysts, like lower parathyroid glands, are remnants of the third pharyngeal pouch. The thymus descends into the midline neck base during fetal life. Remnants in the central neck may present in later life as thymic cysts.

Plunging ranulas

For a description of these, see Chapter 12.

MASSES ASSOCIATED WITH NORMAL STRUCTURES OF THE NECK

Masses associated with the skin

Superficial intracutaneous or subcutaneous masses may be sebaceous cysts, dermoids or lipomas. Final diagnosis and treatment usually involves simple surgical excision.

Masses derived from neural tissue

With masses derived from neural tissue, a definitive diagnosis is rarely made preoperatively. Neurofibromas are usually multiple (unlike schwannoma) and may involve subcutaneous and dermal regions. These can be associated with neurofibromatosis (von Recklinghausen's disease) in which neurofibroma can degenerate to malignancy. Neurofibromas commonly originate from the sympathetic cervical trunk and may be associated with Horner's syndrome. They may also arise from glossopharyngeal, vagus, hypoglossal or spinal accessory nerves, causing associated dysfunction. Occasionally, they may arise from the trunks of the trigeminal or facial nerve. Small neuromas or neurofibromas may be difficult to differentiate from lymph nodes, and often the final diagnosis is made by excisional biopsy. Schwannomas arise in the peripheral nerve sheath. They may arise from cranial nerves, the cervical and brachial plexus or autonomic nerves. They usually present as lateral neck masses that are encapsulated, slow-growing and painless. Treatment is surgical excision. Neuroblastoma is a high-grade neural malignancy that usually presents in children.

Tumors associated with blood vessels or related structures

Tumors attached to or derived from blood vessels or associated structures include aneurysms of the common carotid artery or subclavian artery. Pulsatile masses identified after head and neck trauma should be evaluated with arteriography. Chemodectomas (non-chromaffin paragangliomas) such as glomus tumors or carotid body tumors arise from chemoreceptor bodies. Chemodectomas follow the distribution of paraganglioma tissue in the head and neck. The most common chemodectomas arise from the tympanic paraganglioma bodies in the middle ear, the glomus jugulare at the skull base, the vagal body near the skull base along the inferior ganglion of the vagus and the carotid body at the carotid bifurcation. Carotid body tumors present as a painless slowly growing mass at the carotid bifurcation. Occasionally a bruit may be present. The tumor is not separable from the carotid artery by palpation. The differential diagnosis includes consideration of aneurysm of the carotid, branchial cleft cyst, neurogenic tumor or nodal metastasis fixed to the carotid sheath. Glomus tympanicum tumors and glomus jugulare tumors may be first diagnosed by an appearance of a vascular mass behind the tympanic membrane. Glomus intravagale tumors often grow to substantial size at the skull base before diagnosis.

Other than the glomus tympanicum type, these tumors require arteriography for evaluation, which should usually be performed by a transfemoral route so that the opposite neck may be surveyed. There is a low incidence of bilateral and multiple chemodectomas. This risk is higher in patients with a positive family history of such tumors. The radiologist should be asked to record the venous phase of arteriography, especially with glomus jugulare tumors. The treatment of these tumors is surgical, if possible. Larger unresectable tumors may be controlled for many years with radiation therapy.

Masses within the thyroid gland

For a description of these, see Chapter 17.

Lesions within the esophagus

Occasionally a Zenker's diverticulum will be large enough to present as a mass within the neck. Associated symptoms include dysphagia, food retention and regurgitation. A barium swallow is diagnostic.

Tumors arising from cartilaginous structures

Chondromas and chondrosarcomas may rarely arise from the thyroid or cricoid cartilages. They are firmly fixed to these structures and may present as a mass in the neck, or they may present with respiratory symptoms.

Head and neck nodal metastasis

Squamous cell carcinoma arising from any site in the head and neck can lead to cervical metastasis. Although there are exceptions, certain sites tend to involve certain nodal groups preferentially. A lesion of the nasopharynx often metastasizes to the posterior chain. Oral cavity lesions tend to metastasize to the submandibular gland and high jugular regions. Posterior oropharynx lesions tend to metastasize to the retropharyngeal region, as well as the high and midjugular chain. Lesions of the hypopharynx and larynx tend to metastasize to the mid- and lower jugular chains. Thyroid carcinoma, especially papillary carcinoma of the thyroid, is often characterized by nodal metastasis. Thyroid carcinoma can metastasize to perithyroid nodes, prelaryngeal and pretracheal nodes, paratracheal nodes (recurrent laryngeal nerve chain), as well as mediastinal and mid- and lower jugular nodal regions. Carcinomas arising from the lip and face tend to metastasize to the facial nodal groups as well as submental and submandibular gland regions.

Nasopharynx carcinoma most frequently presents with cervical metastasis. The nasopharynx primary itself may be otherwise asymptomatic. Non-keratinizing and undifferentiated lymphoepitheliomatous forms of nasopharynx carcinoma are associated with Epstein–Barr virus. Fine needle aspiration and open biopsy samples of affected nodes may be assessed with PCR to help establish an appropriate diagnosis. Nasopharyngeal carcinoma, which occurs more frequently in patients of Chinese descent, frequently affects posterior chain nodal groups initially. In a subgroup of patients with head and neck squamous cell carcinoma, the mucosal primary cannot, despite thorough search, be found. Such patients are described as having an occult primary. Regions known to harbor small primaries associated with cervical metastasis are biopsied during panendoscopy. In such patients, these regions include the nasopharynx, the base of the tongue, the tonsil and the pyriform sinus. Salivary gland malignancies, typically carcinomas, may also lead to the development of cervical adenopathy. Nodal metastasis of squamous cell carcinoma of the head and neck is described as the 'N' in the 'TNM' classification system. The designation of nodal size relates to the clinical examination, not the radiographic assessment. The nodal rating system is as follows: N0, no clinically palpable nodes; N1, single node, less than 3 cm; N2a, single node between 3 and 6 cm; N2b, multiple nodes, all less than 6 cm; N2c, bilateral or contralateral nodal disease; N3, nodal mass greater than 6 cm.

Head and neck lymphoma

Lymphoma may present with isolated cervical adenopathy, as an isolated lesion in Waldeyer's ring or in a variety of other sites, including the paranasal sinus, orbit, salivary gland or thyroid. Patients may present with night sweats, fever or weight loss. Fine needle aspiration with flow cytometry can be useful in diagnosing B-cell lymphomas, and are often helpful in identification of T-cell lymphoma. Hodgkin's disease may require additional open biopsy. Treatment for head and neck lymphoma includes regional radiation therapy and chemotherapy, occasionally with bone marrow transplantation. Treatment recommendations are generated after appropriate staging work-up, which often includes blood testing, CT scanning of the chest, abdomen and pelvis, and bone marrow biopsy. Tracheotomy may be necessary for some lymphomas, including those of thyroid origin. Patients with leukemia may present with cervical adenopathy due to accumulation of leukemic cells, as occurs in other organs, including the liver, spleen and bone marrow. This may occur in acute leukemia, as well as in chronic forms such as chronic lymphocytic leukemia (CLL) where lymph nodes may be present and stable over extended periods of time. Leukemias generally present with progressive weakness, fever, joint pain, petechiae, ecchymosis and bleeding (including mouth, bowel and kidney). Other malignancies that may occur in the head and neck, with or without nodal metastasis, include liposarcomas, fibrosarcomas, malignant histiocytoma, rhabdomyosarcoma and hemangiopericytoma.

12

Sore mouth and throat

Gregory W. Randolph

Anatomy of the mouth and throat
Medical history
Examination of the mouth and throat
Infections of the oral cavity
    Aphthous stomatitis
    Herpetic stomatitis
    Varicella
    Herpangina
    Candidiasis
    Acute necrotizing ulcerative gingivitis (Vincent's angina)
    Syphilis
Infections of the pharynx
    Pharyngitis
    Scarlet fever
    Diphtheria
    Gonococcal pharyngitis
    Epiglottitis
    Tonsillitis
    Peritonsillar abscess
    Lingual tonsillitis
    Infectious mononucleosis
    Rare pathogens
    Non-infectious pharyngitis
    Infectious complications
        Ludwig's angina
        Parapharyngeal space infection
        Retropharyngeal infection
Benign oral lesions
    Tongue
    Palate

    Buccal mucosa
    Gingiva and floor of the mouth
Pigmented oral lesions
Inflammatory lesions
    Erythema multiforme
    Pemphigus and pemphigoid
    Behçet's syndrome
    Reiter's syndrome
    Mucositis
    Lichen planus
    Systemic lupus erythematosus
    Necrotizing sialometaplasia
    Other inflammatory lesions
Oral and pharyngeal cancer
    Leukoplakia
    Physical examination
    Work-up of head and neck cancer
    Non-squamous cell neoplasia
Pharyngeal pain
    Pharyngeal burns
    Foreign body
    Glossopharyngeal neuralgia
    Eagle syndrome
    Carotidynia
    Musculoskeletal cervical pain
    Atypical angina
Trismus
Dry mouth (xerostomia)
    Sjögren's syndrome
Non-ulcerative disorders
    Burning tongue syndrome
    Halitosis

ANATOMY OF THE MOUTH AND THROAT

The oral cavity is bounded anteriorly by the lip and extends to the junction of the hard and soft palates (Figure 12.1). It includes the anterior two-thirds of the tongue and the floor of the mouth. The anterior two-thirds of the tongue, or 'oral' tongue, ends posteriorly at the V-shaped line of circular raised circumvallate papillae. The posterior one-third of the tongue is referred to as the tongue base. The tongue musculature consists of three extrinsic muscles (genioglossus, styloglossus and hyoglossus) and three intrinsic muscles (longitudinal, vertical and transverse intrinsic muscles). All of these tongue muscles are supplied by the hypoglossal nerve. With hypoglossal nerve paralysis, the genioglossus, the major protruder of the tongue, is denervated and tongue protrusion on that side is lost. Thus, with unilateral hypoglossal nerve paralysis, the tongue when protruded deviates to the paralyzed side. The floor of the mouth consists of the inferior mucosa between the tongue medially and the mandibular alveolar ridge laterally. The anterior floor of the mouth lies underneath the tongue tip. From the anterior floor of the mouth, the tongue frenulum arises and inserts into the undersurface of the anterior tongue. On either side of the midline tongue frenulum in the anterior floor of the mouth, is the orifice of Wharton's duct of the submandibular gland. Saliva can be expressed from Wharton's duct with submandibular gland massage. The lateral oral cavity consists of the buccal mucosa and the upper and lower alveolar ridges. Adjacent to the second upper molar is the orifice of the parotid gland's Stensen's duct. Saliva can be expressed through this orifice during parotid gland massage. The retromolar trigone consists of the up-sloping posterior oral cavity gingiva which overlies the mandible just posterior to the last mandibular molar. At the apex of the retromolar trigone is the maxillary tuberosity.

The pharynx is divided into the nasopharynx, oropharynx and hypopharynx (Figure 12.1). The oropharynx consists of the soft palate, posterior third of the tongue (tongue base), vallecula, tonsil fossa (including tonsil and anterior and posterior tonsil fossa arches) and posterior oropharynx wall. The anterior and posterior tonsil arches sweep medially to form the distal free edge of the soft palate. The dividing line between the oral cavity (anteriorly) and oropharynx (posteriorly) is the junction of the hard and soft palates superiorly and the circumvallate papillae inferiorly.

The tonsils are supplied by the internal maxillary, facial and lingual arteries. The lingual tonsils are variable and bilateral lymphoid accumulations on the surface of the lateral aspect of the base of the tongue. A ring of lymphatic tissue situated at the entrance to the upper

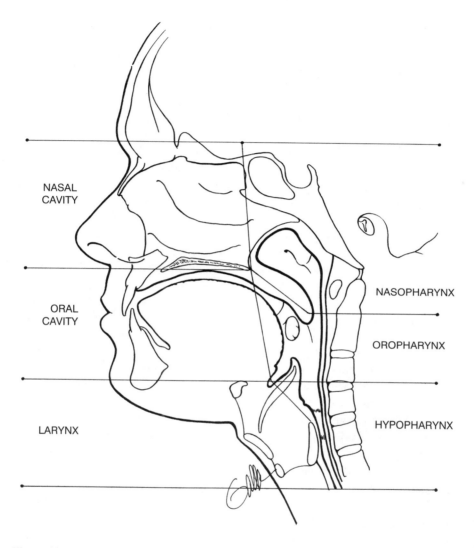

Figure 12.1 Anatomy of the mouth and pharynx. The dividing line between oral cavity and oropharynx is the circumvallate papillae of the posterior tongue

aerodigestive tract is termed Waldeyer's ring. This ring consists of adenoids superiorly, tonsils laterally and lingual tonsils inferiorly. The anatomy of the nasopharynx and hypopharynx is discussed in detail in Chapters 8 and 13.

Sensation in the mouth, including the teeth, alveolar ridges, lips and cheek, is primarily mediated by the trigeminal nerve. Taste and general sensation from the anterior two-thirds of the tongue is mediated via the chorda tympani branch of the facial nerve, which reaches the anterior tongue by way of the lingual branch of the trigeminal nerve. Taste and general sensation of the posterior one-third of the tongue is provided by the glossopharyngeal nerve. Palate sensation is mediated by the trigeminal, glossopharyngeal and vagus nerves. Sensation to the posterior oropharynx is mediated by glossopharyngeal and vagus nerves. Motor function to the palate is mediated by the vagus, except the tensor veli palatini which is innervated by the trigeminal. Pharyngeal motor function is mediated by the vagus and the stylopharyngeus innervated by the glossopharyngeal nerve. Lip and buccal tone is mediated by the facial nerve.

MEDICAL HISTORY

During the evaluation of a patient with oral or pharyngeal pain, the clinician must assess the quality and location of the pain. It is useful to have the patient point to the site of pain. Pain from streptococcal pharyngitis may be localized to the posterior oropharynx. In epiglottitis, pain may be sensed lower in the neck and the patient may point to the thyroid or cricoid cartilages. The temporal course of the pain can also give important clues. Pain from severe tonsillitis or a peritonsillar abscess may develop rapidly, whereas discomfort referable to reflux may be present for many months and have a fluctuant course. The pain referable to an oral carcinoma may develop gradually and slowly progress in intensity. Understanding the impact of the pain on oral intake is critical in decision making regarding the need for admission to the hospital for hydration. The patient should also be questioned regarding the onset of the pain. Was this associated with any specific food such as fish with bones or ingestion of a foreign body? With a chief complaint of sore mouth or throat, we must inquire about other upper aerodigestive tract symptoms including respiratory distress, dysphagia, cough, hemoptysis, voice change, weight loss, odynophagia, ear pain and adenopathy. One should determine whether systemic symptoms that may suggest infection, such as fever and fatigue, are present. HIV status and risk factors should be assessed. Finally, one must question regarding smoking and alcohol intake. Squamous cell carcinoma typically arises in the setting of a significant history of smoking and drinking.

EXAMINATION OF THE MOUTH AND THROAT

During the physical examination of the mouth and throat, the clinician must focus on three main points. Is there any significant asymmetry present? Is there is any significant disturbance to the mucosal lining of the mouth or oral cavity? Is there any palpable abnormality present on examination? The importance of asymmetry cannot be overstated. One tonsil that is larger than the other may indicate a lymphoma. Similarly, a medially displaced asymmetric tonsil fossa may help to identify an occult para-pharyngeal space tumor or peritonsillar abscess. Mucosal lesions to be noted include ulcerative or exophytic lesions suggestive of malignancy. Palpation allows a thorough assessment of the tongue, base of tongue and floor of mouth. Digital palpation of the tongue may identify a unilateral mass of the base of the tongue or midline lingual thyroid. The submandibu-lar triangle can be fully assessed only through bimanual examination. In sialadenitis of the submandibular gland, purulent discharge may be expressed from Wharton's duct with massage of the submandibular gland.

The examination of the mouth and throat should be performed in a purposeful manner. Too often, the mouth and pharynx are examined at a glance. A better approach is to examine each structure within the mouth and pharynx quickly and independently. One way to proceed is to examine the structures quickly in the following order: the buccal mucosa on the right, the right gums and teeth, palate, right tonsil, posterior oropharynx, left tonsil, left buccal mucosa, left gums and teeth, floor of mouth and, with the patient extending his tongue, the posterior one-third of the tongue bilaterally. It is of note that, at the onset of the examination, the identification of trismus (difficulty opening the mouth) can be suggestive of malignancy infiltrating the pterygoid musculature, a peritonsillar abscess causing pterygoid spasm or severe temporomandibular joint syndrome. The buccal mucosa can be examined with one or two tongue blades to stretch the cheek laterally to inspect all aspects of the buccal mucosa as well as the gingival buccal sulcus. Also, the tongue blade can be used to push the lateral aspect of the tongue medially so that the floor of mouth can be fully inspected. A headlight or headmirror (with light source behind the patient's head) is preferable to a hand-held light, as two hands are then available for the examination. For the examination of the hypopharynx and larynx, see Chapter 13.

Typically, when patients are asked to open the mouth, they will also pro-trude their tongue, which often prevents visualization of the posterior oral cavity and oropharynx. Patients can be instructed simply to open their mouth without tongue protrusion. A key maneuver to increase visualization of the posterior oral cavity and oropharynx during the examination is to place a tongue blade approximately two-thirds of the way back on the tongue and push directly downward. This depresses the tongue, does not induce gagging and dramatically increases visualization of the soft palate, bilateral tonsillar fossa and posterior oropharynx wall. If the tongue blade impacts on the posterior one-third of the tongue, posterior oropharynx wall or tonsil fossa region, gagging will probably result. Contact with the soft palate, however, as with indirect mirror examination of the larynx, does not typically induce gagging. The lateral aspect of the posterior tongue is a difficult, but important, region to examine. It is best seen by asking a patient after completion of the initial portions of the examination to protrude his tongue. Any abnormality seen during the head and neck examination should be palpated to assess firmness. The floor of the mouth and submandibular triangle are not fully examined until a bimanual examination is performed. During the bimanual examination, the gloved finger is placed onto the floor of the mouth with the second hand under the mandible in the submandibular triangle. Downward gliding motion of the intraoral finger pushes down the soft tissue of the floor of the mouth and the contents of the submandibular triangle onto the external examining hand, dramatically increasing the sensitivity of the examination in these regions. The base of the tongue should also be palpated with a gloved finger, as the last step in the examination of the oropharynx. The examiner explains to the patient that this last step will probably induce transient gagging.

INFECTIONS OF THE ORAL CAVITY

Stomatitis is any inflammatory disorder of the oral cavity mucosa and is commonly viral, but may be bacterial, fungal or inflammatory. Infectious stomatitis is discussed below.

Aphthous stomatitis

Aphthous stomatitis is the most common form of mouth lesion. Canker sores may occur anywhere, but most commonly present on the lip, buccal and gingival mucosa or adjacent surfaces of the tongue. Such lesions present as a spot of burning pain, one or several small (1–2 mm in diameter, but occasionally up to 1–2 cm) ulcerative lesions that develop red halos with a yellow–gray fibrinous base. Unlike herpetic stomatitis, there is no true vesicular phase. The cause is unknown, but an autoimmune etiology is likely; to date, no virus has been identified. Other putative etiologies include vitamin deficiencies and allergic reactions. A rare subtype of aphthous stomatitis characterized by large ulcerative lesions that occur frequently and persist over extended periods of time is termed Sutton's disease. Many home remedies exist, none of which significantly alters the 2–4-day course of pain, which is followed by several days of healing. The use of anesthetic lozenges may be helpful, as is the application of triamcinolone (Kenalog®, E.R. Squibb & Sons Ltd., Princeton, NJ, USA and Orabase®, HCA, Colgate-Hoyt, Canton, MA, USA). Topical Lidex® (0.5% flucinonide; Medicis, Scottsdale, AZ, USA), Celestone® (betamethasone; Schering Corp., Kenilworth, NJ, USA) rinse or viscous lidocaine can be helpful. Sucralfate slurry and tetracycline oral suspension rinses have also been used. Milk of Magnesia (Roxane Laboratories Inc., Columbus, Ohio, USA) and sodium bicarbonate mouthwashes are old standbys for patients with frequent recurrences.

Herpetic stomatitis

Vesicular erosions that occur secondary to herpes simplex type I or type II are usually 1–3 mm in diameter and typically occur singly or in groups at the mucocutaneous junction of the lip. The vesicles typically coalesce to form yellow–gray painful ulcers 2–10 mm in diameter. Herpes simplex type I infection typically occurs as an oral lesion, but may occur on genitalia. Herpes simplex type II infection typically occurs as genital lesions but can occur in the oral cavity as well. Herpetic stomatitis needs to be differentiated from other common viral stomatitis, including herpes zoster and herpangina (Coxsackie virus). In primary or recurrent herpetic infection, stomatitis may be associated with fever, joint pain and fatigue. Reactivation may be triggered by stress, upper respiratory tract infection or immunosuppression. The virus remains latent in the sensory ganglia corresponding to the previous sites of infection. Lesions, therefore, often recur in the same location as prior infections. The diagnosis is typically made by a characteristic clinical picture; however, viral cultures or viral polymerase chain reaction (PCR) techniques can be used. For viral culture, it is best to swab the vesicular fluid and promptly place the swab in appropriate viral culture medium. The disease is typically self-limiting, usually lasting 4–10 days. Treatment is as needed for symptomatic relief and to diminish the duration of vesicles. Oral acyclovir can be used. Acyclovir may be used at high dose or intravenously in the immunosuppressed patient. Patients with frequent recurrences may be offered prophylactic doses of acyclovir.

Varicella

The oral vesicles and ulcers of varicella (herpes zoster) are found primarily on the mucosa of the hard and soft palate and are distinguishable during the primary infection from other viral lesions by the appearance of the classical vesicles of chicken pox upon the patient's trunk and face. Varicella commonly occurs in epidemics from January to May in children under 10 years of age. Reactivation of varicella/zoster from colonized sensory ganglia is associated with immunosuppression, trauma and steroid use. In the head and neck, such reactivations can result in oral stomatitis without any skin involvement. Such reactivations can be associated with cranial nerve palsies, including palatal or vocal cord paralysis. When reactivation occurs in the ear (herpes zoster oticus or Ramsay Hunt syndrome), vesicles in the ear canal may be associated with facial paralysis, dizziness and sensorineural hearing loss. Evaluation may include acute and convalescent serologies, viral culture or viral identification through PCR. Treatment may include acyclovir, especially if the patient is immunocompromised. Steroids are typically given in the setting of sensorineural hearing loss or facial paralysis associated with herpes zoster oticus.

Herpangina

Herpangina is a summertime viral disease caused by Coxsackie virus group A or B. It typically affects children 6 years and younger, and is characterized by an abrupt onset of fever associated with sore mouth and throat with odynophagia. Its transmission may be associated with summertime communal swimming. There is a characteristic painful vesicular eruption, 1–2 mm in diameter, involving multiple discrete whitish-gray vesicular ulcerative lesions, with a bright red areola located principally on the anterior tonsil pillars, soft palate, buccal mucosa or lip. Herpangina usually requires only supportive treatment and lasts 1–4 days.

Candidiasis

Candidiasis causes oral and pharyngeal pain associated with milky white, slightly elevated lesions. The curd-like white plaque can be scraped with a tongue blade, leaving a red hemorrhagic base. Leukoplakia and lichen planus cannot be removed in this manner. Candidiasis occurs secondary to the fungus *Candida albicans* and can occur at any age. It may also present as angular cheilitis. This occurs especially in the setting of chronic maceration of the skin of the oral commissure from excess salivation or poor salivary control. Candidiasis is usually preceeded by a change in oral flora, for instance following a course of antibiotics or steroids. It can occur frequently in patients on chronic steroid inhalers for asthma. Candidiasis also occurs in patients with a history of radiation therapy to the mouth or throat, during pregnancy and in patients with diabetes mellitus or immunodeficiency (e.g. neutropenic patients or patients with AIDS). Treatment consists of nystatin 4–6 ml four times a day or Mycostatin® (Pharmacia Adria, Columbus, Ohio, USA) oral tablets. Treatment options also include oral ketoconazole or fluconazole. Oral antifungal agents are preferable to topical treatment if the candidiasis is extensive, involves the esophageal mucosa and in the immunosuppressed patient. Such oral antifungal agents may lead to liver dysfunction, so they are used with caution in patients with liver dysfunction (e.g. patients with AIDS with chronic hepatitis B infection). Candidiasis can occur in a chronic atrophic form. In this form, there are no obvious white lesions. Affected patches of mucosa appear atrophic and erythematous and may occur commonly on the tongue dorsum. These can lead to a sensation of burning of the tongue. Median rhomboid glossitis may represent such an atrophic form of candidiasis.

Acute necrotizing ulcerative gingivitis (Vincent's angina)

Acute necrotizing ulcerative gingivitis (also known as trench mouth or Vincent's angina) is a disease affecting young adults and results from a combination of poor dental care and decreased resistance to infection. Before it is diagnosed, acute leukemia, neutropenia and infectious mononucleosis should be considered. The infection occurs secondary to fusiform bacilli and oral spirochetes (including *Borrelia vincentii*), and generally involves the gingiva, tonsils and oral mucous membrane. There is necrosis of the superficial mucosal layer which leads to a gray necrotic pseudomembrane and cervical adenopathy. The patient complains of malaise, a moderate temperature elevation and fetid breath. The infection is sensitive to penicillin and frequent half-strength hydrogen peroxide oral irrigations. Occasionally, the hypopharynx and larynx are involved. The infection is termed noma when it spreads to adjacent soft tissue.

Syphilis

In primary syphilis, the chancre may occur wherever the treponeme first enters the body, for example the lip, tongue or tonsil, approximately 3 weeks after exposure. It usually appears as a single, hard, painless eroded papule, although occasionally there can be multiple lesions. The 'satellite node' is an adjacent large, rubbery, non-tender cervical node. Dark field examination is of no diagnostic value, because of the presence of spirochetes in normal oral flora. Screening serologic tests may be positive, but are often negative until 8–12 weeks have passed; therefore, a negative test must be repeated after 1 month. History of sexual exposure and rising titer is sufficient confirmation for the diagnosis. The primary lesion clears with or without treatment.

Secondary syphilis is characterized by a macular or macular–papular cutaneous rash and lymphadenopathy. Oral lesions consist of gray, raised mucinous patches with discrete borders that are found on the tongue and oral mucosa. During secondary syphilis, screening reagin tests such as the Venereal Disease Research Laboratory (VDRL) test and the rapid plasma reagin card (RPR) test, become positive. A specific treponemal antibody test, such as the fluorescent treponemal antibody absorption (FTA-ABS) test, is reserved for confirmation. Benzathine penicillin G 2.4 million units intramuscularly is generally recommended for the treatment of syphilis. The oral manifestation of tertiary syphilis includes gummatous lesions of the palate. Rhagades, Hutchinson's incisors and mulberry incisors are seen in congenital syphilis.

INFECTIONS OF THE PHARYNX

Pharyngitis

Pharyngitis may be caused by viral, bacterial, fungal or mycoplasmal infection. Viruses that may be associated with pharyngitis include Coxsackie A and B, echo, herpes simplex I and II, rhinovirus, coronavirus, influenza, parainfluenza, adenovirus, measles, Epstein–Barr virus, cytomegalovirus, rubella, smallpox, HIV and chicken pox. The most important bacterial pathogen is β-hemolytic group A streptococcus (*Streptococcus pyogenes*). Other possible bacterial pathogens may include group C and G streptococcus, *Staphylococcus aureus*, *Haemophilus influenzae*, *Moraxella catarrhalis*, anaerobic microbes (*Bacteroides*, *Peptococcus*, *Peptostreptococcus* species), *Mycoplasma*, *Corynebacterium diphtheriae*, other *Corynebacterium* species, *Bordetella pertussis*, *Treponema pallidum* and *Neisseria gonorrhoeae*. See the section on tonsillitis for a discussion of treatment of bacterial pharyngotonsillitis.

Scarlet fever

Scarlet fever results from pharyngitis caused by a strain of *Streptococcus* that elaborates a cutaneous toxin which results in a characteristic skin rash. Treatment is the same as for streptococcal pharyngitis.

Diphtheria

Pharyngeal diphtheria is fortunately now rare as a result of immunization programs. During the infection, *C. diphtheriae* can elaborate a neuromuscular and myocardial toxin. The neural toxin may lead to paralysis of the palate and vocal cord. The characteristic pharyngeal finding in diphtheria is a gray-to-white membrane in the posterior oropharynx. The throat is erythematous and covered by this dirty, gray membrane, which extends from the tonsil to the palate and pharynx. Typically, there is no reactive cervical adenopathy despite the intense pharyngitis. The removal of the pharyngeal membrane results in a raw bleeding surface (see Chapter 13). Airway obstruction may result from this obstructing diphtheric membrane, as well as from associated edema and laryngeal paralysis. Cultures are grown on Loeffler's medium. Treatment is with antitoxin, intravenous penicillin and tracheotomy, as needed.

Gonococcal pharyngitis

Gonococcal pharyngitis (*N. gonorrhoeae*) is manifested by a brightly erythematous inflammatory reaction in the pharynx and the development of irregular superficial whitish-gray ulcers with yellowish fetid exudate 1–2 days after exposure. In the majority of patients affected, the infection, despite the physical findings, produces little in the way of pharyngeal symptomatology. A gonococcal focus in the tonsil is not easily eradicated, and may lead to disseminated gonorrhea with arthritis. Cultures require special handling. Thayer–Martin chocolate agar plates should be swabbed and incubated in a 5% CO_2 environment within 15 min.

Epiglottitis

Patients may complain of sore throat and may describe the discomfort as being lower than that which occurs during a typical sore throat. These patients often present with difficulty managing their secretions and may have a gurgling or wet-type phonation. Usually, they present with some degree of respiratory distress. One should consider epiglottitis in a patient who is describing an atypical sore throat with respiratory distress who has a normal oropharyngeal examination. One must have a high index of suspicion to diagnose epiglottitis by means of fiberoptic nasopharyngoscopy or the changes in the epiglottis evident on a lateral neck film. Examination of the oral cavity with a tongue blade is not recommended, as such a maneuver may predispose the swollen epiglottis to become displaced posteriorly and occlude the airway (see Chapter 15).

Tonsillitis

Acute bacterial tonsillitis is often the result of β-hemolytic group A streptococcal infection. For other bacterial and viral pathogens, see the section on pharyngitis. β-Hemolytic group A streptococcal infection is associated with the development of non-suppurative sequelae: acute rheumatic fever and glomerulonephritis. Acute rheumatic fever occurs in approximately 3% of untreated patients following exudative streptococcal pharyngotonsillitis in studies in military recruit camps, and in slightly less than 1% in pediatric populations. The major manifestations of acute rheumatic fever occur with a latency of approximately 19 days after sore throat and include carditis, polyarthritis, chorea, subcutaneous nodules and erythema marginatum. Cardiac involvement can lead to chronic valvular disease. The clinical manifestations of glomerulonephritis, which occurs with a latency of approximately 10 days after sore throat, include edema, hypertension and a rusty color to the urine. The attack rate can be as high as 10–15% after infection with nephritogenic strains. Prompt antibiotic treatment of the streptococcal pharyngotonsillitis has been shown to decrease the risk of development of acute rheumatic fever, but has no significant effect on the development of glomerulonephritis. While patients with symptomatic acute streptococcal pharyngotonsillitis are at risk of the development of these non-suppurative sequelae, patients who are asymptomatic carriers are not. Therefore, throat culture alone does not distinguish between active streptococcal infection and the asymptomatic carrier state.

In clinical assessment and treatment of pharyngotonsillitis, one must offer treatment to patients with streptococcal pharyngotonsillitis who are at increased risk of acute rheumatic fever if untreated with penicillin. One should also treat patients with bacterial pharyngitis (whether streptococcal or not) who are at risk of development of local and systemic complications of infection, including sinusitis, otitis media, mastoiditis, lateral sinus thrombosis, bacteremia, pneumonia, peritonsillar abscess, retropharyngeal abscess and lateral neck abscess. However, unnecessary treatment with antibiotics should be avoided, given the common viral etiology of pharyngotonsillitis and the risk of induction of drug resistance with indiscriminate antibiotic treatment. Inappropriate antibiotic use is also costly and risks the development of allergic reactions in patients. β-Hemolytic group A streptococcal pharyngotonsillitis is appropriately treated with penicillin VK for 10 days or erythromycin in the penicillin-allergic patient. Broader spectrum antibiotics are not recommended. Alternatively, a single dose of penicillin benzathine 1.2 million units intramuscularly can be considered.

Various approaches have been used in the evaluation and treatment of patients with acute pharyngotonsillitis. 'Rapid strep antigen' detection tests will fail to detect 5–10% of patients with streptococcal infection. Standard throat culture is, therefore, an important part of the evaluation of such patients. One approach is to culture and treat all patients initially and discontinue antibiotics if the culture is negative for streptococcus at 48 hours. Another approach is to perform both a rapid strep antigen test and a throat culture, and treat all patients with positive rapid strep antigen test. In those few patients where the rapid strep antigen test is negative yet the culture is positive at 48 hours, treatment can be started when the culture becomes positive. In discussing the evaluation and treatment of patients with pharyngotonsillitis, two points should be considered. The first is that clinical factors other than rapid strep antigen test and culture data should be included in the decision-making process to treat. Patients who have severe pharyngotonsillitis with decreased oral intake, respiratory distress or evidence of toxicity should be treated. Also, patients who are at risk of the development of progression of infectious symptoms or complications such as sinusitis, otitis media, mastoiditis, bacteremia, suppurative adenitis, or peritonsillar or lateral neck abscess should be treated regardless of rapid strep antigen test and culture data. If the history and physical examination suggest diphtheria, or gonococcal or syphilitic pharyngitis, special culture techniques and treatment are necessary. The second point is that patients should be counseled that, whether they are treated with penicillin or not, ongoing symptoms or the development of new symptoms should prompt repeat evaluation. This will allow for identification and treatment of resistant pathogens, as well as complications such as suppurative adenitis or peritonsillar abscess. Such complications may occur despite a negative streptococcal throat culture.

Patients who harbor β-hemolytic group A streptococcus in their pharynx, and are asymptomatic and without serologic response associated with clinical streptococcal infection, are termed streptococcal carriers. Such patients are not at risk for the development of the streptococcus-associated non-suppurative sequelae of acute rheumatic fever and glomerulonephritis. These patients, as long as they are asymptomatic, do not require repetitive culture and treatment. However, such carriers may have a history of recurrent clinically significant streptococcal infections themselves or in family members. The carrier state is felt to facilitate the development of these recurrent clinical infections. In these cases, suppressive antibiotic treatment of penicillin and rifampin can be considered. If this prophylactic treatment is not effective, tonsillectomy can be considered to lower the streptococcal carrier rate.

Patients who have developed rheumatoid complications of streptococcal pharyngitis are at increased risk for development of recurrent acute rheumatic fever with subsequent streptococcal infections. This risk can be decreased by offering chronic prophylactic antibiotic therapy.

If tonsillitis is frequently recurrent, tonsillectomy may be considered. Patients with seven episodes in 1 year, five episodes per year for 2 years or three episodes per year for 3 years are considered surgical candidates. Tonsillectomy may be recommended with fewer episodes if the episodes of infection are associated with respiratory distress, febrile seizure, abscessed cervical nodes or significant absence from work, or in patients with cardiac valvular disease. Tonsillectomy may also be recommended in patients with obstructive sleep apnea, usually as part of a uvulopalatopharyngoplasty (UPPP). Patients who have had a peritonsillar abscess and are at high risk of recurrent peritonsillar abscess may be offered tonsillectomy. In general, this includes patients who are less than 30 years of age and have had a history of recurrent tonsillitis prior to their initial peritonsillar abscess. Recurrent peritonsillar abscess is less likely in patients over 30 years who have not had a history of recurrent tonsillitis prior to their peritonsillar abscess. Patients should be offered tonsillectomy if they have significant tonsillar asymmetry, to rule out underlying malignancy. Studies have suggested that approximately 6% of patients who have asymptomatic asymmetric tonsils have underlying lymphoma. As noted above, selected patients who are persistent carriers of streptococcus unresponsive to medical management may be offered tonsillectomy. Also, tonsillectomy may be offered to patients with chronic tonsillar debris or tonsillolithiasis. Rarely, patients will be offered tonsillectomy if tonsillar hypertrophy has resulted in a secondary dysphagia or significant speech abnormality.

Tonsillectomy is a safe and successful operation when performed for appropriate indications. In one study of children undergoing adenotonsillectomy, 97% of parents and 87% of referring physicians concluded that the surgery had resolved or greatly improved the medical problem for which the surgery was performed. It is of note that hemorrhage may occur after tonsillectomy and typically occurs with some delay, approximately 7–10 days after surgery.

Peritonsillar abscess

Peritonsillar abscess is an infrequent complication of tonsillitis that can occur unexpectedly, even if the patient is receiving oral antibiotic therapy. It is manifested by a marked swelling of the tonsil and soft palate, which usually occurs several days after the onset of tonsillitis. The physical examination is notable for a marked asymmetric bulge centered at the apex of the tonsil fossa and lateral soft palate. This deviates the uvula to the opposite side. There is deep throat pain radiating to the ear with marked spasm of the surrounding musculature, including the pterygoid muscles, resulting in trismus. Because of the pain and because of the fullness in the lateral soft palate, patients have a full voice described as a 'hot-potato' voice and have difficulty managing their saliva.

The diagnosis of peritonsillar abscess is confirmed with needle aspiration, which also provides material for culture. The abscess is incised and drained after the area is infiltrated with local anesthetic. A no. 15 blade can be used to make a superficial incision through the mucous membrane and superficial muscle of the anterior pillar and lateral palate, and a hemostat is used to spread the wound until the abscess cavity is completely drained. The patient often experiences immediate and marked relief of pain. Patients may be hospitalized for intravenous hydration and intravenous antibiotics, usually penicillin. Repeat probing of the cavity is often necessary, but tonsillectomy (Quincy tonsillectomy) is infrequently necessary at the initial presentation. Rarely, deaths have occurred secondary to peritonsillar abscess from sudden rupture of the abscess and aspiration, or from the gradual progression of the abscess through deep fascial planes to the parapharyngeal space, lateral neck and even mediastinum.

Lingual tonsillitis

The lingual tonsils are rarely infected. When they are, the pathogens do not vary from those causing faucial tonsillitis. Pain and swelling can be either unilateral or bilateral and patients may have difficulty articulating ('hot-potato' voice) and swallowing. In severe cases, the airway may be compromised. The diagnosis is confirmed by mirror examination or fiberoptic examination showing enlarged lingual tonsils, often with some surface exudate. The posterior oropharynx may appear grossly normal. Lingual tonsillitis is treated with antibiotics, proper hydration and management of any airway difficulties. Recurrent infections may require removal of lingual tonsillar tissue with electrocautery or laser.

Infectious mononucleosis

Infectious mononucleosis is a generalized disease caused by the Epstein–Barr virus, typically affecting young adults. Mononucleosis often presents as severe pharyngotonsillitis with white membranous exudate associated with cervical adenopathy (usually posterior chain), splenomegaly and malaise. Infectious mononucleosis can lead to hepatitis. The tonsillitis associated with mononucleosis may be indistinguishable from that produced by group A β–hemolytic streptococcus. Mononucleosis-like syndromes may also be produced by cytomegalovirus, hepatitis A, adenovirus, rubella and *Toxoplasma gondii*. Infectious mononucleosis is associated with an increase in the percentage of atypical lymphocytes in the white blood cell count, and a positive monospot test (Monoplus®, Walpole Laboratories, Cranbury, NJ, USA) or heterophil agglutination test. It is of note that the monospot and heterophil tests may be negative in the first 2 weeks of the illness. As a result, early negative tests may need to be repeated. The condition of a patient with severe mononucleosis pharyngotonsillitis may be improved with a short course of steroids in addition to the usual supportive measures. Superimposed bacterial infections do occur and require antibiotic treatment. Amoxicillin and ampicillin should be avoided, as there is a high incidence of rash in patients with infectious mononucleosis given these agents. The acute phase usually lasts 2–3 weeks.

Rare pathogens

There are many unusual pathogens which can rarely manifest clinically in the oral cavity and oropharynx. Cat scratch disease typically is seen in the head and neck with cervical adenopathy, but can present with pharyngitis. *Actinomyces* normally colonizes the mouth, but can lead to infection with a tendency towards fistulous tracts. Mycobacterial infection (*M. tuberculosis*, *M. bovis*) can rarely affect the pharynx and larynx. Typically, such involvement is associated with active pulmonary disease (see Chapter 13).

Leprosy (*Mycobacterium leprae*) can affect both the nasal cavity and the pharynx. Rhinoscleroma (*Klebsiella rhinoscleromatis*) usually presents as a nasal pathogen, but infection can spread to the pharynx. *Leishmania brasiliensis* has been reported to affect the mouth and throat. Pharyngeal tularemia has also been reported. Rarely, the head and neck can be affected by non-candidal mycoses, including *Cryptococcus neoformans*, *Rhinosporidium seeberi*, *Histoplasma capsulatum*, *Blastomyces dermatitidis* and *Paracoccidioides brasiliensis*. It should be noted that, in a patient with altered immune status (e.g. AIDS or neutropenic patients), oral stomatitis and pharyngeal infections can be severe and caused by a wide variety of unusual pathogens, including *Mucor* and *Aspergillus*.

Non-infectious pharyngitis

Non-infectious pharyngitis is common and should be considered when a patient notes mild symptoms with a chronic and fluctuant course. Factors that may alone, or in combination, lead to non-infectious pharyngitis include smoking, reflux and postnasal drip. Allergies may also lead to an irritated throat. Oral dryness from chronic nasal obstruction with night-time mouth breathing may also contribute to chronic throat irritation.

Infectious complications

Ludwig's angina

Ludwig's angina is a severe, progressive oropharyngeal infection centered in the floor of mouth and submandibular triangle. It often arises from a tooth or submandibular gland. It can be quickly progressive, spreading through fascial planes rather than through lymphatic pathways. When extending to the floor of the mouth and base of the tongue, tongue elevation may occur and threaten the airway. During the physical examination, the patient may be toxic. Submandibular and submental tenderness and swelling with edema of the floor of the mouth are present. Tongue induration and elevation is a late and worrisome finding suggesting impending airway obstruction. Such infection is usually polymicrobial involving *Streptococcus* or *H. influenzae* and anaerobes. Aggressive treatment must be instituted immediately in the form of intravenous antibiotics. Computerized tomography (CT) scanning will often show no discrete collection. Because of the rapid progression possible with this infection, the clinician must have a low threshold for the decision to perform wide external drainage often with tracheotomy. Complications include airway obstruction, neck abscess and mediastinitis.

Infections that arise from the teeth characteristically track to specific fascial compartments, encompassing and helping to identify the problematic dentition. For example, since the posterior mandibular molar roots extend into the mandible below the mylohyoid muscle insertion, infections of these teeth track to the submandibular gland triangle initially. Infections in the more anterior mandibular dentition are encompassed within the mylohyoid and so initially track to the sublingual space and floor of the mouth. Infections of the maxillary molars track to the masticator space which encompasses the masseter muscle.

Parapharyngeal space infection

The parapharyngeal space extends superiorly from the base of the skull, inferiorly to the hyoid bone. Medially is the superior constrictor of the pharynx, and laterally are the parotid gland, mandible and lateral pterygoid. The parapharyngeal space contains the carotid artery and the jugular vein and cranial nerves IX, X, XI and XII. Infections initially in the tonsil, pharynx, draining lymph nodes, posterior mandibular teeth, or deep lobe of the parotid may result in abscess formation in the parapharyngeal space. The physical examination typically reveals medial displacement of the tonsil tissue and adjacent lateral pharyngeal wall. These changes often lead to the development of a 'hot-potato' voice. Trismus usually occurs, as the pterygoid musculature in the parapharyngeal space is intimately associated with the infection. Evaluation includes CT scanning. Treatment includes external drainage, followed by intravenous antibiotics. Complications of parapharyngeal space infections include jugular vein thrombosis, airway obstruction, carotid rupture, cranial nerve palsies and spread of infection along the carotid sheath to the mediastinum.

Retropharyngeal infection

The retropharyngeal space extends along the anterior surface of the vertebral column from the base of the skull to the mediastinum. Laterally, this space is bounded by the carotid sheath. The retropharyngeal space may be involved in infections of the nasopharynx and oropharynx, and often results from secondary abscess formation in retropharyngeal nodes. Patients will describe dysphagia, odynophagia and cervical rigidity, often with a 'hot-potato' voice. Physical examination may show a posterior oropharynx bulge. Complications include sepsis and spread of infection through fascial planes leading to mediastinitis. Treatment involves drainage usually through an external approach, not transorally, with subsequent intravenous antibiotics. Tracheotomy may be necessary.

BENIGN ORAL LESIONS

Tongue

Among the normal findings of an examination of the mouth and throat might be a short, taut frenulum which, if it is of no inconvenience to the patient and does not affect speech, need not be divided. In the geographic tongue there is an area of smooth red depilated surface with a smooth margin which gradually changes over time. Patients are typically asymptomatic. The cause is unknown, and no treatment is necessary. Median rhomboid glossitis is a rather common finding involving a rhomboid area of depilated tongue surface. It is located in the midline, just anterior to the circumvallate papillae. It is asymptomatic and no treatment is required. This form of glossitis probably represents a chronic atrophic form of candidiasis.

The fissured or scrotal tongue is another common variation in the appearance of the glossal surface. Fissured tongue may be responsible for glossitis in patients with poor oral hygiene, resulting from debris in the fissures. It has also been associated with recurrent facial palsy in Melkersson–Rosenthal syndrome, a triad of facial paralysis, facial edema and fissured tongue.

The coated tongue, common among acutely ill and febrile patients, is due to the accumulation of debris on the dorsum of the tongue secondary to dehydration. It is of no specific diagnostic significance.

The hairy tongue is characterized by marked elongation of filiform papillae and may be blackish or brownish in color. The posterior dorsum of the tongue or posterolateral tongue may be involved. Hairy tongue may be associated with chronic irritation from smoking, nutritional deficiencies or secondary candidal infection. Maintenance of good oral hygiene with this disorder can be troublesome. The tongue needs to be physically cleaned several times a day with a soft even-bristled toothbrush and a solution of half-strength hydrogen peroxide and normal saline. Antibiotics should be discontinued and vitamin supplementation should be considered.

Glossitis, with or without angular cheilosis, manifests as a shiny, smooth, reddish tongue. It may be asymptomatic or result in a sensation of burning. Glossitis can be associated with pernicious anemia, vitamin B_{12} deficiency, iron deficiency (Plummer–Vinson syndrome), riboflavin deficiency or nicotinic acid deficiency. Vitamin C deficiency can cause gingival erythema, edema and bleeding.

Small varicosities are commonly present in the floor of mouth, lateral tongue, base of tongue and vallecula. These are considered normal findings in older patients, and have no clinical significance. They rarely, if ever, bleed. Bleeding vascular lesions may be present in the mouth in patients with Osler–Weber–Rendu or Sturge–Weber syndrome.

Traumatic ulcers of the tongue or buccal mucosa are usually self-evident and are associated with dentures, dental fillings or wires.

Palate

Examination of the roof of the mouth may reveal in the central hard palate a bony, firm and sometimes irregular mass which is asymptomatic. This bony growth, torus palatini, looks like an irregular lesion, but is a benign bony excrescence of the palate, without clinical significance. Patients may not have been aware of it until they look for the first time or feel it. This initial awareness is usually accompanied by anxiety, given the size, firmness and irregularity of the lesion. Similar bony irregular outgrowths of the inner aspect of the parasymphyseal mandible abutting the adjacent floor of the mouth are termed torus mandibulari.

Squamous papilloma (small stalked lesions with distal frond-like extensions) are usually asymptomatic and common in the tonsil fossa apex and soft palate. They can be excised easily in the clinic and tend not to recur.

Buccal mucosa

The 'bite line' is a normal variant that can be mistaken for leukoplakia. It is a horizontal white line, slightly raised, on the buccal mucosa that corresponds to the point of junction of the upper and lower teeth. The buccal mucosa meets the interdigitating dental surface here, generating chronic microtrauma with formation of the 'bite line'. Focal dental trauma to the buccal mucosa can lead to a bite fibroma. This represents a pedunculated, mobile, mucosalized, firm lesion of the buccal mucosa, usually adjacent to the bite line. It is easily excised and infrequently recurs, unless trauma continues.

Fordyce granules represent small, yellow papules in the posterior buccal mucosa and are of no clinical significance.

Gingiva and floor of the mouth

An epulis is any gingival tumor. These may represent benign congenital growths, giant cell reparative granuloma or squamous cell carcinoma. Gingival hyperplasia can occur with chronic use of phenytoin. A ranula is a painless floor-of-mouth cyst arising from the sublingual gland. These may, when extensive, extend into the upper neck and present as a neck mass (plunging ranula).

PIGMENTED ORAL LESIONS

Kaposi's sarcoma may occur in patients with AIDS and is seen as a purplish macular lesion, often on the palate or alveolus. Melanosis represents a normal variant of oral mucosa pigmentation and must be differentiated from true mucosal melanoma. Darkly pigmented lesions may also represent staining of the oral mucosa by dental amalgam. Intoxication from a variety of agents can discolor the oral mucosa. These include bismuth, arsenic, lead, mercury and silver. Kawasaki's disease may present with a reddish 'strawberry tongue'. Polycythemia is a bluish to red discoloration of the oral mucosa and tongue.

INFLAMMATORY LESIONS

Erythema multiforme

Erythema multiforme is characterized by erythematous bullous inflammatory lesions of the skin and mucosa. It is mediated by antigen–antibody complex deposition and may be spontaneous, or represent a hypersensitivity reaction to medication or infection, or may develop in response to stress. The skin and mucosal vesicular bullous lesions show concentric annular erythematous rings ('bull's-eye' pattern). Stevens–Johnson syndrome is a severe systemic form of erythema multiforme. It can be complicated by conjunctival and corneal scarring. Treatment includes discontinuation of the inciting agent, corticosteroids, supportive therapy including hydration and antibiotics to prevent superinfection.

Pemphigus and pemphigoid

Pemphigus vulgaris and pemphigoid often begin as extremely painful oral bullae that quickly burst to form superficial ulcerations with mucosal tags. In pemphigus, oral lesions often precede cutaneous manifestations. Pemphigoid results predominantly in mucosal lesions and occurs in an older age group than pemphigus. Although it is non-fatal, marked mucosal conjunctival scarring may occur. The diagnosis is made through biopsy. Biopsy material should be prepared appropriately for direct and indirect immunofluorescence studies for IgG, IgA, IgM and complement. In pemphigus, there is an intercellular deposition of antiepithelial autoantibodies. This causes the intraepithelial bulla formation characteristic of pemphigus vulgaris. In pemphigoid, autoantibody deposition is found only along the basement membrane. This results in the epithelium separating off the underlying basement membrane, generating the subepithelial bullae characteristic of pemphigoid. Treatment for pemphigoid is with topical and injected steroids. If pemphigoid results in severe symptoms or ocular complications occur, oral steroids, immunosuppressant agents (Cytoxan® (Bristol-Myers Squibb Oncology Division, Princeton, NJ, USA), azathioprine and methotrexate) and sulfones may be used. Treatment for pemphigus vulgaris is typically high-dose oral steroids initially, often combined with immunosuppressive agents.

Behçet's syndrome

Behçet's syndrome is a rare, autoimmune vasculitis. It is seen primarily in the Middle East and Orient. It usually presents in young males with recurrent ulcerations of the mouth and genitalia, inflammatory ocular lesions (uveitis), arthritis and vasculitis.

Reiter's syndrome

Reiter's syndrome is a systemic inflammatory disorder occurring in certain human leukocyte antigen (HLA) types, after exposure to venereal or dysenteric illness. Patients present with arthritis, conjunctivitis and urethritis, as well as mucocutaneous lesions of the penis, mouth, palms and soles. Reiter's syndrome is associated with HLA B27, and has been linked to prior *Chlamydia, Mycoplasma, Shigella, Salmonella, Yersinia* and *Campylobacter* infections.

Mucositis

Oral mucositis is associated with chemotherapy and radiation therapy and manifests with patchy erythema and ulceration, with mucosal slough and fibrinous exudate. Treatment includes gentle cleaning with saline and sodium bicarbonate. Topical agents that may be helpful include a combined mixture of Benadryl® (Pfizer, Morris Plains, NJ, USA), Kaopectate®

(The Upjohn Company, Kalamazoo, MI, USA), Milk of Magnesia and viscous lidocaine. Sucralfate slurry may also be helpful. Systemic pain management is essential.

Lichen planus

The oral lesions of lichen planus are generally whitish and can have a variety of specific morphologies. Lesions typically are evanescent and recurrences may be associated with stress. Histologically, there is lymphocytic infiltration of the basal layers with hyperkeratosis. The reticular form consists of a network of fine, white, lacy striae. The plaque form of lichen planus resembles leukoplakia. Reticular and plaque forms of lichen planus may be asymptomatic. Atrophic, erosive and bullous forms also occur. Erosive forms are usually symptomatic. Erosive forms are thought to increase the risk of development of squamous cell carcinoma. Treatment is symptomatic and may include topical or systemic steroids, retinoids or Dapsone USP (Jacobus Pharmaceutical Co. Inc., Princeton, NJ, USA). The erosive form of lichen planus should be differentiated from pemphigus, pemphigoid, systemic lupus erythematosus (SLE) and erythema multiforme.

Systemic lupus erythematosus

Patients with SLE usually have a positive antinuclear antibodies (ANA) test, and may have a positive lupus erythematosus (LE) cell test. This systemic autoimmune disease may result in arthritis, glomerulonephritis and cardiac, lung and mucocutaneous manifestations. The deposition of antigen–antibody complexes results in mucocutaneous inflammatory lesions, which can be seen as erythematous plaques which tend to ulcerate and often heal with scarring. Immunofluorescence may show IgG deposition in basement membrane. Lesions are treated symptomatically with topical or injected steroid and respond to systemic treatment for SLE (systemic steroids and antimalarials).

Necrotizing sialometaplasia

Necrotizing sialometaplasia presents as a worrisome midline palate ulcer. This represents a benign self-limiting condition which is felt to represent soft tissue reaction to salivary gland ischemia. Any non-healing ulcer in this region should be biopsied to rule out squamous cell carcinoma, adenoid cystic carcinoma of the minor salivary glands of the palate, Wegener's granulomatosis or lethal midline granuloma.

Other inflammatory lesions

Wegener's granulomatosis is a necrotizing granulomatous vasculitis which can affect the upper respiratory tract, lung and kidney. Lesions in the head and neck may occur in the nasal cavity, sinus and laryngopharynx. Lesions in the laryngopharynx are typically granular ulcerations. Diagnosis may be obtained through biopsy and through positive antineutrophilic cytoplasmic antibody (ANCA) blood testing. ANCA may be negative in patients with localized disease. Treatment for Wegener's disease includes steroids and immunosuppressive agents.

Crohn's disease is an inflammatory granulomatous disease of unknown etiology affecting primarily the intestine. Rarely, the oral cavity and the pharynx can be involved, with ulcerative lesions.

Sarcoid is a granulomatous disease characterized by hilar adenopathy, frequently with lung, joint and skin findings. Multiple sites in the head and neck can be involved, including ear, nose, salivary gland, oral cavity and laryngopharynx. Biopsy shows non-caseating granulomata. Treatment includes topical or systemic steroids.

Kawasaki's disease is a systemic vasculitis of unknown etiology. Usually, affected children present with fever, conjunctivitis, cervical adenopathy and rash. The lip, tongue and pharynx may be dry, erythematous and swollen. The tongue in Kawasaki's disease has been described as a 'strawberry tongue'.

Dermatitis herpetiformis is a disorder of unknown etiology that presents in young adults with abnormal intestinal absorption, as well as bulla of the skin and oral cavity.

ORAL AND PHARYNGEAL CANCER

Cancer of the upper aerodigestive tract results in significant morbidity, involving respiration, phonation, deglutition and often significant cosmetic issues. Ninety-five per cent of all oropharyngeal cancers are squamous cell carcinoma. Other malignancies include minor salivary gland carcinoma, lymphoma and melanoma. Heavy smoking and alcohol use are strong historical correlates of squamous cell carcinoma. The risk of squamous cell carcinoma is increased with cigarette, cigar and pipe smoking, as well as with chewing tobacco, snuff and betel nut use. Most oral squamous cell carcinomas develop in areas felt to be regions exposed to pooled carcinogens, including the gingival buccal sulcus, the anterior floor of the mouth, the lateral border of the tongue and the anterior tonsil pillar. Other risk factors which have been associated with squamous cell carcinoma include poor oral hygiene, dental trauma, human papilloma virus and chronic reflux. Patients with Plummer–Vinson syndrome have an increased risk of the development of postcricoid squamous cell carcinoma. The overall prognosis of squamous cell carcinoma is poor, with a 50% five-year survival for all patients with oral and pharyngeal cancer. The prognosis declines in patients with larger tumors and tumors with greater invasion, and survival is halved in patients who have metastatic cervical adenopathy. Clearly then, early detection represents a significant goal. Most patients have clear-cut progressive head and neck symptoms and often have identifiable oropharyngeal lesions. Unfortunately, despite the easy visibility of the oral cavity, many lesions are not detected until advanced, especially in patients with significant alcohol use.

Leukoplakia

Leukoplakia is a raised, sharply demarcated whitish patch on the oral mucosa. It may occur as a result of chronic mucosal irritation due to tobacco or alcohol use, or due to poor oral hygiene or dental appliances. Histologically, leukoplakia usually demonstrates epithelial hyperplasia and hyperkeratosis. However, varying degrees of atypia may be present. In fact, leukoplakic lesions may vary from being completely benign to frankly invasive squamous cell carcinoma. Lesions with atypia may become squamous cell carcinoma in the future and therefore represent premalignant lesions. Leukoplakic lesions not directly referable to local irritation which do not resolve with close follow-up are excised. When leukoplakic areas remain after biopsy, oral vitamin A derivatives have been used with good response although toxicity may occur. Repeat excision is necessary for all non-responding lesions. Erythroplakia is a raised, velvety, reddish lesion which has a higher risk than leukoplakia of underlying malignancy, and therefore should be excised when identified. Hairy leukoplakia has been associated with HIV infection, and occurs usually on the dorsum or posterolateral aspect of the tongue. It is felt to be related to chronic Epstein–Barr virus epithelial stimulation with secondary candidiasis. Such lesions may respond to acyclovir, but may recur after cessation of treatment and should prompt HIV testing.

Physical examination

A complete head and neck examination, including mirror or fiberoptic laryngoscopy, is essential. The emphasis is on detecting asymmetry and focal mucosal lesions. Squamous cell carcinoma can often be seen as either a leukoplakic patch, ulcerative lesion (characteristically with heaped-up margins) or as a granular non-mucosalized exophytic mass. Palpation helps to identify the infiltrative margins which can exist significantly beyond the visible lesion. This is especially true in the tongue. Trismus implies malignant infiltration of pterygoid musculature. A 'hot-potato' voice implies mass-like deformation of the palate or posterior oropharynx. A gurgling-type phonation implies hypopharyngeal salivary pooling which may result from esophageal inlet obstruction. The posterolateral tongue, base of tongue and hypopharynx are often difficult areas to examine. Patients with lesions in these areas may present with referred otalgia. The clinician should be persistent in the evaluation of a smoker who has otalgia with a normal ear examination. In such circumstances, there should be a low threshold to referral to otolaryngology. Patients with head and neck squamous cell carcinoma may present with a neck metastasis, and therefore careful examination of the neck is mandatory. Midline cancers (e.g. those arising from the midline base of tongue) may spread to both sides of the neck.

Work-up of head and neck cancer

Tumors of the oral cavity, pharynx and hypopharynx, as elsewhere in the head and neck, are staged according to the TNM staging system. Tumors are assigned a T score 1–4 based mainly on size and invasive characteristics. The N score describes regional cervical nodal involvement. The M score describes the presence of distant metastasis. The depth of invasion, age of patient and co-morbidities, although important, are not taken into account with this system. After a complete head and neck examination, radiographic evaluation is often done. This may involve computerized tomography (CT) or magnetic resonance imaging (MRI) scan of the oral cavity and neck. Such studies may be helpful to determine the extent of the lesion and are typically performed with T2 tumors or greater. CT and MRI help to delineate the extent of the primary tumor, and also allow for search for cervical adenopathy. In general, lymph nodes greater than 1 cm or those with central necrosis are considered suspicious for harboring metastatic disease. A Panorex plain film can be obtained if there is a question of mandibular involvement. Barium swallow can help to delineate the extent of the tumor and can also be helpful in searching for a second esophageal primary. A chest X-ray is usually obtained to rule out metastatic disease and also to search for a second primary. Liver function tests and calcium estimation are often performed.

The next step in the evaluation for head and neck cancer involves panendoscopy and biopsy. Five to 10 per cent of patients with an existing head and neck primary squamous cell carcinoma have a synchronous malignancy in the upper aerodigestive tract. Panendoscopy in the form of examination under anesthesia of the oral cavity and neck, direct laryngoscopy, esophagoscopy and bronchoscopy are, therefore, required in most cases. Neck masses can be evaluated with fine needle aspiration in the clinic preoperatively. Endoscopy allows for the appropriate staging of the tumor, and for obtaining definitive biopsy material.

After staging endoscopy and biopsy information is available, discussions with the patient regarding treatment are initiated. Typically, treatment for oral and pharyngeal malignancies involve surgery and/or radiation therapy. Chemotherapy is an adjunctive treatment and does not represent a primary modality. Because of the complexity and morbidity of surgery and X-ray therapy, a team approach is useful in the treatment of the patient with a head and neck cancer. The team includes speech and swallowing therapy, dentistry and oral prosthesis experts, and nutritionists, in addition to a head and neck surgeon, radiation oncologist and medical oncologist. Prior to treatment, nutritional assessment is essential. Typically, patients with oral and pharyngeal malignancies have had poor oral intake for many months and are nutritionally depleted.

Generally, small tumors (T1, T2) can be treated with surgery or radiation therapy, whereas larger tumors (T3, T4) are treated with both. Often, in patients treated with both modalities, surgery is often offered first so that the decision to treat the field with radiation therapy can be influenced by the surgical pathology. Radiation therapy is most effective when tumors are exophytic rather than infiltrative or ulcerative. For patients with clinically positive necks, surgery is considered necessary in the form of neck dissection. Neck dissection is also contemplated for patients who are staged as N0 if the risk of microscopic disease is greater than 20–30%. Floor of mouth, base of tongue and pyriform sinus are sites associated with a high rate of occult metastasis at presentation. A CT scan of the neck which is read as negative should not necessarily lead one to conclude a neck dissection is not warranted if the patient's primary is associated with a high rate of occult cervical metastasis. Complications of radiation therapy include xerostomia, loss of taste, soft tissue ulceration and osteoradionecrosis of the mandible. Hyperbaric oxygen has been found invaluable to prevent and treat severe radiation-induced complications. There have been significant surgical advances in the complete and safe resection of tumors and reconstruction of the oral cavity and pharynx. Advances include improved preoperative radiographic assessment of the tumor, and appropriate preoperative emphasis on dental and nutrition issues, including alimentation via gastric tube. Intraoperative advances include neural monitoring for neural preservation, improved carotid artery coverage through skin flap design and flap coverage, and introduction of modified and selective neck dissections where appropriate. Postoperative protocols incorporate close follow-up, radiographic surveillance and attention to the potential development of radiation-induced hypothyroidism. Reconstructive options include primary closure, split thickness skin graft, regional pedicled flap closure (e.g. pectoralis major flap) or microvascular free tissue which can include bone (e.g. fibular free flap). Significant improvements in speech and swallowing therapy and prosthetics have improved the quality of life for patients postoperatively. New and exciting developments include the prevention of second primaries with retinoids, as well as advances in photodynamic therapy.

Non-squamous cell neoplasia

Other malignancies occurring in the head and neck include minor salivary gland carcinoma, lymphoma and melanoma. Minor salivary gland carcinoma typically presents as a focal ulcerative mass, often in the palate. This usually represents adeno- or mucoepidermoid carcinoma. Lymphoma typically presents in the tonsil or base of tongue. Patients with asymptomatic asymmetric tonsils have a 6% incidence of lymphoma. Malignant melanoma may present in the nasal or oral mucosa. Mucosal melanoma has a worse prognosis than its cutaneous counterpart. Pigmented lesions may also represent benign melanosis or dental amalgam stain. Kaposi's sarcoma presents as a purplish lesion on the alveolus or palate in patients with AIDS. Parapharyngeal space masses, when large enough, may be evident on physical examination with bulging of the posterolateral oropharynx wall or medial displacement of the tonsil. Such parapharyngeal space masses typically represent deep lobe parotid pleomorphic adenomas, neurogenic tumors (including schwannomas, neurofibromas and paragangliomas) or lymphomas. Lingual thyroid presents as a mass in the midline base of the tongue resulting from arrest of thyroid migration (see Chapter 17). Lingual thyroid may present with respiratory distress, globus sensation or dysphagia, or may be asymptomatic. Treatment usually includes suppressive T4 treatment, or I^{131} ablative treatment. Surgical options are available. Surgery is preferred if malignancy is suspected.

PHARYNGEAL PAIN

Severe throat pain which is not infectious should prompt search for neoplastic disease. This is especially true for pain in the posterior tongue, vallecula, epiglottis and pyriform sinus. Evaluation may include initially a full head and neck examination, occasionally CT scanning and examination under anesthesia with endoscopy.

Pharyngeal burns

Occasionally patients, particularly those with dentures, will develop traumatic pharyngitis secondary to eating hot food. This can result either in a first- or second-degree burn of the posterior pharynx, often in the arytenoid area of the posterior larynx. It is here that hot food is held as the patient decides whether to spit it out, cough or swallow. Patients with burns complain of pain when swallowing and the sensation of a pharyngeal mass due to local edema. In most cases, there is no compromise of the airway. Clear liquids are helpful. Antibiotics and steroids may be necessary for unusually severe burns.

Foreign body

A small foreign body embedded in mucosal musculature of the hypopharynx can result in chronic pain generated by swallowing. As with pharyngeal burns, this occurs more commonly in elderly patients who wear dentures. Small foreign bodies, particularly fish bones, may be difficult to see, and the examining physician should look as much for an area of inflammation as for an actual foreign body. Often a foreign body passes, leaving an abrasion of the pharynx, but because of residual pain the patient will complain of a foreign body. If the patient is able to localize a specific point of pain, and if the examiner is unable to see a foreign body or area of inflammation, a reasonable approach to the problem would be to ask the patient to return in 12–24 hours. If the pain is secondary to an abrasion from a foreign body, it will have cleared. If the foreign body is, indeed, present, there should be some increased inflammation and pain surrounding it, and further diagnostic tests can be undertaken. These tests may include plain films, a barium swallow or CT scan, particularly for those areas that are poorly visualized directly. Endoscopy may be necessary for direct examination and removal of foreign body.

Glossopharyngeal neuralgia

Patients with glossopharyngeal neuralgia experience spasms of very severe, unilateral, boring pharyngeal pain, usually transient, lasting seconds, often triggered by a specific pharyngeal movement such as yawning or swallowing in a certain way. The pain is centered in the base of the tongue, soft palate and tonsil fossa, often radiating deeply to the ear. It occurs most commonly in middle-aged or elderly patients and the cause is unknown. The treatment for persistent cases is sectioning of the glossopharyngeal nerve, if medical treatment is ineffective.

Eagle syndrome

Eagle syndrome is an unusual disorder felt to occur as a result of a long or calcified styloid process or stylohyoid muscle tendonitis. It may occur as a result of scarring post-tonsillectomy. Pain is usually experienced in the tonsillar fossa with radiation to the ear and may flare with swallowing. Pain can be reproduced by palpating the styloid process and scar in the tonsillar fossa. The treatment includes anti-inflammatory medication. Surgical resection of the styloid process through the tonsillar bed can be performed if medical management is ineffective.

Carotidynia

Carotidynia is an idiopathic disorder involving neck pain centered in the carotid bulb region radiating to the ipsilateral ear. Pain can be reproduced by pressing on the carotid bifurcation. Treatment options include non-steroidal anti-inflammatory medication or a short course of steroids. Carotidynia has also been treated by anticonvulsant and migraine medications.

Musculoskeletal cervical pain

A number of musculoskeletal disorders including cervical arthritis and cervical disc disease, which are associated with cervical muscular spasm, can lead to chronic neck pain. A clear-cut history will identify such patients as having neck and not throat pain.

Atypical angina

In patients where there is no other explanation for chronic neck or jaw pain, atypical angina should be considered. Cardiac pain may radiate to the jaw, throat and neck.

TRISMUS

Inability to open the jaw, trismus, may be caused by a variety of different disorders. Severe temporomandibular joint pain, often associated with previous mandibular or facial trauma, may result in trismus. Dental infections and peritonsillar or parapharyngeal abscesses may result in pterygoid muscular spasm and produce trismus. In these circumstances, trismus implies spread of oral infection and should result in prompt referral. Oral, pharynx and base of skull tumors, through pterygoid muscular malignant infiltration, may also produce trismus. Trismus may be produced by tetanus, rabies or other neurologic disorders.

DRY MOUTH (XEROSTOMIA)

Dry mouth (xerostomia) is commonly caused by chronic nasal obstruction and obligatory mouth breathing. Patients will awake thirsty several times during the night. Correction of the nasal obstruction, usually performed surgically by straightening the nasal septum and reducing hypertrophied turbinate tissue, will correct the dry mouth. Dry mouth may also be caused by many medicines, including decongestants, appetite suppressants, antiemetics, diuretics, antispasmodics, antidepressants, tranquilizers, antipsychotic medications, antidiarrheal medications, non-steroidal anti-inflammatory drugs, certain antihypertensives and antihistamines. Patients with collagen vascular disorders (e.g. scleroderma), as well as patients who have received radiation therapy, may also develop xerostomia.

Sjögren's syndrome

Sjögren's syndrome is an autoimmune disease manifested by intermittent lacrimal and salivary gland enlargement (most commonly the parotid), rheumatoid arthritis, keratoconjunctivitis sicca and xerostomia. In patients with dry eyes and arthritis, a complaint of xerostomia should lead to consideration of Sjögren's syndrome. Secondary Sjögren's syndrome is associated with rheumatoid arthritis and lupus erythematosus, while primary Sjögren's syndrome occurs in isolation without a systemic inflammatory disease. Characteristic autoantibodies may be present (SSA and SSB). SSA and SSB are usually present in primary Sjögren's syndrome, while SSA is usually absent in secondary Sjögren's syndrome. Rheumatoid factor, antinuclear antibody and anti-double-stranded DNA may be present.

Although keratoconjunctivitis sicca is the most common symptom of Sjögren's syndrome, xerostomia is the most troubling. A sialogram may demonstrate a characteristic non-obstructive sialectasia. Biopsy of salivary gland tissue (usually minor salivary gland from inside the lip or parotid tail biopsy) typically demonstrates ductal dilatation, periductal infiltrates of lymphocytes and atrophy of acini. Carious destruction of teeth and halitosis are serious consequences of reduced salivary flow. Treatment of xerostomia is symptomatic and involves the following measures: increased fluid intake; sialagogues such as tea with lemon and sugarless hard candy, as well as mouth moisturizers; massage of the glands to keep saliva flowing and to clear plugs from the ducts; and vigorous dental care. Careful surveillance of patients is necessary, given the increased risk of development of salivary gland lymphoma in patients with Sjögren's syndrome.

NON-ULCERATIVE DISORDERS

Burning tongue syndrome

Burning tongue syndrome occurs most commonly in the middle-aged and elderly, especially postmenopausal women, and can be difficult to correct. Local factors, including caries, gingivitis and chronic atrophic candidiasis should be considered. Burning tongue may be a symptom of vitamin deficiency-induced glossitis (including iron, nicotinic acid, B_{12} and folate). One should also consider if the symptoms relate to a specific food, oral medicine or topical medicine such as a specific denture gel or over-the-counter mouthwash.

Treatment options include daily multivitamins, half-strength Milk of Magnesia mouthwashes three times daily, cessation of excessive over-the-counter treatments and consideration of a course of an antifungal agent.

Halitosis

Halitosis can be caused by many different entities, and can be difficult to correct. It may be caused by local or regional infections including dental and gingival infections. It may also be associated with xerostomia. Nasopharyngitis, sinusitis with postnasal drip, ozena, infected nasopharynx cyst, nasal foreign body and pulmonary infections or neoplasia may be associated with halitosis. Patients with tonsillar debris with cryptic tonsillitis, reflux or Zenker's diverticulum may also be affected with halitosis. Certain foods and alcohol can result in bad breath. Halitosis may also reflect certain metabolic disorders. Uremia may lead to a urine-like breath, while diabetic ketoacidosis breath smells like acetone. The breath of a patient with hepatic encephalopathy is described as 'mousy'. In psychogenic halitosis, patients feel that their breath is foul, though others cannot note any abnormality.

13

Hoarseness and the larynx

Gregory W. Randolph

Anatomy and physiology of the larynx
Clinical evaluation
   Acute laryngitis
   Chronic laryngitis
   Reflux
   Hyperfunctional voice disorders
   Polyploid corditis
   Vocal cord polyps
   Vocal cord nodules
   Vocal cord hemorrhage
   Arytenoid granuloma
   Sulcus vocalis
   Laryngeal conversion disorders
   Laryngeal hemangiomas
   Laryngeal cysts
   Laryngeal papillomatosis
   Cricoarytenoid arthritis
   Sarcoid
   Systemic lupus erythematosus
   Wegener's granulomatosis
   Pemphigus
   Relapsing polychondritis
   Laryngospasm
   Laryngotracheal bronchitis
   Laryngeal diphtheria
   Tuberculosis
   Laryngeal candidiasis
   Other mycotic infections of the larynx
      Histoplasmosis
      Coccidioidomycosis

      Paracoccidioidomycosis
      Blastomycosis
    Chondroradionecrosis
    Neurologic disorders
    Spasmodic dysphonia
    Vocal cord paralysis
    Bilateral vocal cord paralysis
    Treatment of vocal cord paralysis
    Superior laryngeal nerve paralysis
    Laryngeal trauma
    Laryngeal cancer
      Leukoplakia
    Approach to laryngeal carcinoma
      Carcinoma *in situ*
      Glottic carcinoma
      Supraglottic carcinoma
      Subglottic carcinoma
Laryngeal surgery
  Microlaryngoscopy
  Tracheotomy and tracheostomy
  Tracheal cannulation
  Cricothyroidotomy
  Total laryngectomy
  Supraglottic laryngectomy
  Hemilaryngectomy
  Supracricoid laryngectomy
  Near-total laryngectomy

ANATOMY AND PHYSIOLOGY OF THE LARYNX

The larynx has three main functions: voice production, sphincteric protection of the airway and production of cough. Voice is generated as exhaled air interacts with the bilateral vocal cords, and is further modified in the throat, nose and mouth. During swallowing, laryngeal elevation, epiglottic deflection and false and true cord closure protect the tracheobronchial tree from ingested materials. Cough is generated through appropriate glottic closure, allowing the creation of transient increased intrathoracic and intra-abdominal pressure. Rapid glottic opening facilitates upward movement of tracheal air and effective cough. Similarly, glottic closure is necessary for lifting, straining and defecation.

The larynx is adjacent to the anterior hypopharynx from the base of the tongue to the upper cervical trachea (Figures 13.1 and 13.2). It is composed of two main cartilages, the thyroid and cricoid cartilages. These can be considered to be two elaborate, evolved tracheal rings. The thyroid cartilage is shield-like. Its superior midline notch is referred to as the 'Adam's apple'. The thyroid cartilage encircles the laryngeal lumen as well as the lateral mucosal recesses, the pyriform sinuses. Below the thyroid cartilage is the second main laryngeal cartilage, the cricoid. The shape of the cricoid is like a ring with the band being anterior and its flat broad plate oriented posteriorly. The cricoid ring represents the only point along the airway where cartilage completely encircles the airway. This subglottic region represents a fixed and narrow point in the airway. Stenosis may form if this region is damaged, as can occur with prolonged endotracheal tube intubation from cuff-induced subglottic injury. Two small pyramidal cartilages, the arytenoids, are sited on the upper edge of the posterior plate of the cricoid. Anteriorly in the midline, from the inner aspect of the thyroid cartilage, arises the epiglottis. The epiglottis extends posterosuperiorly, rising above the level of the vocal cords, and extending into the hypopharynx. Posterolaterally, the epiglottis is continuous with the aryepiglottic folds, which extend posteriorly to the arytenoids. Within the two aryepiglottic folds is the endolarynx, which directly surrounds and forms the laryngeal airway. The false and true vocal cords project into the airway lumen, with false cords superior to true cords. The lateral recess between these folds is termed the ventricle. The ventricle has a small anterior diverticulum, the saccule. On mirror examination, the false and true cords appear as bands. The true vocal cord is approximately 15 mm long. It extends from the inner aspect of the thyroid cartilage in the midline posteriorly to insert on the vocal process of the arytenoid cartilage. The

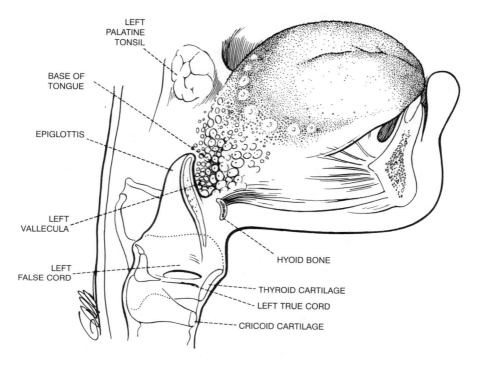

Figure 13.1 Relationship between the larynx and the base of the tongue. The pyriform sinus, vallecula, false cord and true cords can be seen

anterior two-thirds of the cord is membranous, and the posterior one-third is cartilaginous, formed by the vocal process of the arytenoid. The vocal cords arise from the inner aspect of the thyroid cartilage, approximately halfway down the vertical height of the thyroid cartilage.

The laryngopharynx is covered for the most part by respiratory pseudostratified ciliated columnar epithelium. Stratified squamous non-keratinizing epithelium covers the vocal cord, pyriform sinus and lingual surface of the epiglottis. Deep to the vocal cord epithelium lies the vocal ligament, which covers the underlying core of the vocal cord, the thyroarytenoid muscle. The vocal ligament represents the upper free edge of the conus elasticus, a cone-shaped elastic membrane that arises from the cricoid and extends superiorly to the vocal cords.

Lateral to the aryepiglottic folds, but still within the confines of the lateral thyroid cartilage laminae, are the pyriform sinuses (Figures 13.1 and 13.2). The medial wall of the pyriform sinus is the aryepiglottic fold, and the

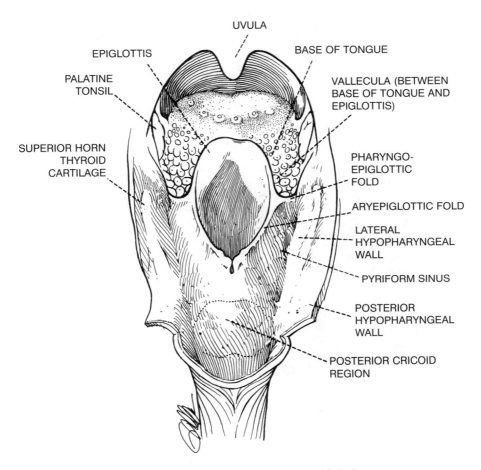

Figure 13.2 Posterior view, showing the base of the tongue and the larynx

lateral wall is the mucosa which covers the medial aspect of the lamina of the thyroid cartilage. The vallecula is the recess formed by the sloping base of the tongue anteriorly and the lingual surface of the epiglottis posteriorly. The pharyngeal segment extending from the base of the tongue superiorly to the cricopharyngeal esophageal inlet inferiorly is termed the hypopharynx. It is divided into the posterior pharyngeal wall, the pyriform sinuses and the postcricoid region (the mucosa that covers the posterior cricoid).

The larynx (Figure 13.3) is divided into three regions relative to the level of the vocal cords: the supraglottis, the glottis and the subglottis. The supraglottis encompasses the area above the vocal cords and includes the epiglottis, false cords, aryepiglottic folds and arytenoids. The glottis

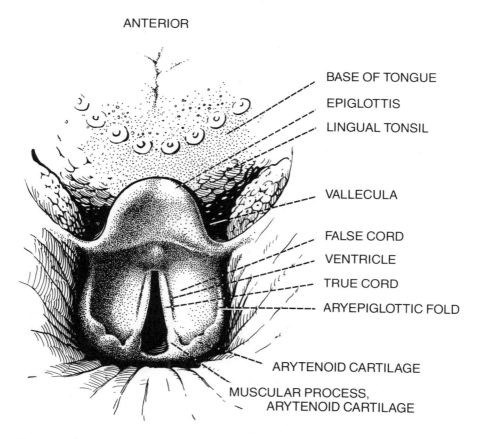

ANTERIOR

BASE OF TONGUE

EPIGLOTTIS

LINGUAL TONSIL

VALLECULA

FALSE CORD

VENTRICLE

TRUE CORD

ARYEPIGLOTTIC FOLD

ARYTENOID CARTILAGE

MUSCULAR PROCESS,
ARYTENOID CARTILAGE

Figure 13.3   The surface anatomy of a normal larynx viewed from above, demonstrating the base of the tongue, the epiglottis, lingual tonsil, vallecula, false cord, ventricle, true cord, aryepiglottic fold, arytenoid cartilage and the muscular process of the arytenoid cartilage

includes the vocal cords and the region immediately below the vocal cords. The glottis is the space between the vocal cords. The subglottis is the region starting 1 cm below the vocal cords and ending in the upper cervical trachea. Just below the inferior edge of the cricoid, the arytenoid cartilages are small, paired pyramidal cartilages that share a synovial joint with the posterior lamina of the cricoid. The muscle of the true vocal cord inserts into the vocal process of the arytenoid. The arytenoid cartilage rotates (i.e. swivels) on the cricoid. The vocal cords are drawn laterally or medially, depending on the direction of arytenoid rotation. The posterior cricoarytenoid muscle, the main laryngeal abductor, arises from the posterior cricoid and inserts on the arytenoid cartilage's muscular process. With this orientation, its contraction causes lateral rotation of the arytenoid cartilage, and therefore abduction of the vocal cord. The lateral cricoarytenoid muscle arises from the lateral cricoid cartilage and inserts onto the muscular process of the arytenoid. Its contraction causes medial rotation of the arytenoid, causing medial movement (adduction) of the vocal cord. Two paired cartilages, the cuneiform and the corniculate, are found just above the arytenoid as small nodular features of the posterior aspect of the bilateral aryepiglottic folds, but are without clear-cut function. The thyroid, cricoid and arytenoid cartilages consist of hyaline cartilage and calcify to some degree with age.

Aside from the posterior cricoarytenoid and the lateral cricoarytenoid muscles already mentioned, intrinsic laryngeal muscles include the thyroary-tenoid or vocalis muscle. This muscle extends from the inner surface of the thyroid cartilage anteriorly to the vocal process of the arytenoid posteriorly. This muscle constitutes the bulk of the vocal cord's substance. Its tension regulates vocal tone. It is considered a vocal cord tensor. The cricothyroid muscle is found on the external laryngeal framework, extend-ing from the anterior cricoid to the anterolateral thyroid cartilage's lower edge. Its contraction tilts the thyroid cartilage forward relative to the cricoid and, along with the thyroarytenoid, serves as a vocal cord tensor. As noted above, the posterior cricoarytenoid muscle serves as the main vocal cord abductor, and the lateral cricoarytenoid muscles as the main vocal cord adductor. Vocal cord adduction is also served by another laryngeal intrinsic muscle, the interarytenoid muscle. Extrinsic laryngeal muscles include the strap muscles (omohyoid, sternohyoid, sternothyroid and thyrohyoid), as well as the stylohyoid, digastric, mylohyoid and middle and inferior pharyngeal constrictors. Extrinsic laryngeal muscles are important in regulating laryngeal motion during deglutition.

The hyoid bone straddles the space between the mandible above and the larynx below. The hyoid and larynx are connected in part through the strap muscles. The hyoid is in turn suspended in part by the suprahyoid musculature. This complex muscular system allows for highly co-ordinated movement of the tongue, hyoid and larynx with deglutition. During this movement, the larynx moves forwards and upwards. One can palpate the laryngeal elevation during swallowing. Tracheotomy can impact on swallow-ing in part by tethering the larynx to the skin and decreasing the impor-tant upward gliding motion with deglutition. The thyroid, and nodules within it which are fixed to the laryngotracheal complex, will elevate with swallowing while regional lymph nodes do not.

Laryngeal lymphatic drainage is primarily to middle and inferior jugular chain nodal beds and to pretracheal nodes. The lymphatic drainage of the vocal cords proper is limited. This is why vocal cord malignancies do not metastasize to cervical lymph nodes early in their development.

Innervation of the laryngopharynx is through the vagus nerve. All intrinsic musculature of the larynx is innervated by the recurrent laryngeal nerves except for the cricothyroid, which is innervated by the external branch of the superior laryngeal nerve. Additional motor function to the lower pharynx and upper esophagus is provided by direct pharyngeal branches. The recurrent laryngeal nerves branch from the vagus nerve in the upper chest and re-enter the neck in the thoracic inlet and extend to the larynx, traveling in or near the tracheoesophageal groove. The recurrent laryngeal nerve on the right travels around the right subclavian and on the left around the arch of the aorta (Figure 13.4). Sensory function at and above the cords is mediated by the superior laryngeal nerve. The superior laryngeal nerve arises from the vagus in the superior neck and extends to the larynx by piercing the thyrohyoid membrane, which runs between the thyroid cartilage inferiorly and the hyoid bone superiorly. In this way, the superior laryngeal nerve innervates the supraglottis. Sensory function below the level of the cords is mediated through the recurrent laryngeal nerve. The vagus nerve receives sensory input from the external auditory canal as well as the hypopharynx; thus, ear cleaning can provoke cough, and otalgia can be caused by cancer in the hypopharynx.

Phonation occurs as a result of the true vocal cords' interaction with the exhaled column of air from the lungs. This interaction results in the development of a true vocal cord mucosal wave. This mucosal wave can be thought of as an oscillating epithelial flutter of the vocal cord mucosa relative to deeper vocal cord structures (thyroarytenoid muscle and vocal ligament). The mucosal wave is modified by the muscular tone of the cord itself and other laryngeal intrinsics impacting on the cords in order to produce voice. The nearly approximated bilateral true vocal cords then oscillate as air moves through the glottis. The pitch is controlled by changes in the length of the vocal cords and the tension of the overlying mucosa. Loudness is proportional to subglottic pressures. Voice is then resonated in the pharynx and nose and articulated by fine motor control of the tongue and lips. A patient with a cleft palate may have normal vocal cord function, but because of the palatal defect will have a voice that has a hypernasal resonance. So, too, the dysarthric patient may have normal vocal cord function, but abnormal articulation, for example, because of neurologic dysfunction of the tongue or lips.

a

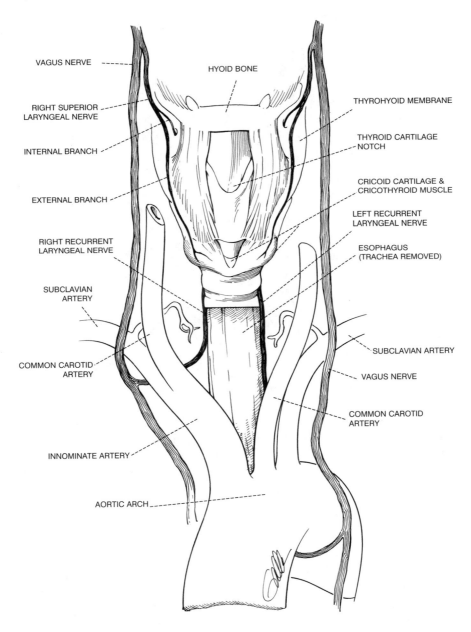

VAGUS NERVE

HYOID BONE

THYROHYOID MEMBRANE

RIGHT SUPERIOR
LARYNGEAL NERVE

THYROID CARTILAGE
NOTCH

INTERNAL BRANCH

CRICOID CARTILAGE &
CRICOTHYROID MUSCLE

EXTERNAL BRANCH

LEFT RECURRENT
LARYNGEAL NERVE

RIGHT RECURRENT
LARYNGEAL NERVE

ESOPHAGUS
(TRACHEA REMOVED)

SUBCLAVIAN
ARTERY

SUBCLAVIAN ARTERY

COMMON CAROTID
ARTERY

VAGUS NERVE

COMMON CAROTID
ARTERY

INNOMINATE ARTERY

AORTIC ARCH

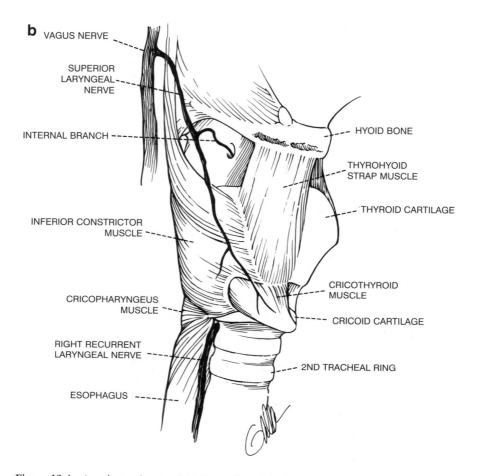

b VAGUS NERVE

SUPERIOR LARYNGEAL NERVE

INTERNAL BRANCH

INFERIOR CONSTRICTOR MUSCLE

CRICOPHARYNGEUS MUSCLE

RIGHT RECURRENT LARYNGEAL NERVE

ESOPHAGUS

HYOID BONE

THYROHYOID STRAP MUSCLE

THYROID CARTILAGE

CRICOTHYROID MUSCLE

CRICOID CARTILAGE

2ND TRACHEAL RING

Figure 13.4 (*see also previous page*) (a) Front view of the laryngopharynx, demonstrating the bilateral superior layngeal nerves, external branch of the superior laryngeal nerves, recurrent laryngeal nerves and vagus bilaterally. (b) Lateral view

CLINCAL EVALUATION

Because of the potential for persistent hoarseness representing an early vocal cord cancer, any patient with a complaint of hoarseness for more than 2 weeks demands complete otolaryngologic and head and neck examination. During the history taking, the specific qualities of the voice disorder should be elicited. Its duration and pattern of onset (e.g. sudden, or gradually progressive) should be noted. Any potential triggering factors should be investigated; these include vocal abuse, concurrent upper respiratory tract infection or exposure to known allergens or toxins. A history of other head and neck symptoms that may occur with hoarseness, especially in the setting of a head and neck malignancy, should be elicited; these include respiratory distress, stridor, cough, hemoptysis, ear or throat pain, dysphagia, odynophagia (pain with swallowing) and weight loss. Additional important points include a history of smoking or alcohol use, which dramatically increases the index of suspicion for squamous cell carcinoma of the larynx in a patient with persistent hoarseness. The patient should be asked about reflux symptomatology and be questioned regarding the normal patterns of vocal use. The bartender, soccer coach and professional singer all have very different patterns of vocal use. Such information is crucial in the management of these patients. A history of past surgery of the thyroid, neck, base of skull or chest should be elicited. Cough is commonly associated with hoarseness. Cough can be due to a number of different etiologies, ranging from various forms of pneumonitis to sinusitis (with postnasal drip), cough variant asthma, reflux, subglottic stenosis or foreign body of the airway.

Disorders in the area of the laryngopharynx and esophagus may cause referred ipsilateral otalgia through cranial nerves IX and X. The most common causes are neoplasms of the epiglottis, pyriform sinus and post-cricoid area. In advanced neoplastic disease, otalgia is considered a negative prognostic sign, because it suggests deep invasion. In a patient complaining of otalgia with a normal ear examination, a careful history should be taken for disorders of the laryngopharynx. A careful examination of the laryngopharynx is performed, particularly of the laryngeal surface of the epiglottis, pyriform sinus and postcricoid region. Appropriate studies, including a barium swallow and computerized tomography (CT) scan of the larynx and neck, are usually not performed unless there is positive symptomatology or unless a physician has a high index of suspicion for disorders in this area.

The quality of the voice must be assessed and documented. Any voice abnormality at all is often referred to as 'hoarseness'; however, voice can be abnormal in many different ways. An attempt should be made to define the exact phonatory disorder. Such observations on the voice may provide diagnostic clues. Is the voice coarse, rough, gravelly or husky, as we might expect if the medial phonatory surface of the vocal cord were irregular? Such vocal cord surface irregularity could be due to an early vocal cord malignancy or to the effect of benign polyploid degeneration. Is the voice weak and breathy, as in unilateral true vocal cord paralysis, where there is persistent glottic patency during phonation with air escape? Is the voice 'wet', gurgling, full or 'hot potato'-like, as with a peritonsillar abscess or a supraglottic tumor mass with supraglottic salivary pooling? Is there is loss of vocal ranges, with weakness and cracking of the voice? Such voice abnormality may occur with the excessive vocal strain of muscular tension dysphonia. Is there an intermittent whispered quality to the voice or complete aphonia, as can be present with psychogenic dysphonia? In the evaluation of such patients, an assessment of respiratory pattern, rate and comfort should also be made.

The physical examination of the larynx is the most important component of the hoarse patient's evaluation. Indiscriminate non-targeted radiographic evaluation is relatively insensitive in the detection of laryngeal pathology and is certainly not a substitute for the physical examination. The physical examination may be performed by indirect laryngoscopy with a mirror in the posterior oropharynx. The skill of the examiner and the gag reflex of the patient will impact on the quality of the examination. A headmirror is used, reflecting light from a source behind the patient's head and allowing the examiner two free hands. The head of the patient is moved slightly forward in a sniffing position and the tongue is pulled forward with gauze. The patient is instructed to breathe through the mouth; the laryngeal mirror, after being warmed to reduce fogging, is introduced into the posterior oropharynx. The mirror is extended posterior to the base of the tongue, slowly back into the uvula and midline soft palate, to reveal the laryngopharynx. The patient is instructed to say 'ee', which brings the vocal cords together. The patient can be instructed to sniff, to bring the two vocal cords apart. Topical anesthetics can be used to facilitate indirect laryngoscopy. Fiberoptic laryngoscopy is an excellent method of laryngeal examination and potentially allows a more prolonged and relaxed examination than that available with the mirror. Fiberoptic laryngoscopy is typically performed with a thin-gauge flexible fiberoptic scope threaded in through the nose after topical nasal anesthesia is provided. The flexible head of the scope is angled downwards behind the palate to visualize the laryngopharynx from the nasopharynx. Formal video strobe laryngoscopy can be performed through the flexible or rigid scopes. Such examination allows detailed information to be gathered regarding the fine details of the mucosal wave of the vocal cord. In selected patients, general anesthesia and direct laryngoscopy can be performed. This allows the most complete laryngeal examination. For example, the pyriform sinus, which can be only partially examined in an awake patient, can be fully examined with direct laryngoscopy. The laryngoscope can also be stabilized by being placed into suspension, and a microscope can be brought in to facilitate a detailed examination. Also, biopsy material can be obtained. With all types of laryngeal examination, the mucosa of the vallecula, epiglottis (lingual and laryngeal surface), supraglottis (false vocal cords, ventricle, aryepiglottic folds, arytenoids), hypopharynx (postcricoid region, posterior hypopharynx wall, pyriform sinuses) and true vocal cords should be closely evaluated for surface or submucosal abnormalities. In addition, vocal cord motion should be assessed, as well as degree of laryngeal or hypopharyngeal pooling of saliva.

The main diagnostic entities as well as the specific structural lesions associated with hoarseness are now reviewed. It should be understood that the vocal cord is subject to a variety of external influences including inhaled allergens, cigarette smoke and medicines, as well as internal factors including reflux, vocal strain and hormonal milieu.

Acute laryngitis

Any disruption to the true vocal cord surface and motion can cause voice disorder. Acute laryngitis represents a common and self-limiting condition, usually associated with either a viral upper respiratory tract infection or acute vocal strain. When occurring as part of an upper respiratory tract infection, hoarseness may be associated with rhinorrhea, cough and mild sore throat. When associated with acute vocal strain such as screaming at a football game, submucosal vocal cord hemorrhage results in vocal cord edema and hoarseness. In both cases, the hoarseness is usually transient and resolves without specific treatment. The vocal cord of the patient suffering from acute infectious laryngitis may be seen to be erythematous, injected and slightly swollen. There may be a scattered sticky mucoid discharge. The larynx injured from recent severe vocal strain may reveal unilateral submucosal vocal cord hemorrhage with slight edema. Treatment is generally symptomatic and includes hydration, humidification and voice rest. Antibiotics are generally unnecessary unless there is evidence of coexistent bacterial pharyngitis. Otolaryngologic consultation should be considered if hoarseness persists for more than 2 weeks, especially in the setting of a history of smoking or alcohol use or other coexistent symptomatology, especially including cough, hemoptysis, severe ear pain or throat pain, odynophagia, dysphagia or weight loss.

Chronic laryngitis

Chronic laryngitis is typically associated with one or more chronic irritants which, over time, lead to laryngeal injury. Such irritants include smoking, other inhalant irritants (such as chemical fumes), chronic reflux, chronic sinusitis with postnasal drip, chronic alcohol abuse and chronic vocal strain. Smoking increases the risk of the development of squamous cell carcinoma of the larynx and also, as a laryngeal irritant, is associated with the development of benign vocal cord changes, including benign leukoplakia and polyploid corditis. These entities are discussed below.

Reflux

The reflux of acidic gastric secretions into the hypopharynx is one of the most common etiological factors in patients with voice disorders. Many other non-specific throat and laryngeal symptoms have been associated with reflux. Such symptoms include chronic sore throat, cough, a globus sensation, chronic throat clearing, laryngospasm and chronic sensation of excessive mucus in the throat. Reflux has also been associated, at least in part, with the development of vocal cord lesions such as leukoplakia or arytenoid or contract granuloma and may, some feel, be associated with the development of laryngeal stenosis in isolated cases. Reflux frequently adds to vocal abuse and smoking in the generation of laryngeal and throat symptomatology. Reflux characteristically varies over time, so symptoms may fluctuate. Only approximately 30% of patients with symptomatic reflux affecting the laryngopharynx may note typical heartburn symptoms. The physical examination findings in these patients are inconstant, but may include erythematous and even slightly edematous arytenoids with redundant interarytenoid mucosa. The sensitivity of this examination finding is not known. A barium swallow may reveal reflux and hiatal hernia or may be negative. Reflux esophagitis may not be present in patients with symptomatic reflux affecting the laryngopharynx. Although the diagnosis can be made with confidence with pH double-probe monitoring over a 24-hour period, often when the history and physical examination are suggestive, empiric treatment is offered. Treatment includes avoidance of aggravating foods (typically chocolate, carbonated beverages, caffeine, alcohol and fatty foods), as well as avoidance of smoking. The head of the bed is elevated to at least 30° and the patient is instructed to refrain from eating for at least 3 hours before going to bed. Antacids or H_2 blockers or hydrogen pump inhibitors are prescribed and follow-up is provided to insure that symptoms abate.

Hyperfunctional voice disorders

Hyperfunctional voice disorders include a number of diagnostic entities in which abnormal hyperfunctional mechanisms of voice production lead to a vicious cycle of microtrauma of the vocal cord and resultant dysphonia. The traumatic change to the larynx in turn leads to the recruitment of excess counterproductive vocal mechanisms characterized by strain and excess muscle tension and glottic compression during phonation. Terms used more or less synonymously to describe this dysphonic state include muscle tension dysphonia, vocal hyperfunction or vocal abuse. Muscle tension dysphonia can be suspected when excessive glottic and supraglottic contraction can be identified during phonation by video laryngoscopy. One example of extreme strain with resultant excess contracture of the larynx with phonation that results in hoarseness is termed dysphonia plicae ventricularis. Here, supraglottic contraction is so great that the false cords are brought to meet in the midline, so that the patient phonates through vibration of the false rather than the true cords. When long-standing and severe, muscle tension dysphonia can lead to vocal cord structural lesions including vocal cord polyploid change (Reinke's edema), vocal cord polyps, vocal cord ('singer's') nodules, arytenoid ulcers and granuloma. Muscle tension dysphonia is not considered a voluntary or psychological disorder and is not considered a neurologic disease or dystonia. Muscle tension dysphonia is generally not associated with other systemic neurologic diseases or dystonias, and is typically amenable (unlike laryngeal dystonias) to voice therapy.

Polyploid corditis

Polyploid corditis, also known as Reinke's edema, typically presents in a middle-aged female smoker with chronic and severe hoarseness. There is bilateral diffuse edema and erythema of the bilateral vocal cords which appear redundant, floppy and bag-like. Polyploid corditis is strongly associated with smoking and reflux. Similar cord changes can be seen in hypothyroidism. Once these relatively profound vocal cord structural changes are in place, significant secondary muscle tension dysphonia may occur. The edematous redundant polyploid tissue represents an abnormal accumulation of myxoid connective tissue elements in the subepithelial layer, which is also referred to as Reinke's space. Beneath this space are the deeper layers of the lamina propria, vocal ligament and vocalis muscle. Initial treatment involves smoking cessation, reflux treatment and voice therapy, with consideration for checking thyroid function tests depending on the clinical presentation. Surgery may be necessary in severe cases or where focal irregularity demands biopsy. Despite the association with smoking and the profound hoarseness, polyploid corditis is not thought to be a premalignant condition. The surgical treatment involves microlaryngoscopy. During such endoscopic surgery, the vocal cord is examined and operated on through a laryngoscope under an operating microscope using specially sized microlaryngeal instruments. A lateral incision is made in the dorsum of the vocal cord. The vocal cord epithelium is carefully elevated without injury to the underlying layers of the lamina propria, and excess myxoid substance is evacuated from Reinke's space, usually with suction. The overlying flap of epithelium is trimmed and redraped so as not to injure the lamina propria or the medial phonating edge of the vocal cord.

Vocal cord polyps

A focal vocal cord polyp should be considered the focal structural manifestation of chronic vocal cord irritation. The main etiologic factors may include smoking, reflux and muscle tension dysphonia. A focal polyp may develop as a result of a focal cord submucosal hemorrhage which then organizes. Polyps are more common in the anterior third of the vocal cord. Even small polyps can, by disturbing the vocal cord phonating medial edge, produce profound hoarseness. When large, polyps can 'ball valve' into the glottis, causing intermittent respiratory distress. The treatment is usually surgical, in the form of microlaryngoscopy. It is critical postoperatively, as with diffuse polyploid corditis, to understand and treat the underlying predisposing etiologic factors to prevent recurrence.

Vocal cord nodules

Vocal cord nodules are also called 'singer's' or 'screamer's' nodes. They can be thought of as a callus of the vocal cord. They are the residual of chronic vocal microtrauma from vocal strain and often occur bilaterally. They occur characteristically at the point of maximal vocal cord vibration during phonation at the junction of the anterior one-third and posterior two-thirds of the vocal cords. They are more common in women and children. There is often a history of excessive vocal strain. They occur typically in children who abuse their voice, and in cheerleaders, bartenders and teachers. The early vocal cord nodule is seen as a focally edematous region. In the setting of ongoing vocal cord microtrauma, this evolves into a thickened fibrosed mature nodule. Treatment is usually aimed at correction of the underlying vocal strain and is infrequently surgical.

Vocal cord hemorrhage

With a discrete vocal cord injury (for example, from screaming at a football game), a vocal cord submucosal capillary may rupture with the subsequent development of submucosal vocal cord hemorrhage. Such hemorrhage may resolve completely with normal vocal cord function, or may lead to vocal cord scarring or polyp formation. Vocal cord hematomas are typically not of sufficient size to produce airway distress. Such hemorrhages are usually treated conservatively with voice rest and humidification.

Arytenoid granuloma

Arytenoid granulomas represent an exuberant focal granular response to laryngeal trauma, such as intubation trauma or chronic microtrauma during phonation in patients with certain vocal styles. Patients trying to project their voice at a lower pitch, as, for example, may occur in executives using an authoritative tone, or patients who chronically clear their throat may be at increased risk for the development of microtrauma and subsequent arytenoid granuloma. There is also an association between chronic reflux and arytenoid granuloma. It is considered that reflux is a cofactor in their development. Granulomas may be unilateral or bilateral, and occur quite characteristically in the posterior vocal cord region at the level of the vocal process of the arytenoid. Symptoms include hoarseness and cough. If the granuloma is large, ball valving into the glottis may occur, with intermittent choking and respiratory distress. Voice change occurring after intubation, especially with odynophagia, also requires consideration of arytenoid cartilage dislocation. The treatment of arytenoid granulomas includes the identification and removal of the inciting laryngeal irritants, and typically includes voice therapy and antireflux measures and medicines. If symptoms and the lesion persist, or if the diagnosis of the glottic lesion is in question, then surgical resection should be considered. It is of note that arytenoid granulomas in their appearance and location can be easily confused with laryngeal granular cell tumors (myoblastomas). There is a high recurrence of arytenoid granuloma after surgery, even with steroid injection at the time of their removal, unless the inciting laryngeal irritants have been adequately identified and treated.

Sulcus vocalis

Sulcus vocalis is a narrow furrow or indentation running along the long axis of the vocal cord, and is best seen during video strobe laryngeal examination. When running along the luminal aspect of the vocal cord, the lesion is called a sulcus vergeture. A sulcus vergeture may interfere with phonatory glottic closure. The treatment is surgical when the sulcus is the source of significant dysphonia.

Laryngeal conversion disorders

The larynx and throat are common somatization targets for patients with active psychological issues. Findings vary, but patients may present with intermittent episodes of respiratory distress, stridor, hoarseness or aphonia, without clear-cut diagnosis. Episodes may be triggered or initially derived from legitimate laryngeal, throat or chest pathology, such as upper respiratory tract infections or asthma. Examination findings vary, but during an episode one may see paradoxical vocal cord motion. Paradoxical vocal cord motion involves adduction with inspiration and abduction with expiration. Also characteristic of, and relatively unique to, laryngeal conversion disorders is intermittent whispered phonation or complete aphonia interspaced with normal phonation. Effective treatment is most readily rendered in the setting of a good patient–physician relationship and primarily involves obtaining voice therapy and appropriate psychological evaluation and counseling.

Laryngeal hemangiomas

Hemangiomas may occur in the pediatric population, most characteristically in the subglottis. Patients may present with a history of croup with respiratory distress. Treatment involves use of the CO_2 laser during laryngoscopy or watchful waiting, as gradual involution can occur over time in some cases.

Laryngeal cysts

Intracordal cysts develop as a result of an obstructed mucous gland or as a result of a congenital lesion. Symptoms become apparent if the cyst is large enough to distort the phonatory surface of the vocal cord. In such circumstances, treatment is surgical. Saccular cysts form from occlusion and enlargement of the saccule, the normal anterior ventricle diverticulum. With significant enlargement of the saccule, it distorts the submucosal surface of the ipsilateral false vocal cord and is termed an internal laryngocele. Internal laryngoceles can progressively enlarge and, with time, extend over the top of the ipsilateral thyroid cartilage and present as a neck mass or external laryngocele. As laryngoceles enlarge, they can lead to progressive hoarseness and even respiratory obstruction. They occur with greater frequency in patients who chronically perform Valsalva maneuvers by playing wind instruments. When significantly symptomatic, laryngoceles may be endoscopically marsupialized or resected through an external neck approach.

Laryngeal papillomatosis

Laryngeal papillomas are a benign papillomatous laryngeal growth associated with the human papilloma virus. Papillomas occur with increased frequency in the children of women with condyloma acuminatum, but can present in adults as well. Papillomas can be multifocal and widespread and can lead to hoarseness and respiratory insufficiency. Despite multiple surgical interventions, papillomas may persist, recur and spread, especially in younger patients. When spreading occurs into the trachea, bronchial tree and lung, the disease is usually fatal. Treatments typically involve laser ablation of the papillomatous regions during laryngoscopy. Tracheotomy is typically avoided, as this tends to facilitate progression of the disease into the tracheobronchial tree. Treatment is usually through the CO_2 laser. Phototherapy and interferon treatment have been investigated. Radiation therapy is avoided, as it tends to lead to the development of squamous cell carcinoma. Despite the potential virulence of pediatric laryngeal papillomas in terms of recurrence, spread and the need for multiple surgical interventions, such pediatric papillomas may also regress at puberty. Adult-onset papilloma is typically more localized and more readily cured.

Cricoarytenoid arthritis

The cricoarytenoid joint is a synovial joint that can be affected by systemic disorders. Cricoarytenoid arthritis usually arises in the setting of severe systemic rheumatoid arthritis. Autopsy studies suggest that 80–90% of patients with severe systemic rheumatoid arthritis demonstrate laryngeal involvement, but only 25% of these patients develop laryngeal symptomatology. Cricoarytenoid dysfunction is also associated with other systemic inflammatory conditions, including various collagen vascular disorders: gout, Reiter's syndrome, Crohn's disease, ankylosing spondylitis, systemic lupus erythematosus (SLE), tuberculosis and syphilis. Patients with cricoarytenoid arthritis present with hoarseness, odynophagia and referred otalgia. Respiratory distress can occur through posteroglottic narrowing from cricoarytenoid fixation and secondary posterior glottic scarring. The physical examination reveals erythematous and edematous arytenoid mucosa with decreased arytenoid and vocal cord mobility. Cricoarytenoid arthritis is treated as for systemic arthritis. Tracheotomy may be needed. Arytenoid procedures (arytenoidectomy and arytenoidpexy) have been performed. Pathology from the cricoarytenoid joint shows synovial thickening and destruction of the joint space with panus formation.

Sarcoid

Sarcoid rarely affects the larynx. Such patients present with pain and a change in the voice that has been characterized as 'honking'. Lesions are usually in the supraglottic region. Affected supraglottic structures are edematous, pale pink and 'turban'-like. Diagnosis can be definitively made by biopsy demonstrating non-caseating granuloma. The treatment is the same as for systemic sarcoid (generally steroids).

Systemic lupus erythematosus

SLE rarely causes acute or subacute laryngitis. Chronic laryngeal SLE manifestations can include chronic hypertrophic laryngitis, supraglottic mucosal ulceration, cricoarytenoid arthritis and transient vocal cord paralysis. Treatment is the same as for systemic disease.

Wegener's granulomatosis

This inflammatory disorder of unknown etiology affects the lung, kidney and upper airway. In the upper airway, preferred sites include the nose, sinus and upper and lower tracheobronchial tree. Histologically, Wegener's lesions are characterized by necrotizing small vessel vasculitis, granuloma and multinuclear giant cells with histiocytes. In the larynx, the subglottis is a site of predilection, which can ultimately lead to subglottic stenosis. Treatment in general is systemic and includes steroids and cyclophosphamide. Tracheotomy may be necessary if there is laryngeal or tracheal stenosis. Laser treatments, tracheal dilatations and injection of steroids have been used. Open surgery is generally not recommended.

Pemphigus

Pemphigus vulgaris is a bullous disease involving the mucosa of both mouth and larynx. Patients are typically elderly and are often of Mediterranean or Jewish extraction. Oral and laryngopharyngeal lesions include bullae and whitish patches of sloughing mucosa. Such lesions are similar to those seen in the mucositis of chemotherapy. The diagnosis can be confirmed by biopsy and appropriate immunofluorescent studies. Histologically, pemphigus shows epidermal acantholysis and bulla formation with the basal layer remaining attached to the dermis. Deposits of IgG and C_3 between cells in the Malpighian layer can be shown on immunofluorescent studies.

Pemphigoid is a closely related clinical entity with slightly different histologic findings with immunoglobulin deposition at the level of the basement membrane. Treatment initially involves systemic steroids and cytotoxic agents. In addition, topical agents and intralesional steroid injections may be helpful.

Relapsing polychondritis

Relapsing polychondritis is a rare autoimmune disease that can involve the cartilage of the ear, the nasal cartilage and the laryngeal cartilage. Resulting loss of support in the laryngeal and tracheal airway results in laryngomalacia. Patients describe a sense of fullness and otalgia with laryngeal and neck erythema and swelling. Treatment includes systemic steroids and cytotoxic agents.

Laryngospasm

The laryngeal glottis reflexively closes with stimulation associated with deglutition. The chemical stimulation of the larynx, which induces glottic closure and systemically induces apnea, bradycardia and bronchoconstriction, is termed the laryngeal chemoreflex. The afferent limb of this reflex is through the superior laryngeal nerve. Laryngospasm is the abnormal or relatively spontaneous transient yet disturbing spasmodic reflex glottis closure. These amount to transient (seconds to several minutes) episodes of respiratory distress, which may include stridor and aphonia. Usually they are not associated with cyanosis or loss of consciousness, and resolve spontaneously. Laryngospasm may occur spontaneously or be triggered by certain foods or by reflux episodes at night. Treatment includes reassurance after a thorough history, examination and evaluation, ruling out other underlying pathology, and may also include reflux treatment as well as avoidance of identified triggering environments or food.

Laryngotracheal bronchitis

Laryngotracheal bronchitis, also called croup when occurring in children, is usually associated with a barking-type cough and hoarseness and can progress to respiratory compromise with stridor. This is usually viral. When occurring in children, it usually occurs in a younger age group than those who are affected with epiglottitis. The infection is centered on the subglottis, which is the most narrowed and fixed point along the airway. Treatment includes close observation, racemic epinephrine (adrenaline) nebulized treatments, steroids, humidification and oxygen (see Chapter 15).

Laryngeal diphtheria

Laryngeal diphtheria presents in non-immunized patients as a quickly progressive, severe laryngopharyngitis. Patients present with throat pain and hoarseness with progressive airway symptomatology. There is a characteristic gray, foul-smelling exudate in the posterior oropharynx and tonsils that bleed with their removal. Culture will be positive for *Corynebacterium diphtheriae* and the Schick test is positive. In addition to throat, voice and airway symptoms, patients may present with cranial neuropathies as a result of diphtherial neurotoxin. Treatment includes intramuscular diphtheria antitoxin, which prevents the development of both polyneuritis and myocarditis. Treatment also includes intravenous penicillin or erythromycin.

Tuberculosis

Laryngeal tuberculosis is strongly associated with advanced pulmonary tuberculosis. The physical examination demonstrates laryngeal erythema with granular or ulcerative change to the mucosa, most characteristically in the posterior larynx. Chronic changes may lead to scarring and subsequent stenosis. If the diagnosis is not apparent through chest X-ray, skin testing and sputum, occasionally laryngeal biopsy can be helpful.

Laryngeal candidiasis

Laryngeal *Candida* is usually seen in conjunction with oral candidiasis and is commonly seen in the same clinical setting, including young children or the immunosuppressed. When occurring in an otherwise normal adult, immunologic work-up including HIV testing may be indicated. The pain and hoarseness associated with laryngeal candidiasis usually quickly resolves with an oral antifungal agent such as fluconazole.

Other mycotic infections of the larynx

Mycotic infections of the larynx, as with tuberculosis, are usually associated with rather severe pulmonary mycotic infections and are more common in patients with altered cellular immunity. Although they were previously confined to certain regions of the country in the USA, because of travel mycotic infections are now found in patients from any region. Mycotic infections of the larynx may present in a variety of ways, ranging from a small granuloma of the vocal cord to extensive inflammatory laryngeal disease with subsequent cicatricial deformities and laryngeal stenosis.

Histoplasmosis

This is usually a benign self-limiting disease that results from *Histoplasma capsulatum*, which is found particularly in soil in the Midwest USA that has been contaminated with poultry droppings. The diagnosis is suggested by chest X-ray films, and is best confirmed by rising titers of anti-*Histoplasma* antibody. Biopsy shows caseating granuloma with pseudoepitheliomatous hyperplasia, which can mimic carcinoma grossly and histologically. When the disorder is self-limiting, no treatment is used. When treatment is required, itraconazole and ketoconazole have been effective.

Coccidioidomycosis

Also known as Valley Fever, this is endemic to the Southwestern USA. It is caused by *Coccidioides immitis*, which is an inhaled soil saprophyte. One week to 1 month after exposure, the patient usually presents with cough, fever and malaise. The disorder is self-limited in 95% of patients, but occasionally a patient will develop a pulmonary abscess or cavitary pulmonary lesion. Diagnosis can be assisted by skin or serologic tests. Most patients require no treatment. Itraconazole and ketoconazole have been used.

Paracoccidioidomycosis

Infection with *Paracoccidioides brasiliensis* is a systemic mycotic infection of South America usually characterized by chronic progressive respiratory symptomatology. Mucosal lesions may occur in the mouth, nose and larynx, and are characterized by edema and granulomatous change. Cervical adenopathy may be present. Diagnosis is through biopsy. Treatment is through sulfa drugs, imidazole compounds or amphotericin B.

Blastomycosis

This is endemic to the Southeastern USA and is caused by *Blastomyces dermatitidis*. Granulomatous lesions develop throughout the body, especially in the lung, skin and bone. Granulomatous lesions in the larynx are characterized by microabscesses with overlying epithelial hyperplasia and can mimic carcinoma. Cultures are diagnostic. Silver stain is positive. Treatment includes itraconazole or ketoconazole.

Other infections reported to affect the larynx are actinomycosis, nocardiosis and infections caused by *Aspergillus fumigatus* and *Cryptococcus*. These infections do not cause laryngeal disease without extensive pulmonary disease. Other infections that rarely affect the larynx include leprosy, syphilis and rhinoscleroma.

Chondroradionecrosis

Chondroradionecrosis of the larynx is the laryngeal equivalent of mandibular osteoradionecrosis. This is considered to represent a radiation-induced ischemic necrosis of the laryngeal cartilage, typically occurring in patients treated with therapeutic levels of radiation therapy for laryngeal carcinoma. Patients present with progressive pain, odynophagia, dysphagia and hoarseness, and can ultimately develop respiratory insufficiency. Physical examination reveals external neck edema and erythema and fetor of the breath. Laryngeal examination reveals erythema and edema and can also demonstrate deep mucosal ulceration. The symptoms of chondroradionecrosis closely mimic the symptoms of recurrent cancer. Magnetic resonance imaging (MRI) and CT scanning in part can help to make the difficult distinction between recurrent laryngeal cancer and chondroradionecrosis. Occasionally, endoscopy and biopsy are necessary. Biopsy risks progression of cartilage necrosis through added cartilage and mucosal injury. Treatment involves elimination of any existing laryngeal irritants, certainly smoking cessation, removal of any existing nasogastric tubes and treatment of reflux. Antibiotics may be offered but typically do not impact significantly on the patient's course. The primary treatment for chondroradionecrosis is hyperbaric oxygen therapy. Hyperbaric oxygen therapy can help to improve symptoms and facilitate healing. End-stage chondroradionecrosis may require laryngectomy.

Neurologic disorders

A variety of neurologic disorders can impact on the laryngopharynx, affecting both voice and deglutition. Such disorders range from systemic neurologic disorders to unilateral vocal cord paralysis.

A variety of myopathies and neuromuscular dystrophies lead to progressive loss of function at the level of the laryngopharynx; these include amyotrophic lateral sclerosis, myasthenia gravis, multiple sclerosis and progressive supranuclear palsy. Myasthenia gravis leads to laryngeal and hypopharyngeal weakness, with dysphagia, dysarthria and dysphonia. Patients note tiredness with eating or phonation and that they need to concentrate intentionally during eating or drinking. The laryngopharynx can be affected by peripheral neuropathies, including a variety of collagen vascular disorders and Guillain–Barré syndrome. Laryngeal and hypopharyngeal symptoms are often prominent in patients with disorders of the brain stem nuclei, including pseudobulbar palsies, stroke (Wallenberg's syndrome), Arnold–Chiari malformation, syringobulbia or brain stem tumors. Cortical disease, including trauma, stroke or tumor, as well as cerebral palsy, may also impact on the laryngopharynx. Systemic dyskinetic disorders, including Parkinson's disease (characterized by decreased loudness, monotone, hoarseness and vocal tremor), essential tremor, Shy–Drager syndrome, multiple system atrophy, various dyskinesias, myoclonus, choreas, dystonias, cerebellar degenerative disorders or stroke may result in laryngeal and hypopharyngeal symptoms. The larynx may, in isolation, be affected by dystonia.

Spasmodic dysphonia

Spasmodic dysphonia is a discrete voice disorder representing a focal laryngeal dystonia. It is associated with other dystonic disorders including, for example, Meige's disease. In its hyperadduction form, it is characterized by a halting, strained, strangled-type voice as a result of uncoordinated excess adduction during phonation. This occurs especially with vowels and occurs intermittently, as distinct from the patient with muscular tension dysphonia. The voice symptomatology is usually less severe, and voice therapy more effective, for patients with muscular tension dysphonia as compared to patients with spastic dysphonia. The abduction form of spastic dysphonia results in voiceless gaps in speech, from the dysregulation of abduction vocal cord motion. Spastic dysphonia is not considered to be psychogenic in origin. Many treatments have been offered. As noted above, voice therapy is typically not effective. Recurrent laryngeal nerve section has been used in the past, but is associated with a higher recurrence rate after section. The current treatment of choice is the injection of small doses of botulinum toxin into the affected laryngeal muscles. Such treatment reduces the excess muscle activity producing chemical denervation, blocking acetylcholine release, and has been used in other head and neck dystonias. The effect of botulinum toxin is limited and retreatment is required, typically every 3–4 months.

Vocal cord paralysis

Classically, with unilateral recurrent laryngeal nerve injury, the affected vocal cord comes to rest in a paramedian position (not fully adducted or fully abducted), but the exact position varies (Figure 13.5). In this position, the glottic airway is not significantly narrowed and airway complaints are rare; however, the opposing cord may not provide adequate glottic closure with phonation. A small remaining glottic gap can persist during phonation. This persistent glottic gap with phonation results in air escape during phonation, causing a weak and breathy voice. The vocal cord surfaces are not irregular and the voice is not truly hoarse. Without adequate glottic closure, an effective cough, which requires transient tight glottic closure in order for subglottic pressures to increase, cannot be mounted. The degree of voice change depends on the exact cord position and the degree of opposite cord compensation.

Unilateral vocal cord paralysis, depending on the exact cord position, can also be associated with significant aspiration as the paralytic cord is unable to protect its half of the glottis from saliva or ingested material, especially liquids. Solids, which are swallowed more easily, are usually not problematic. Paroxysms of coughing may occur during swallowing of liquids or saliva. The degree of symptoms (breathy voice, ineffective cough and dysphagia) with unilateral vocal cord paralysis varies, owing to the degree of injury (paresis versus complete paralysis), the position of the paralyzed cord and the degree of compensation of the opposite cord.

Patients with vocal cord paralysis caused by vagal nerve injury, especially high vagal injury, usually are more symptomatic than patients with isolated recurrent laryngeal nerve injury. This is for two reasons. The first is that vagal injury results in denervation of the external branch of the superior laryngeal nerve, with resulting loss of innervation to the cricothyroid muscle. The loss of this vocal cord tensor amounts to decreased vocal cord adduction. As a result, the affected cord comes to rest in a more lateral

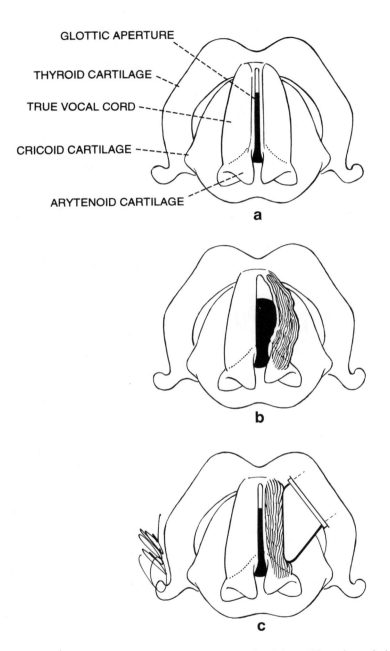

GLOTTIC APERTURE

THYROID CARTILAGE

TRUE VOCAL CORD

CRICOID CARTILAGE

ARYTENOID CARTILAGE

a

b

c

Figure 13.5 (a) Normal glottis with phonation; (b) right vocal cord paralysis, with right paralyzed cord in the paramedian position; (c) right vocal cord paralysis after thyroplasty implant. Note the medialization of the affected paralyzed cord

position, worsening voice quality and increasing aspiration. It is of note that the correlation between the site of lesion and the affected cord position is controversial. The second reason that high vagal lesions result in more symptomatic vocal cord paralysis is that, with superior laryngeal nerve loss, there is sensory denervation of the ipsilateral supraglottis. The combination of an insensate supraglottis and an ipsilateral vocal cord paralysis typically represents a more profound dysphagia than recurrent laryngeal nerve-induced paralysis alone.

Vocal cord paralysis may arise from many different etiologies. Tumor at the base of the skull, in the neck (usually thyroid), or in the mediastinum or chest may injure the vagus or recurrent laryngeal nerve. Similarly, neck and chest trauma, laryngeal trauma as with endotracheal tube intubation and thoracic aneurysm are all associated with vocal cord paralysis. Paralysis may be surgically induced. High-risk surgical procedures include thyroid and parathyroid surgery, carotid endarterectomy and anterior cervical approaches to the cervical spine. A variety of chest and base-of-skull procedures also place the vagus or recurrent laryngeal nerve at risk. Inflammatory disorders of the neck base and mediastinum can result in neural dysfunction. Radiation-induced fibrosis, degenerative neural disorders including bulbar palsies (e.g. polio), demyelinating disease and vascular syndromes (e.g. Wallenberg's syndrome) may cause vocal cord paralysis. Overall, the most common causes of vocal cord paralysis are pulmonary malignancy and surgically induced injury. Approximately one-third of cases ultimately are diagnosed as idiopathic. In such patients, as in patients with Bell's palsy, a viral etiology is suspected. This clearly represents a diagnosis of exclusion.

Bilateral vocal cord paralysis

Bilateral vocal cord paralysis represents a very different constellation of symptoms as compared to unilateral vocal cord paralysis. The bilaterally denervated vocal cords typically come to rest in the midline, demonstrating very little abduction. Typically, bilateral vocal cord paralysis is caused by bilateral thyroid surgery, but it can also be caused by neurologic events. A similar glottic configuration with bilaterally fixed midline cords can be caused by posteroglottic scarring or bilateral cricoarytenoid joint dysfunction. While the voice is usually quite good, respiratory function is compromised. Such patients can present with respiratory distress in the recovery room after thyroidectomy and may require urgent tracheotomy. Unrecognized respiratory distress without change in voice in a patient with a bilateral vocal cord paralysis can result in hypoxia, respiratory arrest, cerebral anoxia and death.

Electromyographic (EMG) intraoperative monitoring of the recurrent laryngeal nerve during thyroidectomy and other surgery that risks the recurrent laryngeal nerve or vagus allows surgeons to assess the functional integrity of the nerve at the end of the surgery. This allows the prediction of postoperative vocal cord function. With such assessment performed at the end of the first side of a planned bilateral thyroid surgery, the loss of significant EMG activity during evoked stimulation of the nerve that is operated on would allow the surgeon to defer contralateral surgery. With such an algorithm, bilateral cord paralysis could not develop during thyroid surgery.

A patient presenting with vocal cord paralysis requires a thorough history, emphasizing any past thyroid, neck or chest malignancy, and a thorough review of past surgical procedures. The physical examination includes a full head and neck examination. Imaging including CT scanning or MRI of the base of the skull, neck and upper chest, including the course of the vagus and recurrent laryngeal nerve, is typically required. In addition, thyroid sonography may be helpful to identify small invasive thyroid lesions. Laryngeal EMG can be helpful to differentiate bilateral vocal cord paralysis from posterior glottic stenosis or arytenoid fixation, and can provide prognostic information regarding the potential for return of function of the vocal cords. Arytenoid dislocation or fixation, cricoarytenoid arthritis and posteroglottic stenosis can result in immobility of the vocal cords without neural paralysis. In such instances, direct laryngoscopy may be required to palpate the arytenoids and inspect the posterior glottis.

Treatment of vocal cord paralysis

A recurrent laryngeal nerve which has been transected at surgery or infiltrated with malignancy will not regain function, but speech therapy can be helpful, by facilitating the patient's own contralateral cord compensation. In nerves that are bruised, stretched, but not transected (i.e. neurapraxic), generally function returns within 6 months, and almost definitely by 1 year. Laryngeal EMG can offer prognostic information regarding the likelihood of resumption of function. If necessary function does not return with speech therapy, or if significant aspiration is present, the patient should be evaluated for surgical correction. The typical problem with unilateral vocal cord paralysis is that the cord is too lateral. Medial repositioning of the vocal cord can be accomplished by endoscopic injection of bulk material (e.g. Gelfoam® (The Upjohn Co., Kalamazoo, MI, USA) or fat) into the substance of the vocal cord, laterally to the vocal cord muscle. Unfortunately, most of these materials are reabsorbed over time. Teflon® (E.I. du Pont de Nemours and Company, Wilmington, DE, USA) has been used in the past, but owing to problems with extrusion, granuloma formation and migration of Teflon, such treatment has been abandoned. Currently, the most effective treatment available for repositioning a paralyzed vocal cord is through transcervical placement of an implant in the larynx deep to the thyroid cartilage, lateral to the vocal muscle. This procedure is called a thyroplasty (Figure 13.5). Inserted prosthestic material can be shaped to appropriate dimensions for correct positioning of the cord, and is stabilized by fixation to the overlying thyroid cartilage lamina.

The problem in bilateral vocal cord paralysis is insufficient glottic patency. Tracheotomy may be necessary to provide sufficient airway. In order to widen the glottis, procedures that lateralize one cord or resect or ablate one arytenoid have been devised. Such procedures can be accomplished endoscopically with laser-assisted arytenoidectomy or cordotomy or through open-cord lateralization procedures. As an unavoidable consequence of such glottic widening procedures, as glottic patency increases, the quality of the voice worsens and the risk of aspiration increases.

Superior laryngeal nerve paralysis

Superior laryngeal nerve paralysis is less common after thyroid surgery than recurrent laryngeal nerve injury. Patients present with hoarseness, vocal fatigue, difficulty projecting their voice or singing and a loss of the higher vocal registers. The physical examination shows rotation of the posterior glottis. The ipsilateral vocal cord is typically lower than the normal vocal cord, and is shorter in length and bowed. Treatment includes voice therapy.

Laryngeal trauma

External laryngeal trauma must be suspected in certain types of injury, including blunt neck trauma (especially motor vehicle accidents) and strangulation injuries. The airway may be lost if hoarseness and early respiratory distress are overlooked in such a patient. In patients with laryngeal trauma, one should have a high index of suspicion of associated cervical spine fracture. Patients with suspected laryngeal trauma should be carefully assessed for hoarseness, respiratory distress, hemoptysis and dysphagia. The physical examination may show loss of normal laryngeal landmarks. Laryngeal tenderness is experienced during the neck examination. In addition, subcutaneous emphysema may be present. This implies penetration of the aerodigestive tract with air forced subcutaneously. In a stable patient setting, the initial evaluation includes transnasal fiberoptic laryngoscopy. Assuming the laryngeal examination demonstrates an adequate airway, additional work-up may include CT scanning, barium swallow and endoscopy. If the airway is compromised, tracheotomy under local anesthesia or careful endotracheal tube intubation with a small endotracheal tube by an experienced physician will be necessary. Unrecognized laryngeal injury may lead in the long-term to vocal cord paralysis, laryngeal or subglottic stenosis and arytenoid fixation.

Endotracheal tube intubation can result in laryngeal injury acutely, or secondary to prolonged intubation, or intubation with an inappropriately sized endotracheal tube. Short-term complications resulting from intubation include poor endotracheal tube placement, upper aerodigestive tract laceration and bleeding, perforation and arytenoid dislocation. Long-term complications associated with endotracheal intubation include arytenoid granuloma, sinusitis, laryngeal, subglottic and tracheal stenosis and vocal cord paralysis. Typically, the subglottic and upper cervical trachea is injured because of mucosal injury induced by the cuff of the endotracheal tube. Cuff-induced inflammation leads to scarring and stenosis. Inflammation with subsequent scarring and stenosis can also occur from the endotracheal tube itself, and may, therefore, occur at the level of the glottis. The risk of such laryngeal and tracheal chronic injury can be reduced by offering tracheotomy to patients who require intubation for more than 2 weeks. Tracheotomy represents a more stable and less injurious method of airway control than transglottic endotracheal tube intubation. Laryngeal and tracheal injury can further be reduced by reducing movement of the endotracheal tube relative to the patient. An appropriate level of sedation and muscle relaxation may be helpful. Laryngeal and subglottic stenosis can also occur from high tracheostomy or cricothyroidotomy, chemical or inhalation burns, and progressive inflammatory granulomatous infection such as tuberculosis.

Laryngeal cancer

The vast majority of laryngeal cancer is squamous cell carcinoma, which arises from the mucosal surface of the larynx and tends to metastasize to regional cervical lymph nodes. When early-stage malignant lesions are large

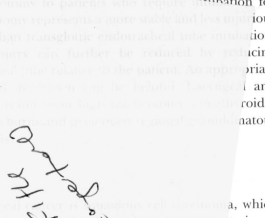

and exophytic or deeply ulcerative and obvious on the physical examination. Early lesions may appear initially as leukoplakic plaques and may be asymptomatic or may present with hoarseness if strategically located on the luminal surface of the vocal cord. The 5-year cure rate is over 90% for such small, early vocal cord lesions, with laryngeal and voice preservation. Once the lesion enlarges and metastasizes to the cervical regional lymph nodes, cure rates are typically halved. This emphasizes the need to examine the vocal cords of any patient with significant hoarseness of 2 weeks' duration or more. This is especially important for patients with a history of significant smoking and alcohol use.

Leukoplakia

Focal leukoplakic lesions of the vocal cord may be benign, precancerous or frankly malignant. Histologically, a lesion may be hyperplastic (i.e. characterized by thickened epithelium) or keratotic. A keratotic lesion involves the development of keratin on the normally non-keratinized stratified squamous epithelium of the vocal cord. Keratosis may be associated with varying degrees of atypia. Atypia is graded according to the degree of abnormal nuclear changes in epithelial cells. Lesions of increasing atypia carry an increased risk of carcinoma development. Such patients need to be followed closely. Atypia is also graded according to the degree of change and the thickness of epithelium. Leukoplakia, therefore, is a clinical description of a lesion with a white, thickened patch of epithelium. Erythroplakia is a clinical description of a lesion that is raised, plaque-like and reddish. Erythroplakia carries a higher risk than leukoplakia of underlying malignancy. Hyperplastic and keratotic lesions of the vocal cords typically result from chronic irritant exposure to smoking, alcohol, vocal strain, chemical irritants and reflux. Close observation is necessary to insure that such lesions resolve, after any identified irritants are removed. If the lesion is especially suspicious or persists, biopsy is recommended. Approximately 2–10% of patients having had keratotic lesions biopsied ultimately develop carcinoma. This is more likely if the keratotic lesions demonstrate atypia. Close follow-up is therefore required.

Approach to laryngeal carcinoma

For purposes of cancer staging and prognostication, the larynx is divided into three regions. The supraglottic region is that portion of the larynx that includes the epiglottis, aryepiglottic fold and false vocal cords. The subglottic region is the area extending from about 1 cm below the vocal cords to the undersurface of the cricoid. The final region is the glottis or true vocal cords.

The bulk of important information in the work-up of laryngeal carcinoma comes from the physical examination of the head and neck. Tumor extent is judged, vocal cord mobility is assessed and the neck is examined for lymphadenopathy. Supraglottic carcinoma is characterized by early and bilateral nodal disease. Glottic carcinomas are slow to involve the regional cervical lymph nodes and are typically detected early. After the physical examination, radiographic evaluation usually involves chest X-ray, neck CT scanning and barium swallow. The next most important step is panendoscopy. Here, the patient undergoes general anesthesia. The laryngopharynx can now be fully manipulated and rigorously inspected in a way impossible in the awake patient. Biopsy can also be obtained. The remainder of the upper aerodigestive tract can be thoroughly inspected, including the tracheobronchial tree. Since cigarette smoke and alcohol, the main carcinogens involved in the development of squamous cell carcinoma of the laryngopharynx, both induce widespread field changes, approximately 15–20% of patients with a known larynx carcinoma have a second squamous cell carcinoma primary present in the upper aerodigestive tract. This underscores the importance for panendoscopy. Once endoscopy is complete and biopsy information is available, treatment options can be reviewed with patient and family.

Carcinoma in situ

This term denotes atypia of the full thickness of the epithelium and an intact basement membrane, without subepithelial invasion. Treatment involves removing the affected portion of vocal cord epithelium endoscopically, along with close follow-up. Radiation therapy is typically reserved for patients with multiple recurrences or who have in follow-up developed invasive squamous cell carcinoma.

Glottic carcinoma

Over 75% of invasive carcinomas of the larynx arise on the true vocal cords. It is fortunate that in these instances hoarseness is an early and persistent symptom. Indirect examination of the larynx will readily demonstrate even a small lesion involving one or both vocal cords. The tumor will therefore be discovered before it has deeply invaded the laryngeal musculature or metastasized. One treatment option involves radiation therapy. A common course of radiation therapy may involve 6500 rad given over 6 weeks. In general, patients tolerate radiation therapy of this type well. After the resolution of initial radiation-induced laryngopharyngitis, the patient's voice returns to near-normal. Alternatively, if there is a minimally invasive lesion, endoscopic resection can be effective if invasive disease can be encompassed without significant resection of the vocalis muscle.

Patients with advanced laryngeal carcinoma may present with transglottic lesions. This implies that glottic, supraglottic and potentially even subglottic regions are involved at presentation. Such advanced lesions can be treated with induction chemotherapy and radiation therapy, with close follow-up, with the hope that the disease can be controlled with laryngeal preservation. Standard treatment options for such patients also include laryngectomy and neck dissection with postoperative radiation therapy, if indicated by evidence of deep invasion or spread in the surgical pathology of the specimen.

Patients with recurrence of early glottic carcinoma after radiation therapy can be effectively treated by removal of the affected cord through a vertical laryngectomy (Figure 13.6).

Supraglottic carcinoma

Approximately 25% of carcinomas of the larynx involve the supraglottis. Squamous cell carcinomas involving this area represent a greater hazard to the patient than those that develop in the glottis, because tumors here do not cause hoarseness until a very late stage of development. For this reason, they may remain undetected until the tumor has become bulky enough to be felt as a mass or to cause pain, generally referred to the ipsilateral ear. Also, these tumors tend to metastasize to cervical lymph nodes early and can, if located towards the center of the supraglottis, result in bilateral nodal metastases.

Small tumors (1–2 cm in size) can be treated effectively by radiation therapy to the supraglottic larynx and to the sites of predilection for cervical metastasis. Generally, if there is gross nodal disease prior to radiation therapy, the patient should be offered neck dissections at the completion of radiation therapy. Such small supraglottic lesions can also be treated surgically by resection of the supraglottic larynx (Figure 13.6). This surgery is reserved for patients who are in good general health and have good pulmonary reserve. Treatment options for more advanced supraglottic carcinoma are similar to those for transglottic carcinoma.

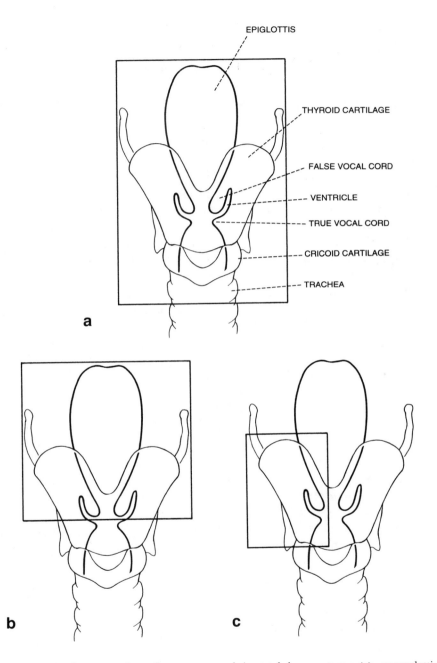

EPIGLOTTIS

THYROID CARTILAGE

FALSE VOCAL CORD

VENTRICLE

TRUE VOCAL CORD

CRICOID CARTILAGE

TRACHEA

a

b

c

Figure 13.6 Demonstration of areas resected in total laryngectomy (a); supraglottic laryngectomy (b); and hemilaryngectomy (c)

Subglottic carcinoma

Carcinoma of the subglottic larynx tends to be a silent tumor and causes little or no symptomatology until symptoms of respiratory obstruction become apparent. The principal modes of therapy are radiation, chemotherapy and surgery. Unfortunately, the failure rate, owing to local recurrence, is high.

LARYNGEAL SURGERY

Microlaryngoscopy

Direct laryngoscopy is the most common surgical procedure performed on the larynx. It is used for examination and biopsy as well as for the removal of leukoplakia, polyps, granulomas and papillomas. These procedures are performed through an L-shaped laryngoscope that is placed into the mouth and fixed into position through suspension. An operating microscope is then used to improve visualization of laryngeal structures through the laryngoscope. Microlaryngeal instruments greatly facilitate the removal of small lesions of the vocal cord with minimal injury. The CO_2 laser has also been helpful for removal of small lesions of the larynx with great precision.

Tracheotomy and tracheostomy

When there is a compromised airway secondary to tumor, edema or hemorrhage, a tracheotomy is necessary. Tracheotomies are temporary and are generally removed when the immediate airway problem has resolved.

There is some confusion in the literature regarding the terms 'tracheotomy' and 'tracheostomy'. Tracheotomy is a temporary opening made through the skin of the neck and carried through the anterior wall of the trachea. Tracheostomy is a permanent stoma created by sewing the margin of the trachea to the cervical skin; it is commonly performed after transecting the trachea during laryngectomy. Aside from transient upper airway obstruction, tracheotomies may be placed if intubated patients are expected to be intubated beyond 2 weeks. Tracheotomy allows endotracheal tube removal, decreasing the risk of induced airway injury. The tracheotomy represents a more stable and less injurious way of maintaining the airway and is better tolerated by the patient. Other indications for tracheotomy include the requirement of patients for ongoing intense pulmonary toilet. A tracheotomy allows for aggressive tracheal suctioning of the tracheobronchial tree. Tracheotomy may also be indicated in patients with severe obstructive sleep apnea.

Tracheotomy tubes (Figure 13.7) are available in different sizes with or without inner cannulas, and can be cuffed or uncuffed, and with or without fenestration. The inner cannula allows for luminal cleaning of the trachea without removal of the entire tracheotomy tube. A cuff is required if supported ventilation is necessary. When inflated, the cuff effectively seals off the lower airway and places it in continuity with the ventilation system. Patients cannot speak with such a system, as long as the cuff is inflated. Cuffs are inflated through a separate narrow tube, usually with a syringe. For patients at risk of aspiration, the cuff can be inflated during meals. It is also effective to prevent passage of blood from above, as with recently biopsied laryngeal tumors. It should be noted that for patients with ongoing severe aspiration inflated cuffs will not completely avoid aspiration. Tracheotomy tubes that are inordinately large or with excess cuff pressure can injure the tracheal wall and lead to tracheal damage, both tracheal stenosis and tracheomalacia. Tracheotomies can also deform and stenose the tracheal segment through which they are introduced and can, if high, also lead to subglottic stenosis.

Patients with a tracheotomy, especially if cuffed, can progressively lose glottic function through disuse over time and become dependent on the tracheotomy. It is best in patients with tracheotomies, depending on the clinical situation, to promote glottic function to avoid this dependence. The smallest uncuffed tube that the patient will tolerate will promote glottic airflow and function. Also, fenestrated tracheotomy tubes promote glottic airflow. Fenestrated tubes that fit improperly can irritate the trachea and lead to granulation tissue at the level of the fenestration. Speaking valves can be attached to the outer tip of the tracheotomy tube. These open with inspiration, allowing good tracheal air inflow, and close with expiration. Expired air is thus directed up the trachea, around the sides of the intraluminal aspect of the tracheotomy tube, and to the glottis. A fenestrated tube further facilitates this airflow. Overall, the speaking valve increases subglottic pressure and can reduce aspiration. It improves glottic airflow, allowing phonation without digital occlusion of the tracheotomy tube. Short-term tracheotomy complications include bleeding, pneumothorax, pneumomediastinum and tracheoesophageal fistula. Long-term complications can include subglottic and tracheal stenosis, tracheoesophageal fistula, bleeding, obstruction secondary to secretions or granulation tissue and dysphagia (secondary to laryngeal tethering). A consequence of tracheotomy is a significant loss of nasal humidification, which must now be externally provided. Without this, the tracheotomy tube will lead to tracheitis, a vicious cycle of tracheal drying, crusting and bleeding, with thick secretions and an irritative cough.

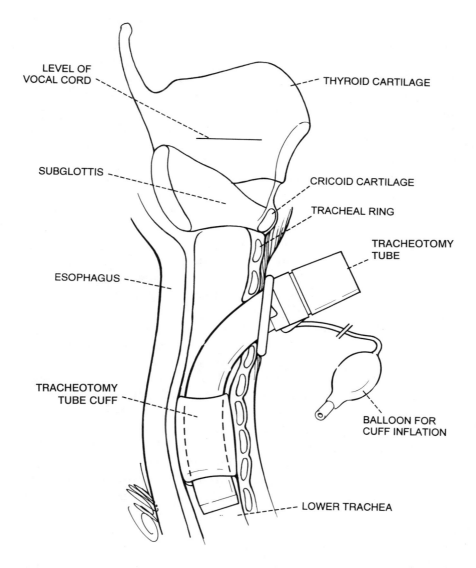

Figure 13.7 Tracheotomy tube in place – side view, demonstrating inner cannula and cuff

Tracheal cannulation

This is an alternative to the use of a formal tracheotomy tube. A commonly used form of tracheal cannula is the Montgomery® (Boston Medical

Products, Westborough, MA, USA) cannula. A cannula is a straight silicon tube with a small lip on the inner edge. This inner aspect of the tube extends into the trachea; the lip fits onto the inner surface of the anterior tracheal wall. On the outer (skin) aspect of the cannula, a Silastic® washer is placed over several rib-like rings on the cannula. The washers hold the cannula in a stable position relative to the skin, subcutaneous tissue and trachea. Because there is very little within the airway, the cannula is generally well tolerated. For patients with cannulas placed for obstructive sleep apnea, the cannula can be capped during the day, allowing normal phonation, and uncapped at night.

Cricothyroidotomy

This is a technique available in those rare instances when an immediate airway is required, endotracheal intubation is not available and there is insufficient time for a formal tracheotomy. During a standard tracheotomy, the airway is entered usually at approximately the second to third tracheal ring in order to leave undisturbed the upper cervical trachea and sub-glottic region with its propensity for stenosis. In order to access the second to third tracheal rings, typically the vascular thyroid isthmus needs to be identified and transected. During cricothyroidotomy, the vascular region of the thyroid isthmus is avoided and the airway is accessed through the relatively avascular cricothyroid membrane. It is not unexpected that, since the airway is entered quite high relative to the cords, cricothyroidotomy is associated with increased rates of subglottic stenosis compared to tracheo-tomy. During cricothyroidotomy, the operator quickly palpates the neck anatomy, identifying the thyroid notch and subsequently the cricoid ring anteriorly. The cricothyroid membrane is a relatively depressible interval between the lower edge of the thyroid cartilage and the upper edge of the cricoid. In the midline a vertical skin incision is made, and a second incision is made through the subcutaneous tissues in this area. A horizontal incision is made through the cricothyroid membrane just above the cricoid, and the airway is accessed, typically with a small endotracheal tube. Usually, the cricothyroidotomy is converted to a formal tracheotomy to avoid the poten-tial for laryngeal and cricoid damage and subsequent subglottic stenosis.

Total laryngectomy

The most frequently performed form of laryngectomy is the total larynec-tomy (Figure 13.6). This procedure is performed for extensive glottic, supraglottic, or subglottic tumors of the larynx; if there is metastatic neck disease, it is typically combined with a neck dissection. Because of the propensity of supraglottic tumors to metastasize to the regional cervical lymph nodes, surgeons will often perform prophylactic neck dissections in this setting. Consequences of this type of surgery for the patient are, in general, poorly understood. Care must be taken to ensure that the patient understands the changes that will occur. Most patients can adapt to the loss of the larynx. Patients should be counseled that, while communication is quite feasible through a number of different techniques, postoperatively, the voice as they know it will be lost permanently. Loss of voice is coupled with the disfigurement represented by the stoma at the base of the neck which can affect self-image. Since total laryngectomy involves separating the nose and mouth from the lungs and trachea, the patient loses the ability to blow his nose, whistle and to converse while eating. Patients are also unable to swim. Because the larynx serves to stabilize the chest during the Valsalva maneuver, the loss of this function causes decreased ability to lift heavy objects. All of these problems need to be thoroughly discussed preoperatively with the patient and his family. Many laryngectomy patients are reformed alcoholics and the stress of this postlaryngectomy syndrome can result in a resumption of old drinking patterns.

With good training, approximately half the patients who undergo laryngectomy will develop esophageal speech satisfactorily enough to converse on the telephone and with strangers without embarrassment. Some patients, though, because of the anatomical structure of the remaining cervical esophagus, are incapable of developing adequate esophageal speech. One alternative is the use of a vibrator placed against the hypopharynx wall or through a small plastic tube extension into the corner of the mouth. Such vibrations produced are articulated by the patient's throat and mouth into discernable speech. The tone of this speech is monotonous and tends to draw attention to the laryngectomee. As a result, many patients feel uncomfortable with such devices.

A number of surgical procedures have been developed that attempt to re-establish the ability to speak in the laryngectomy patient. A fistula is created between the trachea and esophagus so that, if the tracheal stoma is occluded, some peristomal tracheal air is forced through the fistula into the esophagus, causing the upper esophagus to vibrate, allowing the patient to produce speech through articulation of the air by the throat and mouth. Typically, a small puncture-type fistula is created just above the stoma in the midline, connecting the suprastomal trachea with the esophagus, and a small Silastic® valve is placed. With digital occlusion of the valve, the tracheal air column is allowed through the valve into the upper esophagus. A variety of sophisticated devices and procedures are currently being researched for such patients, including electronic speech generation and experimental transplantation.

Supraglottic laryngectomy

This is a procedure (Figure 13.6) that removes the structures of the larynx above the true vocal cords. The vocal cords themselves are conserved. This type of conservation surgery is possible because the lymphatic flow from the supraglottic portion of the larynx does not extend to the glottis. Resection margins, although close along the glottic margin, can be obtained.

Patients must be carefully evaluated before undergoing the surgery. They must have good pulmonary function in order to allow them to withstand the initial postoperative aspiration and to permit them to cough material free from the tracheobronchial tree. They must also be willing to endure several weeks of relearning to swallow without the benefit of the normal supraglottic structures to protect the lower airway. These patients, having maintained their voice without tracheotomy tube or laryngectomy stoma, avoid many of the difficulties associated with total laryngectomy.

Supraglottic laryngectomy is indicated for lesions of the supraglottic larynx including the epiglottis and aryepiglottic fold. Both vocal cords and anterior commissure must be free of disease. Supraglottic laryngectomy can include one arytenoid and extend into the vallecula and the base of the tongue. Supraglottic laryngectomy is contraindicated if the disease extends to the apex of the pyriform sinus, paraglottic space or to both arytenoids.

Hemilaryngectomy

The vertical or hemilaryngectomy (Figure 13.6) is reserved for patients with glottic tumor, usually a postradiation recurrence that is limited to one side of the glottis. The tumor must not be associated with vocal cord fixation or extension to the paraglottic space, the subglottic region, the ventricle or the false cord. Patients are left with a weak and breathy voice, but they usually have no particular difficulty in swallowing, and can make themselves well understood. They require only a temporary tracheotomy.

Supracricoid laryngectomy

This more extensive laryngectomy is suggested for tumors involving both vocal cords anteriorly, or anterior commissure lesions. It is contraindicated if there is arytenoid involvement or subglottic or epiglottic extension. The thyroid cartilage and upper cricoid are resected, preserving the epiglottis and bilateral arytenoids. It allows resection of anterior glottic lesions with the paraglottic space, and allows for preservation of speech and deglutition.

Near-total laryngectomy

Conservation laryngeal surgery is pushed to its limits in the near-total laryngectomy. The procedure is designed as a voice-preserving procedure for advanced unilateral laryngeal carcinomas in selected cases as an alternative to total laryngectomy. The near-total laryngectomy amounts to an extended hemilaryngectomy with cricoid resection, preserving the contralateral posterior laryngeal segment including one arytenoid, the posterior aspect of the vocal cord and the recurrent laryngeal nerve. This preserved segment is fashioned into a stomal hypopharyngeal shunt. The procedure is designed for transglottic carcinomas with paraglottic space involvement and vocal cord fixation. It is contraindicated if bilateral vocal cords are fixed or there is involvement of the posterior larynx (post-cricoid or interarytenoid region). The patient is left with a permanent tracheostomy. Speech is maintained through digital manipulation of air traveling from the stoma through the preserved shunt into the hypopharynx.

14

Dysphagia

Gregory W. Randolph

Physiology
History
Examination
Differential diagnosis
Treatment

The intake of food is as fundamental to life as it is enjoyable. We take for granted this tremendously complex and ordered neuromuscular function, which the burden of our warm-blooded nature necessitates several times a day. The significant and prolonged disruption of swallowing represents a devastating problem for our patients. Dysphagia, problematic swallowing, has recently received greater attention, in part due to advances in evaluation, including, importantly, the modified barium swallow. The modified barium swallow has allowed greater sensitivity in the detection of dysphagia and has greatly facilitated the treatment of swallowing disorders. Often, dysphagia occurs in a setting of other changes in the laryngopharynx that can be manifest as a change in respiratory pattern and/or voice. Patients and physicians often overlook swallowing problems in the setting of coexistent respiratory or voice complaints. The physician must, therefore, specifically inquire about swallowing function.

PHYSIOLOGY

Normal swallowing involves a complex integration of voluntary and involuntary sequential neuromuscular events of the mouth, posterior oropharynx, hypopharynx, larynx and esophagus.

Lip and buccal motor tone is mediated by the facial nerve, while sensation in these areas is mediated by the trigeminal nerve. The hypoglossal nerve provides innervation for all intrinsic and extrinsic muscles of the tongue, including the genioglossus, hyoglossus and styloglossus. Sensation to the anterior two-thirds of the tongue is mediated by the lingual nerve, a branch of the third division of the trigeminal nerve. The lingual nerve also conveys taste sensation from the chorda tympani of the facial nerve to the anterior two-thirds of the tongue. Sensation and taste from the posterior one-third of the tongue is conveyed by the glossopharyngeal nerve. Palatal motor innervation is primarily via the vagus nerve and the muscles including levator veli palatini, palatopharyngeus, salpingopharyngeus and palatoglossus. The third division of the trigeminal nerve innervates the tensor veli palatini. Sensory innervation of the palate is via the second division of the trigeminal, the glossopharyngeal and the vagus nerves. The muscles of mastication (masseter, temporalis, lateral and medial pterygoid muscles) are innervated by the third division of the trigeminal nerve. Motor function of the pharynx is primarily via the vagus nerve and the muscles, including the palatopharyngeus, salpingopharyngeus, palatoglossus and superior, middle and inferior constrictors. The stylopharyngeus muscle is innervated by the glossopharyngeal nerve. Pharyngeal sensation is mediated primarily by the glossopharyngeal and vagus nerves, which jointly form the pharyngeal plexus. Additional oropharyngeal sensory innervation is provided by the trigeminal nerve. The suprahyoid muscles, the geniohyoid and hyoglossus are innervated by the hypoglossal nerve, while the facial nerve innervates the posterior belly of the digastric and the stylohyoid. The anterior belly of the digastric and the mylohyoid are innervated by the trigeminal nerve. The strap muscles (sternohyoid, omohyoid, sternothyroid and thyrohyoid) are innervated by the hypoglossal nerve.

Swallowing can be divided into oral, pharyngeal and esophageal phases (Table 14.1). The voluntary oral phase begins with chewing, lubrication and bolus formation. The oral phase concludes when the bolus is moved posteriorly to the tonsil pillars through coordinated movement of the lip, tongue and buccal muscles. The involuntary pharyngeal phase of swallowing is triggered by the movement of the bolus beyond the tonsil pillars. During the pharyngeal phase, the bolus moves from the tonsil pillars to the upper esophageal sphincter. As the bolus moves back, the soft palate closes the nasopharynx and the base of the tongue pushes the bolus back into the pharynx. The pharynx responds with sequential contractions of the superior, middle and inferior constrictor muscles. As the bolus enters the pharynx, the suprahyoid musculature contracts and the larynx elevates. As the larynx moves upwards and forward, the epiglottis is deflected posteriorly, covering the glottis and diverting the bolus laterally away from the glottis. The false and true vocal cords close and respiratory function is temporarily halted. As the larynx elevates, the cricoid moves

Table 14.1   The phases of swallowing

Oral phase (voluntary)	Mastication, lubrication
	Lip, cheek, tongue bolus formation
	Bolus presentation to posterior oropharynx at tonsil pillars
Pharyngeal phase (involuntary)	Bolus pushed by tongue into pharynx, with nasopharynx closure by soft palate
	Sequential superior, middle and inferior constrictor contraction
	Laryngeal elevation with suprahyoid muscle contraction, epiglottis deflection, false and true cord closure
	Cricoid anterior motion, cricopharyngeus relaxation, bolus presented to upper esophageal sphincter
Esophageal phase (involuntary)	Upper esophageal sphincter opens, bolus enters esophagus
	Peristaltic movement to lower esophageal sphincter

upwards and forward, and cricopharyngeus tone decreases, opening the upper esophageal sphincter. The involuntary esophageal phase starts with the upper esophageal sphincter opening, and involves sequential peristaltic movement of the bolus down the esophagus, through the lower esophageal sphincter and into the stomach.

The upper esophageal sphincter, formed by the cricopharyngeus muscle and the lower fibers of the inferior constrictor, is closed at rest through active sphincteric contraction. It opens in response to decreased vagal tone and through anterior cricoid displacement brought about by suprahyoid muscular contraction during the pharyngeal phase of swallowing.

HISTORY

Dysphagia can be difficult for a patient to describe. Often, swallowing difficulties are described briefly with 'I can't swallow', 'it gets stuck', or 'it makes me choke'. The clinician who is skilled and patient enough to elicit the exact sequence of problems occurring during swallowing may be rewarded with important diagnostic clues in the patient with dysphagia. This is especially true when one considers the orderly sequence of discrete steps into which swallowing can be divided (Table 14.1). To start, the clinician asks simply what exactly happens to the food or liquids being swallowed. Where is the progress halted? Does the bolus stop, then go down? Does the patient need to 'wash it down' with sips of liquid, or cough or vomit the bolus? Does the problem occur only with solids, or liquids, or both? Does swallowing prompt the cough, as with aspiration or pain (i.e. odynophagia), as with infectious or neoplastic disease? The onset, duration and course of dysphagia should be reviewed. Has the dysphagia been progressive? Has the dysphagia caused the patient to change his or her diet, and is there weight loss? Is there is a history of intermittent aspiration pneumonia? Are there other associated symptoms, including respiratory distress, cough, hemoptysis, ear or throat pain, hoarseness, globus sensation or reflux symptoms? A history of smoking and alcohol use will dramatically increase the index of suspicion of squamous cell carcinoma of the upper aerodigestive tract. Is there a history of foreign body ingestion? Foreign body ingestion should always be kept in mind in both the pediatric and the geriatric populations presenting with dysphagia. Is there a history of disease of the larynx, pharynx or esophagus including inhalational or chemical burn, history of dilatation or radiation therapy? Is there is a history of past surgery (e.g. thyroid surgery) that may be important in the functioning of the laryngopharynx? Since dysphagia may be a manifestation of a neurologic or systemic inflammatory disorder, a thorough review of systems should be obtained. The patient should be questioned regarding changes in concentration, vision, headache (focal or diffuse), numbness or weakness, dysarthria and skin changes or arthralgia.

In general, dysphagia with liquids and difficulties associated with managing saliva may suggest neurologic impairment, whereas dysphagia with solids suggests (at least initially) a structural problem. A history of weight loss is an important diagnostic clue, suggesting that the dysphagia is severe. Patients with Zenker's diverticulum typically describe delayed regurgitation of ingested foodstuffs and a gurgling sensation in their neck. Patients with dysphagia from neoplastic or infectious etiologies typically describe odynophagia as well.

Aspiration may occur through premature delivery of the bolus to the pharynx, a dyscoordinated pharyngeal phase, poor laryngeal elevation and closure, or excess post-swallow pharyngeal residue. Patients may note that liquids are more difficult to handle and prompt a cough. However, aspiration may occur without cough. Detection of such 'silent' aspiration requires clinical vigilance if pulmonary complications are to be avoided. When a patient has a history of upper aerodigestive tract surgery, including tracheotomy, ongoing severe aspiration must prompt consideration of tracheoesophageal fistula, a potentially life-threatening entity that is sometimes difficult to recognize.

Globus (also known as globus hystericus) is a ball- or lump-like sensation in the midline throat, and is a common otolaryngologic complaint most often seen in middle-aged women. If the remainder of the clinical examination is negative, the patient with isolated globus sensation may be treated for gastroesophageal reflux and offered reassurance. If there is no change following this treatment, barium swallow and further evaluation should be undertaken.

EXAMINATION

The head and neck examination forms the basis of the initial evaluation of the patient with dysphagia. During the oral examination, lip, tongue and palate mobility, tone and strength should be assessed. Fasciculations may suggest degenerative neurological disease. Dentition should be evaluated. Evidence of glossitis or angular cheilitis may indicate vitamin deficiency. The nasopharynx, hypopharynx and larynx should be examined with a fiberoptic scope and/or nasopharyngeal and laryngeal mirrors (see Clinical evaluation section in Chapter 13). The laryngopharynx should be assessed carefully for evidence of lesions, salivary pooling or reflux. Vocal cord motion should be assessed. The examination should search carefully for any asymmetries suggestive of infectious or neoplastic disease. Ingested dyed material, either liquid (methylene blue), soft solid or solid, may be given to the patient, and can be followed during fiberoptic laryngoscopy. Such evaluation may be helpful in the assessment of the passage of a bolus and the degree of residual pooling, and may also identify aspiration. During the neck examination, the degree of laryngeal and hyoid elevation with swallowing should be assessed. This is an inherent part of the complete thyroid examination (see Anatomy and physical examination section in Chapter 17). The neck examination should also include assessment of neck scars, which may indicate past surgery. A full cranial nerve examination should be performed in the patient with dysphagia, with emphasis on trigeminal, facial, glossopharyngeal, vagal and hypoglossal nerves. The importance and sensitivity of 'gag reflux' is not known. Aided with clues from the history and physical examination, additional work-up is instituted as needed. The routine barium swallow helps to rule out obstructive pathology in the esophagus below the level of evaluation during the routine otolaryngologic examination. In this way the barium swallow is an excellent complement to the general otolaryngologic physical examination. A modified barium swallow (also known as a fluoroscopic video pharyngoesophogram) is performed jointly by a swallowing therapist and a radiologist. In this study the patient is given barium material of various consistencies (liquid, paste and solid) and swallowing phases are repetitively observed and recorded on video tape. The study, therefore, allows the swallowing therapist and radiologist jointly and repetitively to review the swallowing phases. Additionally, if a swallowing disturbance exists, therapeutic maneuvers can be instituted and their effects evaluated. Typical maneuvers include a change in head position, a change in bolus quality or volume, or the introduction of a timed cough. The modified barium swallow can identify problems in oral bolus formation and dyscoordination between the oral and pharyngeal phases of swallow with premature pharyngeal spillage, and can assess the degree of laryngeal elevation, post-swallow residua and nasopharyngeal regurgitation. Importantly, this study can detect the extent of aspiration, and whether or not the patient mounts an effective cough in response to aspiration. The modified barium swallow may be especially useful in patients with neuromuscular disease or patients who have had head and neck surgery or radiation; it is useful for the assessment of the degree of aspiration and the effectiveness of instituted swallowing maneuvers. Such studies can be performed serially to monitor a patient's progress and response to treatment.

Certain patients with dysphagia may require endoscopy, including direct laryngoscopy, esophagoscopy and bronchoscopy, depending on the history, examination and initial studies. Thin esophageal webs, for example, may not be seen on routine barium swallow, but can be identified and lysed during rigid esophagoscopy. Additional evaluation in patients with dysphagia may include computerized tomography scanning (CT) or magnetic resonance imaging (MRI) if mass lesions are identified on the initial evaluation. Manometry may be helpful if esophageal dysmotility is considered. Double pH probe evaluation may be helpful to diagnose reflux definitively. An electromyogram (EMG) of the laryngopharynx may be helpful in selected patients with neuromuscular dysphagia.

DIFFERENTIAL DIAGNOSIS

Dysphagia can be classified by the phase of swallowing most affected (oral, pharyngeal or esophageal). For example, a patient with hypoglossal paralysis will have a disordered oral phase. No information regarding the degree of impairment or etiology is conveyed. Causes are outlined in Table 14.2. Dysphagia carries a broad differential diagnosis. Structural lesions that may interfere with swallowing include large tonsils and palatine or lingual tonsils. Acute infection may lead to the development and progression of dysphagia in these circumstances. Neoplastic masses, whether in the oral cavity, larynx, hypopharynx or thyroid, may also cause dysphagia through obstruction and pain. Surgery of the laryngopharynx, including tracheotomy, may tether the larynx and impair swallowing. Cranial nerve injury during surgery of the head and neck may also lead to the development of dysphagia. Fibrosis associated with past radiation therapy may also impair laryngeal elevation. Congenital lesions such as cleft palate or tongue tie may be readily apparent on the physical examination; however, congenital esophageal webs or diverticula may not be apparent on initial evaluation. Congenital tracheoesophageal fistulas associated with varying degrees of esophageal atresia typically present early after birth. Usually there is an esophageal remnant that is connected to the tracheobronchial tree. Treatment is surgical. The history usually leads one to suspect chemical inhalation injury or foreign body ingestion; however, children may not offer a clear-cut history of foreign body ingestion, requiring a high index of suspicion in this age group. Other structural lesions including vascular anomalies, Zenker's diverticulum and cricopharyngeal spasm can usually

Table 14.2 Causes of dysphagia

Structural
Mass
  palatine and lingual tonsil hypertrophy, other oral masses
  laryngopharynx, thyroid masses
Treatment-induced
  tracheotomy, other surgery of the laryngopharynx, radiation therapy
Congenital
  cleft palate, tongue tie, esophageal stricture, web, ring, atresia, diverticula
Chemical/inhalational injury or foreign body
Vascular
  dysphagia lusoria (Bayford's syndrome), double aortic arch, aortic aneurysm
Zenker's diverticulum
Cricopharyngeal spasm

Infectious
  laryngopharyngitis, tonsillitis, candidiasis, Chagas' disease
  peritonsillar abscess, Ludwig's angina, retro/parapharyngeal/lateral neck abscess
  angioneurotic edema

Neurologic
Regional
  vocal cord, palate paralysis
  cricopharyngeal spasm
  achalasia
  presbyesophagus
  esophageal spasm
Systemic
  bulbar palsy, cerebrovascular accident, polio, cerebral palsy/head injury, multiple sclerosis,
    amyotrophic lateral sclerosis, myasthenia gravis, Parkinson's disease, diabetic and
    alcoholic neuropathy

Metabolic
  iron (Plummer–Vinson's syndrome), vitamin B_{12} and folate deficiencies
  xerostomia

Inflammatory
  Sjögren's syndrome
  reflux
  inflammatory disease: dermatomyositis, scleroderma, rheumatoid arthritis, cricoarytenoid
    arthritis and other collagen vascular disorders

Congenital
  ocular pharyngeal dystrophy

be readily identified with a barium swallow. Zenker's diverticulum typically presents in elderly men as an outpocketing of the lower pharynx directly above the cricopharyngeus. This may be due to a loss of integrity of the muscular layers in this area, as well as an excess cricopharyngeal tone. Food and saliva fill the diverticulum and may spill into the hypopharynx, leading to intermittent regurgitation of food and aspiration. The treatment is surgical, either removing the sac or suspending the sac superiorly so that it no longer fills. Endoscopic approaches have been performed, taking down the wall between the esophagus and Zenker's sac.

Infections of the laryngopharynx lead to dysphagia primarily through odynophagia. Abscesses, including peritonsillar, retropharyngeal para-pharyngeal and lateral neck abscesses, may, in addition to odynophagia, make swallowing difficult through a mass effect. Angioneurotic edema can lead to dysphagia because of edema of the laryngopharynx.

A variety of neurologic disorders can adversely affect swallowing. These include regional disorders that directly and focally impact on the laryngo-pharynx. Examples include unilateral and bilateral vocal cord and unilateral palate paralysis, cricopharyngeal spasm achalasia, esophageal spasm and presbyesophagus. Unilateral vocal cord paralysis typically results in liquid dysphagia (see the section on vocal cord paralysis in Chapter 13). High vagal lesions lead to more profound dysphagia secondary to an insensate hemisupraglottis. Dysphagia is also compounded if a vagal lesion is combined with dysfunction of the glossopharyngeal or hypoglossal nerves. Cricopharyngeal spasm represents a failure of the sphincter to relax during the end of the pharyngeal phase of the swallow. This may be an isolated entity or part of a diffuse neuromuscular disorder. Achalasia results from a degeneration of the myenteric neural plexus of Auerbach with failure of the lower esophageal sphincter to relax at the end of the esophageal phase of the swallow. Patients describe feeling full after a meal, with retrosternal or epigastric discomfort and food regurgitation. Cough and aspiration may occur. Treatment is through esophageal dilatation or Heller's procedure.

Many neurologic disorders can affect the laryngopharynx and present with dysphagia. These include bulbar and pseudobulbar palsy, polio, cerebrovascular accident, cerebral palsy, head injury, multiple sclerosis, amyotrohic lateral sclerosis, myasthenia gravis, Parkinson's disease and diabetic and alcoholic neuropathies. Although patients with dysphagia secondary to neuromuscular disease may have a wide range of specific neurologic diagnoses, they tend to share certain historical and physical examination features. This tends to separate them from patients with dysphagia secondary to infections, or inflammatory, structural or neoplastic entities.

Usually, patients with neuromuscular dysphagia describe slowly progressive dysphagia which is much more profound to liquids than to solids. Solid food tends to stick together and usually is more easily managed by the neurologically impaired throat. The physical examination in such patients may be characterized by decreased muscular tone and poorly coordinated movement of the lip, tongue, pharynx or larynx. On physical examination, these patients may have dysarthria or evidence of nasal regurgitation, and they may demonstrate difficulties in managing their own secretions and may demonstrate gurgling during phonation.

Patients with Plummer–Vinson's syndrome may present with iron deficiency anemia, glossitis, hypothyroidism and dysphagia. This occurs more commonly in women than in men, and is more common in patients of Scandinavian descent. Dysphagia is caused by postcricoid fibrosis and upper esophageal web formation. Symptoms may improve with iron replacement. Esophageal webs may be dilated. The increased risk of postcricoid squamous cell carcinoma requires ongoing vigilance in the follow-up of these patients. Xerostomia from any cause may lead to dysphagia. Severe xerostomia is often related to radiation therapy but may also be associated with Sjögren's syndrome, a variety of medicines and bulimia.

A variety of systemic inflammatory conditions may present with dysphagia. Dermatomyositis, a form of polymyositis, involves both skin and muscle, and presents with reduced esophageal peristalsis. Such patients may be treated with steroids. In scleroderma, there is a progressive sclerosis involving the esophagus with a secondary loss of flexibility and normal muscular contraction. This preferentially affects the distal two-thirds of the esophagus. A rare autosomal dominant disorder, ocular pharyngeal dystrophy, is more common in patients of French Canadian ancestry. Cricopharyngeal spasm and ptosis are the two main manifestations. Such patients respond well to cricopharyngeal and inferior constrictor myotomy.

TREATMENT

In systemic disorders with dysphagia (e.g. myasthenia gravis, Parkinson's disease), dysphagia typically improves with treatment of the underlying systemic disorder. Swallowing therapy may also be helpful. The patient may be followed clinically or with sequential modified barium swallows. Stenosis of the esophagus may be treated with dilatation. Stenosis of the laryngopharynx, if sufficiently severe, can be surgically corrected. In patients with significant laryngeal tethering, lack of laryngeal elevation and laryngeal suspension, a surgical lifting of the larynx to the hyoid or mandible can be helpful. Patients with prolonged tracheotomy may benefit from conversion to a small fenestrated tracheotomy tube with a speaking valve. This allows increased glottic airflow, the recruitment of any ongoing glottic function and increased subglottic air pressures, which may be helpful in prevention of aspiration.

Dysphagia from significant isolated cricopharyngeal spasm such as in patients with ocular pharyngeal dystrophy or in patients with Zenker's diverticulum may be significantly helped by cricopharyngeal myotomy. Cricopharyngeal myotomy is probably of less value when cricopharyngeal dysfunction is part of a more global regional pharyngeal muscular dysfunction. The condition of patients with pre-existing severe reflux may worsen after cricopharyngeal myotomy. Zenker's diverticulum, when sufficiently large and symptomatic can be treated surgically with excellent results.

Swallowing therapy may provide a set of recommendations that can be helpful in patients able to incorporate the suggestions. An example of such a set of recommendations or swallowing hints is the 'supraglottic swallow', in which a patient who is aspirating after supraglottic laryngectomy tucks his chin inward, coughs, swallows, then coughs again. This maneuver and sequence of coughs reduces aspiration. For patients with neuromuscular disorders of the laryngopharynx and esophagus, swallowing therapy and diet modification can be helpful. For example, a patient with unilateral vocal cord paralysis may aspirate less if thickening agents are added to the ingested liquids.

In some patients with severe dysphagia associated with aspiration, safe oral intake may not be possible. Gastrostomy tube alimentation may be necessary. In patients with intractable aspiration, laryngeal diversion or closure procedures, including laryngectomy, may be considered.

15

Airway evaluation

Gregory W. Randolph

Acute airway emergency: initial assessment
Airway management
   Infections of the airway
      Epiglottitis
      Acute spasmodic croup
      Bacterial tracheitis
      Pertussis
      Diphtheria
   Acute laryngeal angioedema
   Respiratory obstruction in the newborn infant
   Chronic respiratory obstruction in a child
      Laryngomalacia
      Foreign body of the airway
      Vascular compression of the trachea
      Laryngeal cysts and laryngoceles
      Laryngeal papillomatosis
      Congenital laryngeal webs
      Subglottic hemangioma
Neoplastic airway obstruction
   Malignant lesions
   Benign neoplastic airway obstruction
      Lingual thyroid
      Laryngocele
Airway stenosis
Laryngeal paralysis
Thyroid disease and the airway
Neck and airway trauma

ACUTE AIRWAY EMERGENCY: INITIAL ASSESSMENT

The assessment of a patient with airway obstruction requires integration of a targeted, but complete, history and focused physical examination to identify the site and magnitude of obstruction expeditiously (Figure 15.1). During this assessment, one must always monitor the overall status of the patient, assessing the patient's respiratory comfort, degree of respiratory effort and peripheral oxygenation. The patient with airway obstruction may be agitated as a result of fear or from hypoxia; however, the patient who lacks agitation, especially a patient who is frankly lethargic, may be significantly obstructed and hypercapnic. The initial global assessment also includes vital signs, pulse oximetry and identification of stigmata of trauma to the head and neck. The cervical spine is evaluated and stabilized as needed. The patient with significant airway distress will typically avoid talking and frequently assume positioning to allow for maximal airway diameter. For example, a patient with epiglottitis may lean forward to allow anterior swollen supraglottis tissues to fall forward. Patients with severe croup, where subglottic edema is circumferentially distributed, may not demonstrate such a positional preference. The presence of skin hemangioma in the pediatric stridorous patient increases the risk of subglottic hemangioma. Neck scars (e.g. thyroidectomy, carotid endarterectomy or anterior approach to the cervical spine) in a patient with upper airway obstruction may give clues as to the source of the stridor.

The history in a patient with airway obstruction is, depending on the magnitude of the obstruction, typically brief and focused. The time course of the stridor is important. Airway symptoms typically first manifest in the setting of neuromuscular relaxation associated with sleep. A history of preceding infection (symptoms of sore throat, cough, fever, odynophagia and dysphagia), head and neck trauma, foreign body ingestion or new medicine, should be sought. Upper aerodigestive tract cancer, most commonly squamous cell carcinoma, usually develops in an older patient with a history of extensive smoking and drinking, although the absence of these historical features certainly does not rule out malignancy. Lymphoma of the upper aerodigestive tract or thyroid carcinoma may occur in younger patients with no history of smoking or drinking. Patients with head and neck malignancy, when asked, will typically relate associated symptoms occurring prior to the development of frank respiratory insufficiency. All such patients should be asked for a complete head and neck review of symptoms including weight loss, cough, hemoptysis, dysphagia, odynophagia, change in voice, otalgia, throat pain, emesis and hematemesis.

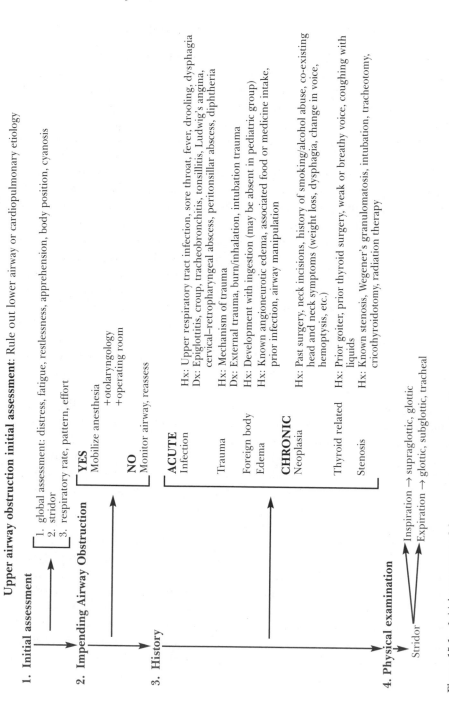

Figure 15.1 Initial assessment of the upper airway – an algorithm

Upper airway obstruction initial assessment: Rule out lower airway or cardiopulmonary etiology

1. Initial assessment
1. global assessment: distress, fatigue, restlessness, apprehension, body position, cyanosis
2. stridor
3. respiratory rate, pattern, effort

2. Impending Airway Obstruction

YES
Mobilize anesthesia
   +otolaryngology
   +operating room

NO
Monitor airway, reassess

3. History

ACUTE
Infection — Hx: Upper respiratory tract infection, sore throat, fever, drooling, dysphagia
Dx: Epiglottitis, croup, tracheobronchitis, tonsillitis, Ludwig's angina, cervical–retropharyngeal abscess, peritonsillar abscess, diphtheria

Trauma — Hx: Mechanism of trauma
Dx: External trauma, burn/inhalation, intubation trauma

Foreign body — Hx: Development with ingestion (may be absent in pediatric group)

Edema — Hx: Known angioneurotic edema, associated food or medicine intake, prior infection, airway manipulation

CHRONIC
Neoplasia — Hx: Past surgery, neck incisions, history of smoking/alcohol abuse, co-existing head and neck symptoms (weight loss, dysphagia, change in voice, hemoptysis, etc.)

Thyroid related — Hx: Prior goiter, prior thyroid surgery, weak or breathy voice, coughing with liquids

Stenosis — Hx: Known stenosis, Wegener's granulomatosis, intubation, tracheotomy, cricothyroidotomy, radiation therapy

4. Physical examination

Stridor
Inspiration → supraglottic, glottic
Expiration → glottic, subglottic, tracheal

During the initial assessment of the patient with airway obstruction, the examiner must take a brief moment to listen to the patient's breathing. Normal respiratory effort is always silent. Stridor, the spontaneous sound made by the patient with significant airway obstruction during breathing, always implies turbulent airflow through a stenotic airway segment. Stridor can be used to help identify location and magnitude of the airway obstruction. A high pulse oximeter reading, while welcome information, should not deter the clinician from aggressive evaluation and treatment of a patient with stridor. Variations in airway caliber can result in a variety of different upper airway sounds. Snoring represents palatal vibration in a narrowed oropharynx chamber during sleep and occurs more frequently in patients with narrow oropharyngeal diameters (e.g. in patients with a long uvula or palate or large tonsils), and in patients who are obese or have nasal obstruction. In general, owing to the relaxation of the upper aerodigestive tract during sleep, most patients with airway obstruction will initially present during sleep. A snoring-like respiratory sound can be present in awake patients with airway obstruction centered in the posterior oropharynx. This can occur in patients with significantly hypertrophic and acutely infected tonsils, large peritonsillar abscess or a large obstructive oropharyngeal or tongue base mass. Patients with lesions in the posterior oropharynx will frequently also have a full, muffled or 'hot potato'-like voice.

Frank stridor is described as being either inspiratory or expiratory, or both. The type of stridor relates to the site of airway obstruction. Isolated inspiratory stridor occurs as a result of restriction of the airway at the level of the vocal cords (glottis) and above (supraglottis), as these regions collapse inward under the force of inspired air. Severe infections with edema or tumors of the supraglottis (i.e. epiglottis, aryepiglottic folds, false vocal cords) typically present with inspiratory stridor. Such supraglottic lesions will also typically affect the hypopharynx's ability to manage handling of saliva. As a result, these patients will have a gurgling, muffled type of phonation. If saliva is significantly affected, drooling will occur. Obstruction at the level of the true vocal cords, or immediately below in the subglottis, typically results in stridor that is mixed inspiratory and expiratory, with the inspiratory component predominating. Lesions of the true vocal cords causing obstruction at the level of the glottis will typically also affect the voice, usually significantly (for example, in vocal cord squamous cell carcinoma). An exception is bilateral vocal cord paralysis, which can occur after thyroid surgery, where the denervated vocal cords come to rest in the midline obstructing the airway. With bilateral vocal cord paralysis, despite the vocal cords' abnormal midline positioning, the true vocal cord surfaces themselves are normal and voice quality is good.

Isolated expiratory stridor is seen in intrathoracic (e.g. tracheal) obstruction. Inspiration is silent and the voice is typically normal. When stridor is present, important diagnostic clues can be obtained by determining the relationship of the stridor to positional changes, sleep and eating.

Laboratory and radiographic evaluation is considered in selected patients without impending airway obstruction after a targeted history and physical examination. In selected patients with stable airways, lateral neck films may help to identify epiglottitis or a retropharyngeal abscess. Lateral neck and chest X-rays can also identify radio-opaque foreign bodies. Deviation of the tracheal air column seen on routine chest X-ray can help identify large and obstructing goiters. However, the degree of tracheal compression can be underestimated in such studies. In all patients with significant tracheal deviation on chest X-ray who are stable, axial computerized tomography (CT) scanning is mandatory. Pulse oximetry can be quickly obtained in most patients with airway obstruction, but it must be understood that hypoxia is a very late finding in airway obstruction, and the overall clinical status of a patient is tremendously more important than the reading on the pulse oximeter. Arterial blood gas status can be determined in stable patients in whom CO_2 retention is suspected. It must be kept in mind, however, that a patient with impending airway collapse may have normal arterial blood gas measures. Similarly, flow volume loops, while quantifying the degree of airway obstruction, are not useful in the acute management of airway obstruction. Changes in flow volume loop profiles in patients with upper airway obstruction typically start to become apparent when the luminal aperture is diminished by at least 80%. Again, the important information in a patient with airway obstruction is the minute-to-minute global assessment of respiratory effort and pattern, with emphasis on the identification of fatigue, restlessness, apprehension, stridor, body position and cyanosis.

AIRWAY MANAGEMENT

In the obtunded patient with respiratory obstruction, the initial maneuver is to facilitate an oral airway through jaw thrust, bringing the tongue forward and providing a preliminary mask oral airway. In the setting of known trauma, there is an obvious need to clean the mouth and pharynx of obstructing blood and foreign bodies such as teeth. In this setting, one must always consider protection of the cervical spine with a collar, avoiding extensive neck flexion, extension or rotation. If the initial mask airway is insufficient, an attempt at intubation transorally can be made. Alternatively, a rigid bronchoscope can be placed through the larynx and ventilation provided through the bronchoscope.

If intubation attempts fail, tracheotomy can be performed urgently. If time permits, local anesthesia can be provided and a vertical incision overlying the upper cervical trachea just below the cricoid in the neck base, just above the sternal notch, can be made. The strap muscles are parted in the midline and the first several tracheal rings are identified. The thyroid isthmus, which typically overlies this region, is clamped and tied, as are any overlying blood vessels. An incision through the second to third tracheal rings is made. This incision is spread with a hemostat and an endotracheal tube or tracheotomy tube can be inserted, providing an airway. Tracheotomy can be performed urgently ('slash tracheotomy') where skin and soft tissues are quickly divided and the airway entered and obtained with pressure and suction providing for hemostasis as best as can be done during the brief procedure.

A cricothyroidotomy (see Chapter 13) is an alternative to urgent tracheotomy. The cricothyroid membrane is identified in the small interval between the lower edge of the thyroid cartilage and the upper edge of the cricoid cartilage in the midline. A transverse incision is made through the cricothyroid membrane with a blade and the airway is entered. The entry site is widened with a hemostat, and an endotracheal tube is placed. The cricothyroid membrane is a relatively avascular site, so urgent entry to the airway here results in less bleeding than at the standard site for tracheotomy, the upper cervical trachea with its overlying thyroid isthmus. However, with cricothyroidotomy the airway is entered higher, actually within the larynx, than with a formal tracheotomy. Cricothyroidotomy brings with it a higher risk of laryngeal injury in general, and subglottic stenosis specifically. If cricothyroidotomy is performed, conversion to a standard tracheotomy should be performed within several days to decrease the risk of subsequent laryngeal injury and stenosis.

In a patient with upper airway obstruction and respiratory distress who is reasonably stable, it is best to obtain otolaryngology and anesthesia assistance. One must keep in mind that airway obstruction, especially when resulting from infection, may occur rapidly. The time course of airway obstruction cannot always be predicted from one's initial assessment. In patients who are judged to be candidates for intubation or tracheotomy, but who are reasonably stable, it is best to obtain additional information, usually in the operating room, with transnasal fiberoptic laryngoscopy.

This can be performed with a patient wide awake and alert, sitting up in the operating room. In this way, otolaryngology and anesthesia personnel can examine the larynx and discuss optimal management if time permits. Occasionally, a fiberoptic bronchoscope can be threaded into the larynx and an endotracheal tube slid down over the scope and into the airway. Helium–oxygen mixtures (80% helium, 20% oxygen; 'heliox') can be used in the initial management of patients with upper airway obstruction. The low density of the helium component of the mixture allows better flow past obstructing lesions and facilitates distal oxygen delivery.

Infections of the airway

Upper airway obstruction may occur to some degree in a patient with acute pharyngotonsillitis, when the acute infection with edema is superimposed upon pre-existing tonsillar hypertrophy. This is especially common in infectious mononucleosis, when acute tonsillar enlargement can be extreme. Symptoms may be especially prominent initially at night, when the surrounding pharyngeal muscular tone is reduced. Oropharyngeal obstruction may be worsened by coexistent nasal congestion through intranasal turbinate edema and adenoidal hypertrophy and inflammation. In cases of extreme tonsillar enlargement with respiratory distress, hospital admission, intravenous steroids and antibiotics usually suffice.

Peritonsillar abscess typically causes severe unilateral sore throat, edema of the soft palate or superior tonsil fossa, a 'hot potato' voice and trismus. Occasionally, the edema associated with peritonsillar abscess may result in airway distress (see Chapter 12). Similarly, lingual tonsillitis may reduce the airway, although its typical symptoms involve sore throat and odynophagia (see Chapter 12). Parapharyngeal and retropharyngeal abscess and Ludwig's angina can all reduce the airway (see Chapter 12).

Epiglottitis

Epiglottitis may occur in the pediatric or adult patient, and is denoted by painful throat and respiratory distress developing over hours. The patient characteristically develops a muffled voice, odynophagia and gradual airway obstruction. Children affected by epiglottitis are usually between 3 and 6 years of age, and will assume an erect sitting position with their neck hyperextended and jaw protruded in order to keep the laryngeal airway open. Such children typically refuse to drink. Drooling is common because of odynophagia. This clinical picture is associated with elevated temperature, pulse and respiratory rate. Dehydration and exhaustion often follow shortly thereafter. Epiglottitis can rapidly progress to complete airway obstruction, so regardless of the patient's initial clinical status, careful and frequent monitoring is essential.

In the case of a severely ill and obtunded child, examination of the pharynx and larynx should be made only in the operating room. For patients who are less acutely ill, a clinical suspicion of acute epiglottitis is best confirmed by a lateral neck film. The lateral neck film in epiglottitis classically shows an epiglottic 'thumb print', identifying the enlarged lateral profile of the epiglottic tip. Examination of the pharynx should be performed only when emergency airway equipment is available. The introduction of a tongue depressor in a patient with epiglottitis can result in backward displacement of the swollen epiglottis and precipitate complete airway obstruction. Epiglottitis can be viral or bacterial, with the most common bacterial pathogen being *Haemophilus influenzae* type B, followed by pneumococcus and group A streptococcus. In approximately 40% of cases, bacterial cultures are negative. The incidence of epiglottitis has been reduced subsequent to the widespread introduction of immunization against *H. influenzae* type B. Antibiotics typically employed for epiglottitis include ampicillin and chloramphenicol, cefuroxime and ampicillin sulbactam. Steroids are usually also given to reduce epiglottic edema.

The establishment of a nasotracheal airway or tracheotomy should not be delayed in children with severe epiglottitis. Respiratory arrest due to sudden obstruction of the laryngeal introitus by an enlarged epiglottis can occur very unexpectedly. Nasotracheal intubation should be established almost without exception in all children under 5 years of age who have epiglottitis. The pediatric airway should be managed jointly by otolaryngology and anesthesia in the operating room. After the airway is established, epiglottic and blood cultures can be obtained.

A related condition involves inflammation of more than one portion of the supraglottis and is termed supraglottitis. Clinical management is similar in epiglottitis and supraglottitis. Adults with mild acute epiglottitis or supraglottitis can often be monitored without intubation or tracheotomy, with fiberoptic laryngoscopy. Studies in adults with epiglottitis have shown that the following clinical features suggest that formal airway intervention through endotracheal intubation or tracheotomy will be needed:

(1) Severe initial respiratory distress with stridor and erect body position;

(2) Rapid clinical course with less than 12 hours between the onset of symptoms and the development of respiratory distress;

(3) The presence of tachycardia on initial assessment;

(4) Positive bacterial blood or throat culture.

Acute spasmodic croup

Acute spasmodic croup occurs in young children between the ages of 1 and 3 years of age. It is unusual over the age of 7. Croup is considered to be primarily viral in etiology, and is typically associated with parainfluenza virus type I. Croup is characterized by severe inflammation with edema and thick mucus centered in the subglottis. The subglottis is formed by the circumferentially complete cricoid cartilage, which is the most narrow point in the upper airway. Croup manifests clinically with a barking-like cough, stridorous respiration, hoarse voice, chest retractions and occasionally intermittent cyanosis. The acute onset or attack can occur without any significant prodrome, often in the middle of the night. The child is often afebrile and has no signs of obvious infection. In the vast majority of cases, only moderate respiratory distress occurs. The most effective treatment is humidification and mucolytics. At home this is best achieved by running the shower with steam inhalation. Occasionally, children will develop respiratory distress with marked retractions and cyanosis, and a depressed sensorium. Such patients require hospitalization. Anteroposterior and lateral neck films may show marked subglottic edema, called the 'steeple sign'. This refers to the upwardly sloping profile of the subglottic mucosa that corresponds to the subglottic mucosal edema. In the hospital the child is placed in a cooled mist tent and intravenous hydration is begun. Oxygen administration is helpful, but obscures cyanosis as a finding. Nebulization of racemic epinephrine (adrenaline) can be administered for 5–10 min/hour over the first 3–4 hours until symptoms improve. Once racemic epinephrine is given, however, close monitoring in the hospital is required, as patients may initially respond to the first treatment and then rebound. Steroids are often considered to reduce subglottic mucosal edema. Intravenous antibiotics can be considered to avoid secondary bacterial infection, such as streptococcus, staphylococcus and pneumococcus. Appropriate antibiotics include ampicillin sulbactam and cefuroxime. Respiratory depressants such as sedatives and opiates are contraindicated.

Children who fail to improve on the above-noted regimen may require insertion of a nasotracheal tube, which should be placed in the operating room. Patients with croup may manifest laryngeal supraglottic edema. Patients demonstrating agitation, cyanosis, lethargy, increased pulse or respiratory rate or CO_2 retention despite treatment should be nasotracheally intubated. In general, endotracheal intubation is avoided if possible, to avoid worsening of subglottic irritation from the cuff of the endotracheal tube. Such cuff-induced trauma in the setting of pre-existing subglottic mucosal inflammation may lead to the development of subglottic stenosis. During intubation, search for foreign bodies should be performed, as foreign body aspiration in a child can mimic croup.

The differential diagnosis of respiratory distress and severe cough in children includes, in addition to croup, epiglottitis, bacterial tracheitis, foreign body, an infected laryngeal cyst, retropharyngeal abscess, laryngeal papillomatosis and diphtheria. Croup can be distinguished from epiglottitis in that it typically occurs in a younger age group. Patients with croup do not usually prefer the leaning-forward position often seen in patients with epiglottitis where the edema is centered in the anterior supraglottis. Usually, patients with croup are hoarse and have less odynophagia than patients with epiglottitis. In pediatric patients with recurrent croup, evaluation between episodes should be undertaken to rule out underlying subglottic stenosis.

Bacterial tracheitis

Bacterial tracheitis is a clinical entity easily confused with croup. This entity is caused by a bacterial infection of the tracheal mucosa characterized by edema, excess purulent discharge with cough and respiratory distress. Cultures typically reveal *Staphylococcus aureus* or *Streptococcus pneumoniae*. Appropriate antibiotics with steroids and humidification are effective.

Pertussis

Bordetella pertussis (a.k.a. whooping cough) is an acute, highly communicable disease occurring primarily in the pediatric population. However, adults and adolescents may become infected if prior immunization has not been effective. Pediatric patients are at higher risk of severe disease than adults or adolescents. Following a catarrhal phase, a paroxysmal cough phase develops. The inspiratory gasp after a coughing paroxysm generates the 'whoop'. A plane lateral neck film may show narrowing of the lateral subglottis ('steeple sign') as with croup. The diagnosis is typically made clinically, but can be confirmed with nasopharynx culture (on chocolate agar), or the disease can be serologically diagnosed. Antibiotics, typically erythromycin, are most effective if started before the paroxysmal cough phase is reached. Prophylactic treatment is indicated for individuals exposed to infected patients.

Diphtheria

Diphtheria (see Chapter 12) during a major outbreak in the 1700s led to the death of 2–3% of the population in the northeast USA. It is now rare, involving primarily the unimmunized. Clinical infection is very rare in an immunized person. *Corynebacterium diphtheriae* is carried in airborne respiratory secretions. Diphtheria produces severe pharyngeal infection characterized by a leathery pharyngeal membrane and serosanguineous nasal discharge. Exotoxin production includes a neurologic toxin elaborated within days of the onset of pharyngeal discomfort. This toxin leads to soft palate paralysis, other cranial neuropathies and ultimately peripheral motor and sensory changes. As throat symptoms improve, a cardiotoxin can also be produced which can lead to myocarditis and arrhythmia. The diphtheric pharyngeal membrane is white to gray, and can occur in the pharynx and entire tracheobronchial tree. Extensive diphtheric membrane can thus lead to obstruction and suffocation. Pharyngeal infection is associated with soft tissue edema and prominent cervical adenitis, the so-called diphtheric 'bull neck'. Diagnosis is made through culture on Loeffler's medium. Treatment includes penicillin and diphtheria antitoxin.

Many other infectious and inflammatory conditions can lead to upper airway obstruction (see Chapters 12 and 13). These include tuberculosis, syphilis, infection with *Klebsiella rhinoscleromatis*, laryngeal chondritis, laryngeal and tracheal radiochondronecrosis, glanders (*Pseudomonas mallei*), leprosy (*Mycobacterium leprae*) and a variety of mycotic infections, including blastomycosis, histoplasmosis, candidiasis, actinomycosis and coccidioidomycosis. Inflammatory conditions that can affect the upper airway include pemphigus, Wegener's granulomatosis, sarcoid and cricoarytenoid arthritis.

Acute laryngeal angioedema

Acute laryngeal edema is most frequently the result of food or inhalant allergy. Laryngeal edema is also part of an anaphylactic response to insect sting injury. Such edema may also occur in response to medicines including antibiotics, morphine, codeine, iodinated intravenous contrast dye or angiotensin-converting enzyme (ACE) inhibitor antihypertensives. The ACE enzyme inhibitors have been associated with chronic cough as well as acute laryngeal edema, even with significant delay after the initiation of antihypertensive treatment. The ACE inhibitor-related edema is associated with increased bradykinin and decreased angiotensin II levels.

Angioneurotic edema of the larynx and upper airway can occur in inherited and acquired forms. Angioneurotic edema of the upper aerodigestive tract is a well-demarcated, non-pitting edema affecting the face, lips, tongue and other mucous membranes, and can result in airway obstruction, especially when affecting the tongue, posterior oropharynx and larynx. Angioneurotic edema can also affect abdominal viscera. Acquired angioneurotic edema can be associated with B-cell lymphoma, immune complex disease (serum sickness) and systemic lupus erythematosus. Inherited angioneurotic edema occurs as an autosomal dominant deficiency of C1 esterase inhibitor. Such deficiency allows complement cascade reactivity after otherwise minor provocation such as minor trauma (e.g. dental work, intubation), infection or emotional stress. The complement reaction results in histamine release followed by swelling and edema secondary to increased vascular permeability. Work-up includes C1 esterase inhibitor and complement levels. In the USA there are approximately 1200 persons affected with this autosomal dominant genetic disorder. Among such persons, mortality rates can be high. Physicians should be alerted to the patient who reports episodes of mucosal and subdermal edema without apparent reason, occurring initially during the teenage years. Such angioneurotic edema episodes can involve the abdominal viscera, and can be symptomatically manifest as abdominal cramping, pain and vomiting. In the respiratory tract, such episodes can cause vague episodes of coughing followed by atelectasis with pleural effusion. Acute treatment of angioneurotic edema of the airway involves subcutaneous epinephrine, intravenous steroids, racemic epinephrine nebulized treatments, antihistamines and close airway monitoring with intubation used as needed. Inherited angioneurotic edema can be treated with danazol (which provides androgen stimulation of C1 esterase inhibitor levels), fresh frozen plasma (FFP) and ε-aminocaproic acid. In patients with inherited angioneurotic edema, avoidance of inciting trauma and stress is best. Prophylaxis during mandibular surgery or dental procedures can be achieved with FFP and ε-aminocaproic acid.

Respiratory obstruction in the newborn infant

A newborn infant, for the first few months of life, is an obligate nasal breather, and obstruction of the nose will result in apnea. Causes of nasal obstruction in the neonate include bilateral choanal atresia, encephalocele, tumors of the nose and nasopharynx and nasal cavity stenosis. Respiratory obstruction in the infant that originates in the oropharynx may be due to macroglossia, small mandible (such as in Pierre Robin syndrome), or the presence of an oral or neck tumor, such as a large cystic hygroma, dermoid or hemangioma. Laryngeal obstruction of the airway in a newborn infant may be due to a large congenital web of the larynx, subglottic stenosis or hemangioma, bilateral vocal cord paralysis, congenital atresia of the larynx, laryngotracheal cleft or tracheoesophageal fistulas.

Chronic respiratory obstruction in a child

Laryngomalacia

Laryngomalacia is by far the most common laryngeal anomaly in young children and is the most common cause of chronic respiratory obstruction. It is not a disease; rather it is an anatomic variation in the structure of the larynx in children up to 2 years of age. Typically, laryngomalacia presents within the first few months of life and improves usually after 1 year of age. Children with laryngomalacia may have a folded Ω-shaped epiglottis. The epiglottis and aryepiglottic folds are excessively flaccid during inspiration and are pulled into the introitus of the larynx, resulting in intermittent airway narrowing. The stridor in these children is intermittent and will improve or clear if the child is turned from the back onto the abdomen. A thorough history is important, including a history of any feeding difficulties. While in adults respiratory insufficiency involving the upper airway is often first manifest while sleeping or during upper respiratory tract infection, young children typically present with stridor that worsens with feeding. The cry of a young child, if hoarse, may suggest pathology of the vocal cords. A weak cry in a child can suggest vocal cord paralysis. When symptoms are severe and persistent, these children can be evaluated with fiberoptic laryngoscopy and, when necessary, direct laryngoscopy and bronchoscopy. The treatment for laryngomalacia is usually observation. Rarely, tracheotomy and excision of supraglottic redundant tissue (epiglottis and aryepiglottic folds) are performed.

Foreign body of the airway

Airway obstruction due to an aspirated foreign body kills up to 3000 patients per year in the USA, with the highest incidence occurring in the very young. Another peak occurs in the elderly, perhaps related to edentulous deglutition or coexistent mental status changes, some of which may be related to sedative medicines and alcohol. The most frequent foreign body that affects the airway is the peanut. Other common foreign bodies include teeth, popcorn, coins, a balloon or fragments of plastic toy. A foreign body that is lodged in the airway will obviously result in sudden onset of coughing, choking and wheezing. However, a foreign body that is large enough to enter the upper esophagus and become lodged there can, if strategically positioned, indent the posterior wall of the trachea and present with airway obstruction as well. Most commonly, aspiration of a foreign body occurs in young children ranging in age from 6 months to 4 years. Not infrequently, the intake of the foreign body is unwitnessed, and the initial symptomatic period is short and followed by a relatively symptom-free period in which the child may be normal except for intermittent periods of croupy cough and wheezing. If the foreign body aspiration is undiscovered for a long time, it may result in focal atelectasis and pneumonitis with fever, cough and occasionally hemoptysis. Foreign bodies of vegetable origin such as nuts, peas and beans, as well as batteries, will cause significant local edema and have a tendency to cause a greater inflammatory response than inert foreign bodies. Patients with undetected foreign bodies may carry the diagnosis of asthma; these patients have been treated for prolonged periods of time with steroids and antibiotics.

A child with croup should be considered to have a foreign body in his lower respiratory tract until proven otherwise. Physical examination may show localized wheezing or decreased breath sounds, or be perfectly normal. Inspiratory and expiratory chest X-rays and fluoroscopy may be required to make a proper diagnosis of a foreign body. The mediastinum may be shifted towards the object with inspiration. Atelectasis may be present in the lung distal to the foreign body.

An adult patient with a laryngeal foreign body typically will not reach the emergency room for treatment. The Heimlich maneuver should be tried at the scene once or twice. If this fails to clear the foreign body, the patient should be placed supine, and the physician should make a quick attempt to remove the foreign body with the fingers or with forceps if they are available. If the airway remains completely obstructed, a cricothyroidotomy or emergency tracheotomy can be accomplished (see Chapter 13).

Vascular compression of the trachea

Vascular compression of the trachea is not an uncommon cause of stridor in an infant. It is usually caused by an anomalous right innominate artery or much less commonly by a double aortic arch or pulmonary vascular sling. The symptoms usually begin very early in life and range from mild stridor and wheezing to severe bouts of dyspnea. Feeding problems are associated with respiratory complaints. Differential diagnosis includes tracheomalacia and tracheal compression from non-vascular masses including thymic or thyroid lesions. Diagnosis is made by a combination of radiologic and endoscopic studies. Surgical correction of the vascular anomaly is the treatment of choice.

Laryngeal cysts and laryngoceles

Laryngeal cysts and laryngoceles result from invaginations of the mucous membrane of the larynx, usually from the ventricular area. They typically produce a mass effect in the false cord and aryepiglottic fold. The diagnosis can be made by X-ray studies and laryngoscopy. Most laryngeal cysts can be endoscopically marsupialized.

Laryngeal papillomatosis

Patients with laryngeal papillomatosis symptomatically present with hoarseness or weak cry, as the true vocal cords are usually preferentially affected. Progressive papilloma mass can result in airway obstruction. Laryngeal papillomatosis can occur in any age group and is associated with the human papilloma virus. While children present with more multifocal disease, which may initially be progressive, such disease, often regresses at puberty. Treatment involves endoscopic CO_2 laser ablation. Interferon has also been used. Tracheotomy is avoided, as it has been associated with increased risk of tracheobronchial spread of papillomas.

Congenital laryngeal webs

The majority of laryngeal webs are partial and are located between the true cords. They result in a weak or hoarse cry and stridor with crying. Occasionally, laryngeal webs can occur more superiorly between the false cords. In these cases, children are stridorous but have a normal cry. The treatment is division of the web endoscopically. Dilatation may be necessary in order to prevent reformation.

Subglottic hemangioma

Hemangiomas may occur in the subglottic larynx and result in airway narrowing. Children with hemangiomas that are large enough to cause partial obstruction have stridor. Plain films may show subglottic deformation. Direct laryngoscopy reveals the presence of a vascular tumor. The diagnosis should be made by visual examination during laryngoscopy, not biopsy. A further clue to the diagnosis of subglottic hemangioma is the presence of cutaneous hemangiomas elsewhere in the body.

Most subglottic hemangiomas increase in size over the first 3–4 months of life, and then often spontaneously regress after 2 years of age. One initial satisfactory method of treatment is tracheotomy and conservative monitoring of the hemangioma, as they regress on their own. Subglottic hemangioma has also been treated by CO_2 laser ablation.

NEOPLASTIC AIRWAY OBSTRUCTION

Malignant lesions

Malignancy of the upper aerodigestive tract may present with respiratory symptoms. The most common malignancy of the upper aerodigestive tract is squamous cell carcinoma. Squamous cell carcinoma lesions may present as large obstructing lesions when arising from the base of the tongue, the hypopharynx and the larynx. Lymphoma and thyroid carcinoma affecting the upper aerodigestive tract may also present with respiratory symptoms, and may occur in a younger age group than patients with squamous cell carcinoma.

Most patients with squamous cell carcinoma of the head and neck have a history of extensive smoking and alcohol intake. A full head and neck review of symptoms, including assessment of weight loss, cough, hemoptysis, sore throat, otalgia, dysphagia, odynophagia or change in voice will usually result in the identification of a clustering of symptoms that may have been present for weeks to months prior to the development of frank respiratory symptoms. Many rarer forms of neoplasia of the upper aerodigestive tract may occur and result in respiratory symptoms, including laryngeal chondromas, neurofibromas, leiomyomas, angiofibromas, myomas, hemangiomas, chemodectomas and granular cell myoblastomas.

Benign neoplastic airway obstruction

Upper aerodigestive tract obstruction may occur from many benign lesions.

Lingual thyroid

If thyroid embryologic migration arrests completely, a lingual thyroid results without tissue in the normal orthotopic site (see Chapter 17). This tissue manifests as a base-of-tongue mass and can present with respiratory embarrassment, dysphagia or hemoptysis. Patients can be studied with CT scanning and I^{123}-scanning. Patients may be managed with T4 hormonal suppression, radioactive iodine (I^{131}) ablation or surgical excision.

Laryngocele

A laryngocele is an air-filled dilated laryngeal saccule, a small laryngeal invagination that arises from the laryngeal ventricle between the true and false cords. An internal laryngocele which is contained within the endo-larynx presents as a submucosal mass in the false cord region. If an internal laryngocele extends superior to the thyroid cartilage, it presents as an external neck mass, an external laryngocele. Although a laryngocele is initially air-filled, it may evolve to form a mucocele or mucopyocele if infected. Patients usually present with hoarseness secondary to laryngeal deformation from the mass, and may develop, if the airway is impacted upon significantly, respiratory embarrassment. Evaluation is through radiographic imaging in the form of a CT scan or magnetic resonance imaging (MRI). The treatment of an internal laryngocele is usually endoscopic laser marsupialization. External laryngoceles are treated by external resection.

Occasionally, benign laryngeal pathology, including vocal cord polyps and arytenoid granulomas (see Chapter 13), can be large enough to 'ball valve' within the glottis and result in intermittent obstructive symptoms.

AIRWAY STENOSIS

Stenosis of the airway may occur at any level, but the majority of significant upper airway narrowing occurs in the larynx and trachea. Laryngeal steno-sis is subdivided into supraglottic (above the vocal cords), glottic (at the level of the vocal cords) or subglottic (below the vocal cords).

Supraglottic stenosis (laryngeal inlet stenosis) can result from chemical injury (e.g. lye), thermal/inhalation burns, external trauma or scarring associated with a chronic inflammatory or infectious disorder (e.g. tuberculosis or pemphigus). Treatment usually involves tracheotomy with resection of the epiglottis and associated stenotic supraglottic tissue.

Glottic and subglottic stenosis are more common than supraglottic stenosis.

Glottic stenosis may occur from narrowing associated with scarring from endotracheal tube-related trauma or endoscopic instrumentation, from external trauma, cricoarytenoid joint dysfunction or from bilateral vocal cord paralysis. Treatment usually involves tracheotomy and cord lateralization with arytenoidectomy through laryngofissure.

Subglottic stenosis may be congenital or acquired. Congenital stenosis in turn may be membranous, involving mucosal or submucosal tissues (i.e. normal cricoid cartilaginous structure), or cartilaginous (i.e. insufficient cricoid cartilage structure). Acquired subglottic stenosis may arise from intraluminal subglottic injury secondary to endotracheal tube cuff trauma, external trauma, high tracheotomy, or cricothyroidotomy with cricoid injury and subsequent narrowing. Endotracheal tube injury is more likely if the endotracheal tube is too large for the airway or is left in for longer than 2 weeks. Regional inflammatory disorders such as Wegener's granulomatosis, pemphigus, sarcoid, amyloidosis, rhinoscleroma, mycotic infections, syphilis or leprosy can also result in subglottic stenosis. Reflux into the hypopharynx and larynx probably represents a cofactor in the development of subglottic stenosis.

Subglottic stenosis can be corrected endoscopically with laser ablation in rare circumstances when it is caused by a thin web or subglottic hemangioma. For most complex cases of subglottic stenosis, open repair through laryngofissure is required. In the case of submucosal scarring, stenotic mucosal and submucosal regions are excised and the exposed underlying cartilage is augmented by grafts to reline the laryngeal lumen. Periods of stenting are usually necessary if the grafted segments are extensive. In cases where the cartilaginous framework is insufficient, cricoid cartilage division and grafting can expand the laryngeal lumen at the level of the cricoid. Typical donor sites include the hyoid bone, the rib or septal, auricular or thyroid cartilage. Subglottic stenosis may also be treated with tracheocricoid resection with thyrotracheal anastomosis.

LARYNGEAL PARALYSIS

Laryngeal paralysis is discussed in Chapter 13. With unilateral vocal cord paralysis, the airway is typically not significantly affected. This is because the affected cord is usually laterally positioned to some degree, and the opposite cord has normal mobility. Thus, the glottic airway is not significantly compromised in the typical case of isolated unilateral vocal cord paralysis. An exception to this is unilateral vocal cord paralysis in an elderly patient. In such a patient, the mobility of the opposite cord may be reduced, perhaps as a result of chronic cricoarytenoid dysfunction. In such a patient, unilateral vocal cord paralysis may manifest with airway symptomatology. Etiologies for adult unilateral vocal cord paralysis are reviewed in Chapter 13. In children, laryngeal paralysis can be associated with cardiac and great vessel anomalies, ductus ligation procedures and birth trauma.

Bilateral vocal cord paralysis typically affects the airway. As the bilaterally paralyzed cords come to rest in the midline, respiratory function degrades and the patient develops stridor which is typically inspiratory more than expiratory. The voice, however, is typically quite good. Bilateral vocal cord paralysis may be due to bilateral recurrent laryngeal nerve injury secondary to thyroid surgery or thyroid cancer, or may be associated with neck trauma. Bilateral mediastinal or base-of-skull malignancy, severe inflammatory disorder, intracranial disease with increased intracranial pressure or degenerative neurologic processes, including brain-stem stroke, can result in bilateral vocal cord paralysis. Bilateral vocal cord paralysis in the child may be associated with Arnold–Chiari malformation, meningomyelocele or birth trauma. Patients with bilateral vocal cord paralysis present with respiratory distress and are treated initially with intubation and tracheotomy. Ultimate treatment to widen the glottic level airway involves lateralizing one-half of the glottis which, to some degree, sacrifices the voice for airway improvement. Techniques include arytenoidectomy, vocal cord lateralization (endoscopic or open) or transverse laser cordotomy. It is important to note, prior to treatment, whether bilateral midline immobile cords is due to bilateral vocal cord paralysis or bilateral vocal cord fixation/tethering caused by either posterior glottic scarring or bilateral cricoarytenoid joint dysfunction. Such bilateral cricoarytenoid joint dysfunction may be associated with advanced age, cricoarytenoid arthritis, external beam radiation or reflux. It may also occur in the setting of chronic bilateral vocal cord paralysis with secondary cricoarytenoid joint scarring and fixation from immobility.

THYROID DISEASE AND THE AIRWAY

Thyroid disease can affect the airway in many ways. Thyroid cancer or thyroid surgery can affect one or both recurrent laryngeal nerves with unilateral or bilateral vocal cord paralysis (see above and Chapter 13).

Thyroid cancer, when invasive, can diminish the laryngeal and tracheal airway. Benign disease can, through airway deviation and compression, significantly affect the airway. The airway may be affected in the neck or with substernal goiter in the chest. Such deviation and compression can occur slowly with significant narrowing of the airway without symptoms. Airway symptoms may occur rapidly once the airway is narrowed beyond a certain critical diameter. In benign goiter, hemorrhage within a nodule can frequently lead to the development of such critical narrowing and the acute development of symptoms. In patients with large cervical or substernal goiters, one must assess for any airway symptoms such as chronic cough, nocturnal dyspnea, choking episodes or positional respiratory distress. In this setting, radiographic evaluation should not be limited to chest X-ray, which can underestimate the degree of airway compression. Axial CT scanning of the neck and chest is mandatory. All substernal goiters and cervical goiters that generate airway symptoms, as well as those that are asymptomatic but show radiographic evidence of significant airway deviation or compression, should be resected. Thyroid hormone suppression and I^{131}-ablation treatments are not reliably effective modalities when considering the airway. Surgery is almost always performed through standard thyroid neck incision and is generally tolerated well.

NECK AND AIRWAY TRAUMA

In an obtunded trauma patient, the airway may be obstructed as a result of loss of tone and collapse, or from blood, teeth or mandibular fracture with posterior displacement of the tongue. Initial management includes cervical spine stabilization in any patient with significant head and neck trauma. In the trauma patient who is obtunded, once the cervical spine is stabilized, jaw thrust is performed and the oropharynx is examined to clear the oral airway. An anesthetic ventilation bag is then used to provide mask ventilation with jaw thrust maintained. If the mask oral airway is inadequate, endotracheal tube intubation is attempted. Nasotracheal intubation in patients with head and neck trauma should be considered carefully, given the possibility of fracture of the cribiform plate and roof of ethmoid. An airway can also be obtained through rigid bronchoscopy and ventilation through the bronchoscope. If such attempts fail or are impossible, cricothyroidotomy or emergency tracheotomy can be performed. Laryngeal and tracheal trauma can result in significant disruption of the laryngotracheal airway by mucosal edema, hemorrhage and bilateral vocal cord paralysis, as well as by frank cartilaginous disruption of the airway. Cartilage fracture, especially anterior cricoid fracture, can be displaced with 'anterior cricoid pressure' during such difficult intubations, and result in loss of airway. Laryngeal trauma may also occur through traumatic intubations with mucosal disruption, bleeding and arytenoid dislocation. Laryngeal obstruction may occur in a patient with inhalational or chemical airway burn, as may occur with thermal burn, crack or other drug inhalation, or ingestion of lye.

A history of the mechanism of injury is important in the motor vehicle accident patient. A history of sitting in the front or back seat, speed and whether the patient was restrained or unrestrained is important. A full upper airway review of symptoms should be obtained if time permits, including the presence of hemoptysis, which suggests mucosal laceration, the presence of hoarseness, which suggests vocal cord pathology and the presence of odynophagia, which suggests arytenoid injury or dislocation.

In the patient with external trauma, the neck examination may show ecchymosis, swelling and loss of the normal laryngeal and tracheal contour. The finding of crepitus (subcutaneous air) helps to identify upper aerodigestive tract disruption and requires complete definitive work-up, usually including airway and esophageal endoscopy, chest X-ray and esophogram. If a leak is suspected, gastrogaffin generates less soft tissue inflammation, whereas barium is better tolerated if aspiration is present. In any patient with signs of significant neck trauma, one must check for pulse and cranial nerve abnormalities. Soot at the nares or mouth in the thermal burn patient implies upper airway burn.

In patients with significant laryngeal trauma with impending airway obstruction, tracheotomy, laryngoscopy and esophagoscopy are usually performed. Performing tracheotomy initially, usually with local anesthesia, helps to avoid further laryngeal injury through intubation. In children with laryngeal trauma who are not candidates for tracheotomy under local anesthesia, rigid bronchoscopic intubation is best. In patients with minor laryngeal trauma, such as small lacerations or small areas of ecchymosis who have a good airway, observation with voice rest, steroids, antibiotics and antireflux measures are sufficient. The airway in these circumstances should be monitored by repetitive flexible fiberoptic laryngoscopy. Laryngeal CT scanning can also be used to guide further therapy. On fiberoptic examination, the larynx should be checked for edema, ecchymosis, hematoma, mucosal lacerations, exposed cartilage and vocal cord mobility. Also, the anteroposterior diameter of the larynx is assessed. Shortening of the anteroposterior diameter of the larynx can suggest arytenoid dislocation, posterior displacement of the epiglottis or significant cartilaginous displacement. If cartilage fractures are significant or are displaced, they can be reduced with or without laryngofissure. With anterior commissure injury or extensive cartilaginous injury, laryngeal stenting is usually performed. During surgery, lacerations are repaired, cartilage is covered and fractures are reduced.

16

Salivary gland disorders

Gregory W. Randolph

Anatomy and physiology
Major salivary glands
  Parotid gland
  Submandibular gland
  Sublingual gland
Minor salivary glands
Diagnostic strategy for disorders of the salivary glands
  Clinical history
  Physical examination
Categories of salivary gland disorders
  Acute inflammatory disorders
    Mumps
    Acute bacterial sialadenitis
    Chronic obstructive salivary gland disease (strictures and stones)
  Chronic progressive inflammatory disorders
    Benign lymphoepithelial lesion of the salivary glands
    Granulomatous infiltration of the salivary glands
    Metabolic disorders
    Xerostomia
  Discrete mass within the salivary gland (salivary neoplasm)

ANATOMY AND PHYSIOLOGY

The daily salivary output of approximately 1500 ml is formed in both major and minor salivary glands. The parotid, submandibular and sublingual glands are termed major salivary glands. In addition, there are multiple small minor salivary glands found in the oral cavity, including the tongue, soft palate and nasopharynx. Major and minor salivary glands are exocrine glands. Saliva is low in sodium and high in potassium and contains a number of enzymes including amylase and lysozymes, as well as mucin and IgA. Saliva is important in digestive function, not only by containing digestive enzymes such as amylase, but also by providing for lubrication of the food bolus through the mouth and throat. Saliva also helps to prevent dental caries and possesses antibacterial properties. The parotid gland produces a predominantly serous saliva while the sublingual glands produce a predominantly mucinous, more viscous saliva. The submandibular gland produces a mixed secretion. Minor or accessory salivary glands produce a primarily mucinous saliva.

MAJOR SALIVARY GLANDS

Parotid gland

The normal parotid gland is barely palpable. It is located on the lateral aspect of the face and extends superiorly to the zygomatic arch, inferiorly to the level of the mandible, posteriorly to the cartilage of the external auditory canal and anteriorly to approximately the anterior margin of the ascending ramus of the mandible. Clinically, the gland is divided into superficial and deep lobes by the branches of the facial nerve, which innervate the muscles of facial expression. The two lobes are interconnected between the branches of the facial nerve, and anatomically there is not a true discrete lobular structure. The tail of the parotid gland represents a variably developed lobule of parotid tissue that extends posteroinferiorly over the angle of the mandible into the neck. The facial nerve exits the base of the skull at the stylomastoid foramen (at the junction of the external auditory canal anteriorly and the mastoid process posteriorly) and extends downwards to ramify at the posterior surface of the parotid gland. Within the gland, the nerve divides into its five main branches: temporal, zygomatic, buccal, mandibular (ramus) and cervical. The deep lobe of the parotid abuts the parapharyngeal space. Therefore, masses in the deep lobe of the parotid can indent the lateral oropharynx wall in the tonsil fossa region, and affect the mandible's pterygoid musculature, leading to trismus. The parotid salivary duct (Stensen's duct) extends from the anterior aspect of the gland lateral to the masseter muscle and pierces the buccinator muscle, opening into the mouth through the buccal mucosa at approximately the level of the second maxillary molar.

Salivary secretions are regulated by the autonomic nervous system. The preganglionic parasympathetic fibers originate in the inferior salivatory nucleus and reach the parotid gland by way of the ninth cranial nerve. The ninth cranial nerve crosses the middle ear space as Jacobson's nerve, exits the tympanic cavity as the lesser superficial petrosal nerve and synapses at the otic ganglion. Postganglionic fibers follow the auriculotemporal branch of the third (mandibular) division of the trigeminal nerve to innervate the gland. Sympathetic innervation of the parotid gland derives from the carotid plexus.

Submandibular gland

The submandibular gland lies in the submandibular triangle and is normally palpable. In the aged, it may become ptotic, firm and quite discrete, often falsely identified as a pathologic neck mass. Superiorly, the gland extends under the mandible, inferiorly it overlays the digastric muscle and anteriorly it extends medially to the mylohyoid muscle (Figure 16.1). The submandibular salivary duct (Wharton's duct) originates on the medial surface of the gland between the mylohyoid and hyoglossus muscles, crosses the lingual nerve and opens at a papilla in the anterior floor of the mouth lateral to the frenulum of the tongue. The ramus mandibularis (the lowest facial nerve branch in the face), which innervates the lower lip, loops down over the mandible and runs on the fascia over the submandibular gland, and hence can be injured during submandibular gland surgery. The hypoglossal nerve lies just deep to the submandibular gland and digastric muscle as it extends anterior and upward to provide motor function to the tongue. The lingual nerve (sensory to the tongue and the floor of the mouth) loops downward to the submandibular gland and is crossed by Wharton's duct as it extends to the floor of the mouth.

The salivary secretion of the submandibular gland is under autonomic control. Preganglionic parasympathetic fibers originate in the superior salivatory nucleus and extend in the nervus intermedius and chorda tympani divisions of the facial nerve. These fibers, after exiting the middle ear through the petrotympanic fissure, run with the lingual nerve to synapse in the submandibular ganglion. Sympathetic innervation of the submandibular gland originates from the carotid plexus.

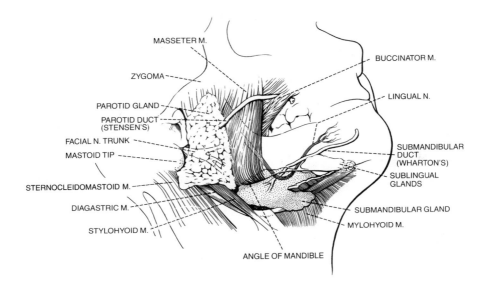

Figure 16.1 Anatomy of the parotid and submandibular glands

Sublingual gland

The sublingual gland is located in a submucosal plane in the anterior floor of the mouth and extends anteriorly along the medial aspect of the mandible to the midline. There are usually multiple sublingual duct orifices in the floor of the mouth, just posterior to the orifice of Wharton's duct. The autonomic nerve supply is shared with the submandibular gland.

Histologically, the major salivary glands are composed of glandular acini, intercalated ducts, striated ducts and finally expiratory ducts. Myoepithelial cells surround the acini and possess contractile properties. Acinar cells actively transport sodium into the lumen of the acini. Salivary composition is further modified in the striated ducts.

MINOR SALIVARY GLANDS

It has been estimated that there are between 500 and 1000 minor salivary glands in the oropharynx, tongue, soft palate and nasopharynx, with the greatest concentration being in the hard and soft palate. These are not under obvious autonomic control.

DIAGNOSTIC STRATEGY FOR DISORDERS OF THE SALIVARY GLANDS

A wide variety of inflammatory, infiltrative, obstructive and neoplastic disorders may affect salivary gland tissue. The physician must develop a diagnostic strategy that helps to separate these lesions into smaller categories to allow selection of further diagnostic procedures. For example, although radiopaque sialography may be diagnostic in cases of suspected strictures or stones, it is contraindicated in acute suppurative sialadenitis.

A working diagnosis, whether specific or relating to a broad category of disorders, is made on the basis of clinical history and an initial examination.

Clinical history

The clinical history is an essential element in assessing salivary gland disorders. The patient's complaint is almost always of a fullness or mass within the salivary gland tissue that may or may not be painful. The following elements of the history should be determined:

(1) How long has the mass or fullness been present? Development over a course of hours suggests an obstructive and perhaps infectious disorder, whereas a mass that enlarges slowly over months or years may suggest some infiltrative or neoplastic disorder. Also, what was associated with the onset of the problem? Coexistent virus-like symptoms may suggest viral parotitis, whereas the existence of significant dehydration and smoking may be associated with reduced salivary flow, ductal plugging and subsequent frank bacterial sialadenitis.

(2) Does the fullness or mass fluctuate in size? Intermittent obstruction will often cause great variations in the size of the mass, whereas neoplastic disorders progressively enlarge in size. Postprandial swelling suggests duct obstruction with a stone or stricture.

(3) Is there pain? Infectious and other inflammatory disorders often cause pain whereas benign neoplastic disorders are generally painless unless they cause secondary obstruction. Malignancies of the salivary glands may cause pain, especially when advanced.

(4) What is the general health of the patient? Are there acute or chronic illnesses that may relate to the salivary gland disorder? For example, suppurative parotitis is most commonly seen in a debilitated, poorly hydrated patient with poor oral hygiene; or the medical history may

suggest that a rapidly enlarging mass within the parotid gland may be a local manifestation of lymphoma or leukemia. Enlargement of the gland may also occur in metabolic disorders, including alcoholism, cirrhosis, endocrinopathy, diabetes mellitus and malnutrition. Systemic granulomatous diseases such as tuberculosis and sarcoidosis may also affect salivary gland tissue. HIV disease may be associated with a diffuse multicystic parotid enlargement, as well as with salivary gland lymphoma.

Physical examination

The following questions help the physician to determine the physical characteristics of the salivary lesion and to assign it to a specific category of disease process:

(1) Is the swelling or enlargement localized to one gland, or are several glands involved? Multiple gland involvement, even to varying degrees, suggests systemic illnesses such as endocrinopathy or inflammatory disorder (e.g. Sjögren's syndrome).

(2) Does the mass or swelling constitute a diffuse increase in the size of the gland or does the swelling represent a nodule or mass within the anatomical confines of the gland? A diffuse increase suggests an inflammatory disorder such as infectious or obstructive disease, Sjögren's syndrome, endocrinopathies or infiltration of the gland as is occasionally seen in leukemia. On the other hand, a mass within, but not filling, the anatomical confines of the gland suggests a neoplasm or in rare cases granulomatous infiltration. A well-encapsulated mass that is easily mobile and possesses a smooth contour suggests a benign lesion or a lymph node; a more infiltrative, poorly mobile, irregular mass suggests a malignant lesion. Facial nerve paresis or paralysis in the presence of an irregular or poorly mobile infiltrative lesion of the parotid gland is further evidence of malignant disease.

(3) Is there a stone? If so, it may be revealed by palpation of the duct which is often best accomplished by bimanual examination. During bimanual examination, one hand pushes inwards in the region of the anterior parotid duct, and the other hand in the mouth palpates the buccal mucosa overlying the distal course and orifice of Stensen's duct. For submandibular stones, bimanual examination, as for floor-of-mouth lesions, is employed. One hand externally palpates over a broad

surface the submandibular gland region from posterior to anterior, while the forefinger of the opposite hand palpates the floor-of-mouth mucosa from above. In this way, large stones in the submandibular gland hilus and Wharton's duct are trapped between the examining fingers.

(4) What is the quality of the fluid that can be expressed from Stensen's or Wharton's ducts? In the setting of acute bacterial sialadenitis with or without stone, either pus or no drainage whatsoever (if the duct is completely obstructed) can be obtained. With viral parotitis, although Stensen's duct orifice may be erythematous, clear saliva will be expressed. To express and visualize parotid gland secretions, an examiner must look into the mouth at the Stensen's duct orifice (adjacent to the second maxillary molar), by holding a tongue blade just in front of it, tenting out laterally the buccal mucosa. As this is done, the remaining hand externally presses firmly on the parotid gland, starting posteriorly behind the ascending ramus of the mandible, and moving forwards. For expressing and visualizing submandibular gland secretion, an examiner must ask the patient to lift the anterior tongue upwards, exposing the anterior floor of the mouth. The submandibular gland is palpated, starting posteriorly and extending anteriorly, as the anterior floor-of-mouth Wharton's duct orifice is inspected. If there is significant salivary pooling in the anterior floor of the mouth, dabbing the region intermittently with an absorbent gauze is helpful.

Once a specific working diagnosis has been reached, or at least a category of disease process has been identified, a decision is made as to the need for radiographic, cytologic or serologic studies.

CATEGORIES OF SALIVARY GLAND DISORDERS

On the basis of history and examination, the salivary gland disorder can be placed into one of three diagnostic categories: acute inflammatory disorders, chronic progressive inflammatory disorders and salivary gland masses.

Acute inflammatory disorders

In acute inflammatory disorders, the clinical history typically consists of an abrupt onset, pain, tenderness and erythema over the gland. Fever may be present.

Mumps

Mumps is recognized as a systemic illness with an obvious predilection for children. One or more of the major salivary glands may be involved. The involved gland is diffusely and acutely swollen and tender to palpation. Trismus and fever are common. In contrast to bacterial sialadenitis, in which purulent material is expressed from the salivary gland duct, salivary secretions expressed from the duct will be clear. Serum amylase concentration is elevated, and the diagnosis may be confirmed by serologic tests if necessary. Many viruses may produce mumps-like acute sialadenitis, including Coxsackie A virus, cytomegalovirus, influenza A virus, enterovirus, echovirus, polio virus, adenovirus, parainfluenza virus and lymphocytic choriomeningitis virus. In true mumps, there is a 14–21-day prodromal phase after contact prior to the development of symptoms. Mumps occurs most commonly in the 4–5-year-old age group. Mumps may be complicated by encephalopathy, pancreatitis, sensorineural hearing loss, orchitis or oophoritis. Treatment is with warm compresses, hydration, oral irrigations, salivary gland massage, the use of sialagogues, including lemon drops, and antibiotics, if there is a suspected secondary bacterial superinfection.

Acute bacterial sialadenitis

The typical clinical setting for acute bacterial sialadenitis involves an aged individual with chronic illness, poor oral hygiene and dehydration. There is marked tenderness, pain and swelling, usually involving the entire gland. There may be overlying skin erythema. The parotid gland is most commonly involved, but the submandibular gland may also be affected. Palpation of the gland while observing the duct orifice may reveal purulent material, which can be sent for Gram stain and culture. Frequently, the white blood cell count is elevated, and the patient is febrile. The duct should be palpated for the possible presence of a stone. Sialography should not be performed when an infectious process is suspected, to avoid spreading the suppurative process and causing further inflammation of the duct lining by sialography dye.

Parenteral antibiotics are required in the treatment of acute, severe bacterial sialadenitis and are selected on the basis of culture and Gram stain. The most common organism is *Staphylococcus aureus*, followed by pneumococcus. Correction of dehydration and improvement of oral hygiene are important adjuncts to treatment. If no improvement is observed in 5 days of appropriate antibiotic therapy, the possibility of an abscess should be considered. Fascial covering and the septation pattern of the parotid gland may prevent discovery of fluctuance by palpation until the abscess breaks into a subcutaneous plane. An abscess requires surgical drainage. Parotitis may progress medially to involve the deep lobe of the parotid as a parapharyngeal process. As this occurs, trismus may occur, owing to the proximity of the pterygoid musculature. The tonsil fossa region may be pushed medially and bulge asymmetrically into the posterior oropharynx. Submandibular gland sialadenitis may extend beyond the gland to spread to the soft tissues of the adjacent floor of the mouth and the tongue. When the infectious process significantly involves the floor of the mouth and the undersurface of the tongue, the process is termed Ludwig's angina. This is a rapidly progressive infectious process that can arise initially from submandibular gland sialadenitis or from dental infections. The lingual inflammation, edema and elevation associated with Ludwig's angina may lead to rapid airway obstruction. One of the earliest signs that submandibular gland sialadenitis is progressing towards Ludwig's angina is the development of floor-of-mouth watery edema. In Ludwig's angina, computerized tomography (CT) scanning often shows a phlegmon in the floor-of-mouth submandibular gland region and may not show a frank abscess; however, the clinician must have a very low threshold for deciding to perform extensive external drainage as well as tracheotomy.

Although rarely present, chronic drainage from skin sinus tracts to underlying nodules of the parotid or submandibular gland region suggests actinomycosis. Sulfa granules may be identified during histologic examination of such drainage. Rarely, tuberculosis, as well as atypical tuberculosis, brucellosis and cat scratch disease, can result in chronic parotid and periparotid lymph node inflammation.

Severe or recurrent episodes of sialadenitis frequently lead to duct stricture, especially in the submandibular gland. Such stricture formation often leads to a recommendation for surgical excision of the submandibular gland. Acute suppurative sialadenitis may be caused by obstruction of the duct by neoplasm or an infiltrative process such as Sjögren's disease. Therefore, once the acute inflammatory process has resolved, the possibility of a predisposing disorder should be considered.

Chronic obstructive salivary gland disease (strictures and stones)

Partial obstruction of the ducts of the salivary glands may cause recurrent, often postprandial, painful swelling of the affected gland. Such an obstruction may be caused by stone formation or stricture within the duct. Approximately 90% of all stones occur in Wharton's duct, presumably because of the more mucinous and viscous saliva produced in the submandibular glands. The swelling resolves over minutes or days. Occasionally, a patient will say that he can taste or feel sand-like material within his mouth as the stone or fragments of it are intermittently shed. Salivary calculi are usually unassociated with any other systemic disorder, other than gout. In gout, salivary gland stones are typically uric acid, not calcium phosphate, which occur in the majority of cases of sialolithiasis. Between attacks, the involved gland will be normal. A stone in Stensen's or Wharton's duct may be detected by bimanual palpation. The calculi may be sufficiently calcified to render them radiopaque. A dental occlusive view often best demonstrates a stone in the submandibular gland. A CT scan is the gold standard for detecting calcified salivary gland stones. Salivary gland stones are frequently multiple. The majority of submandibular gland stones are radiopaque, but parotid gland stones can frequently be radiolucent. Contrast sialography is useful in demonstrating the cause of obstruction, but should not be performed when the gland is acutely inflamed. Sialography is performed by injecting contrast dye into Stensen's or Wharton's orifice, outlining the ductal arborization. Subsequent plain films or CT scanning is performed. Sialography can be helpful in assessing the status of the ductal system, and can be informative in terms of identification of strictures, non-calcified stones and the loss of distal fine ductal branches associated with chronic sialadenitis. In general, magnetic resonance imaging (MRI) and CT scanning are superior for evaluating overall salivary gland architecture.

Occasionally, a stone can be removed transorally if it lies in the distal salivary duct. In other cases, a stone may be broken up by probing the affected duct. Distal strictures may be corrected by simple surgical procedures. In cases of chronic sialadenitis without dilatable strictures or stones which can be removed, patients are managed by hydration, sialagogues, massage and antibiotics when symptoms flare. If these measures fail, duct ligation or tympanic neurectomy (for the parotid gland) can be offered. If all else fails and the patient is still significantly symptomatic, surgical excision of the gland is considered. In glands removed for chronic sialadenitis, there is acinar loss, lymphocytic infiltration, a loss of the fine distal ductal system and ectasia of the remaining ductal system.

Chronic progressive inflammatory disorders

Benign lymphoepithelial lesion of the salivary glands

A benign lymphoepithelial lesion of the salivary glands is a set of chronic degenerative changes in salivary gland histology that can occur in several settings. Classically, these findings include a lymphoreticular infiltrate, ductal acinar atrophy and epimyoepithelial islands with cyst formation. These findings are probably the common endpoint histologically in several salivary gland degenerative diseases characterized by decreased salivary flow and relative salivary gland duct obstruction.

When a benign lymphoepithelial lesion occurs focally in a salivary gland without multifocal lesions or bilateral parotid involvement, it is felt to represent an end-stage lesion resulting from chronic focal sialadenitis. When benign lymphoepithelial lesions occur multifocally throughout the gland bilaterally with prominent cyst formation, they have been associated with HIV disease. Treatment of bilateral multifocal cysts associated with a benign lymphoepithelial lesion in HIV disease can be treated with aspiration, with or without sclerosis, antiviral chemotherapeutic agents and low-dose radiation therapy. Surgery is infrequently necessary. HIV disease has also been associated with a variety of salivary gland neoplasms, including non-Hodgkin's lymphoma and Kaposi's sarcoma of the parotid. Therefore, one must approach a palpable parotid lesion in a patient with HIV disease with caution. HIV disease must be considered in the differential diagnosis in any patient who presents with bilateral gland enlargement.

A benign lymphoepithelial lesion is also the histologic finding in Sjögren's disease. It is considered to be a systemic disorder whose major manifestations are in the salivary glands. Diagnosis of Sjögren's disease can be made by biopsy of the tail of the parotid or a minor salivary gland in the lip. The usual clinical history for a patient with Sjögren's disease is chronic intermittent diffuse enlargement of one or more salivary glands. Fluctuation in size of the gland is common. The gland may at times also be somewhat tender or painful. Superimposed chronic suppurative sialadenitis may also occur, owing to the chronic changes in the ductal system. Classic findings in Sjögren's syndrome include the triad of keratoconjunctivitis sicca resulting from lacrimal gland involvement, xerostomia with a history of salivary gland swelling and an associated connective tissue disorder, usually rheumatoid arthritis. Systemic lupus erythematosus, scleroderma and polyarteritis are other associated diseases. Sjögren's disease may occur as a primary disease without associated systemic disease and, in this setting, is termed Mikulicz disease. Secondary Sjögren's disease occurs in the setting of systemic inflammatory disease, typically rheumatoid arthritis. The etiology of Sjögren's disease is unknown, but may involve an autoimmune basis. SSA and SSB autoantibodies help to characterize Sjögren's syndrome (see Chapter 12).

Contrast sialography demonstrates sialectasia, a non-obstructive ductal dilatation, and delayed emptying of contrast material from the duct structures. In advanced Sjögren's disease, sialectasia may progress to the formation of intraparenchymal cavitary lesions.

The treatment for Sjögren's syndrome is directed towards improving the remaining salivary gland function. Massage in the direction of normal salivary flow, good hydration and sialagogues are helpful in maintaining salivary flow and preventing obstruction. If recurrent infections occur, removal of a gland may be necessary. Patients with Sjögren's syndrome may develop salivary gland lymphoma, Waldenström's microglobulinemia, pseudolymphoma and hypergammaglobulinemia. Ongoing follow-up and work-up of any clinical change in salivary gland architecture is, therefore, warranted. We see again the similarity between Sjögren's disease and Hashimoto's disease of the thyroid.

Granulomatous infiltration of the salivary glands

The usual clinical picture for granulomatous infiltration of the salivary glands involves one or more slowly enlarging nodules within the parenchyma of the salivary gland.

The most important aspect of diagnosis is to differentiate these lesions from true neoplasms. A clinical history that includes some other signs of granulomatous disease such as tuberculosis or sarcoidosis may suggest a diagnosis. Sarcoid of the parotid primarily affects granulomatous involvement of intraparotid lymph nodes and, to a lesser extent, the parotid parenchyma. Patients present with salivary gland enlargement and fever. Angiotensin-converting enzyme (ACE) level is elevated in 80–90% of patients. Parotid involvement by sarcoidosis with transient facial paralysis and uveitis is termed Heerfordt's syndrome (uveoparotid fever) and is treated with steroids.

Metabolic disorders

Metabolic disorders cause bilateral symmetric involvement of the salivary glands. There is diffuse generalized enlargement, rather than a discrete mass within the gland. In some cases, this may be associated with fatty infiltration and, in others, glandular acinar hypertrophy. The parotid gland is typically the most severely affected. The salivary glands are commonly affected in alcoholism, with or without cirrhosis, chronic starvation, diabetes mellitus, hypothyroidism, renal disease, systemic lipoproteinemia and obesity. Bulimia can also be associated with bilateral diffuse parotid gland enlargement.

Sialography will demonstrate normal ductal structure. If the underlying disorder can be reversed, some resolution of salivary gland enlargement may occur.

Though not as avidly as the thyroid gland, salivary gland tissue does trap and secrete iodine from the blood into the saliva. This can result in a chemical sialadenitis after I^{131} administration. This usually does not occur after small scan doses (1–5 mCi), but can occur after higher thyroid remnant ablative doses (30–50 mCi) or higher doses for metastatic disease (100–150 mCi). Treatment here is supportive with hydration, massage and sialagogues. Other agents can induce parotid inflammation, including thiourea, thiocyanate, methimazole, isoproterenol, phenylbutazone and phenothiazine. As well as iodine, salivary gland tissue also concentrates technetium. Certain parotid tumors (Warthin's and oncocytomas) can avidly take up technetium; however, technetium scans as diagnostic tests are performed infrequently in the era of fine needle aspiration.

Ptyalism (excess salivation) can be induced by a variety of agents including mercury and pilocarpine, and can occur in a variety of conditions including rabies, stomatitis, pregnancy and seizure disorder. Bilateral tympanic neurectomies (parasympathetic denervation to the parotid gland), bilateral parotid duct rerouting and bilateral submandibular gland resection have been advocated for refractive cases.

Xerostomia

After external beam radiation therapy, salivary gland function decreases, leading to chronic xerostomia. Xerostomia is difficult to treat despite the availability of a multitude of saliva substitutes or stimulants. Chronic radiation-induced xerostomia can lead to halitosis and carious destruction of the teeth (see Chapter 12).

Discrete mass within the salivary gland (salivary neoplasm)

Any mass within the parotid or submandibular gland mandates complete work-up and often excision. A wide variety of benign and malignant neoplasms may arise from the epithelial or stromal components of the salivary gland (Table 16.1). Although approximately 80% of all salivary gland tumors arise in the parotid gland, the incidence of malignancy is much lower in the parotid gland than in the submandibular, sublingual or minor salivary glands. Only 10% of parotid tumors are malignant, whereas 50% of tumors arising in other minor or major salivary glands are malignant.

A history of radiation therapy increases the risk of development of pleomorphic adenoma and mucoepidermoid carcinoma. Smoking may increase the risk of Warthin's tumor. A history of wood and furniture

Table 16.1   Neoplasms of the salivary glands

I.   Neoplasms of epithelial origin
    a.   Benign
        1.   Benign pleomorphic adenoma (mixed tumor)
        2.   Monomorphic adenoma
        3.   Warthin's tumor (papillary cyst adenoma lymphomatosis)
        4.   Oncocytoma
        5.   Benign lymphoepithelial lesion
    b.   Malignant
        1.   Carcinoma ex-pleomorphic adenoma/malignant mixed
        2.   Mucoepidermoid carcinoma (low, intermediate and high grade)
        3.   Adenocarcinoma
        4.   Adenoid cystic carcinoma
        5.   Acinic cell carcinoma
        6.   Squamous cell carcinoma
II. Neoplasms of stromal origin
    a.   Benign
        1.   Lipoma
        2.   Neuroma
        3.   Hemangioma
        4.   Lymphangioma
    b.   Malignant
        1.   Lymphoma
        2.   Sarcoma
        3.   Rhabdomyosarcoma
III. Metastasis to parotid or intraparotid lymph node
        1.   Renal cell
        2.   Lung
        3.   Breast
        4.   Colorectal
        5.   Skin (sebaceous cell carcinoma, melanoma, squamous cell)

industry occupational exposure increases the risk of minor salivary gland neoplasia. The most common benign salivary gland tumors are pleomorphic adenoma and Warthin's tumors, followed by monomorphic adenoma and oncocytoma. The most common malignant tumors of the salivary glands are mucoepidermoid carcinoma and acinic cell carcinoma, followed by adenocarcinoma, adenoid cystic carcinoma and malignant mixed tumors. Tumors originating in the deep lobe of the parotid gland may present as parapharyngeal masses intraorally. In children, hemangioma and lymphangioma are the most common benign masses. CT scanning and MRI are both excellent in terms of anatomic delineation, with an MRI scan perhaps being superior in delineation of the parapharyngeal space and intracranial extension.

A history of a painless mass slowly enlarging over years generally suggests the presence of benign neoplasm. A rapidly progressive painful mass or one that causes facial paresis suggests malignancy. An easily mobile mass with smooth contour suggests the presence of a benign lesion, whereas a poorly mobile infiltrative lesion suggests malignant disease. The existence of regional adenopathy also suggests malignancy. It is of note that, during physical examination of the parotid, a prominent transverse process of the atlas can be misdiagnosed as a parotid mass.

First branchial cleft cysts (type I and type II) can manifest as parotid region masses. First branchial cyst tracts may extend from the external auditory canal to the preauricular region (type I) or submandibular gland region (type II). The associated tracts can have a close but variable relationship with the intraparotid facial nerve branches. Parotid cysts may also represent dermoids if they are superficial, or cysts associated with benign lymphoepithelial lesion. Warthin's tumors often have cystic components. A ranula is an infiltrative floor-of-mouth cyst that arises from the sublingual glands.

The presence of a mass just inferior to the angle of the mandible is a frequent differential diagnostic problem. The clinician must decide whether the mass is a neoplasm within the tail of the parotid or cervical adenopathy. Because the parotid space is lateral to the mandible, a mass within the parotid tail, except one that is deeply infiltrative, can be moved superiorly and laterally over the mandible. Because a cervical node is inferior to the mandible, a node in the anterior cervical triangle cannot be drawn up over the mandible. CT or MRI scanning may also delineate the exact position of such a mass and its relationship to the parotid. Fine needle aspiration usually allows for a definitive preoperative diagnosis to be made. This allows for discussion of non-surgical options in a patient with a benign Warthin's tumor and allows for appropriate preoperative discussion and surgical preparation when a malignancy is diagnosed.

Lymph nodes are present within and on the capsule of the parotid gland. These nodes represent the first echelon nodal basin for the upper face, periorbital region, anterior scalp and external auditory canal, and so can be involved with cancers in these regions, such as squamous cell carcinoma, melanoma and sebaceous cell carcinoma. The limited number of nodes within the deep lobe of the parotid drain the external auditory canal, middle ear, soft palate and posterior nasal cavity. Rarely, parotid lymph nodes may be involved in distant metastases, including renal cell carcinoma, breast, lung and colorectal cancers. Periparotid lymph nodes may also become involved in lymphoma or leukemia.

Infections, usually skin cellulitis or conjunctivitis, in the upper face, periorbital region and anterior scalp can lead to parotid region adenopathy. Rare infectious agents associated with specific oculoglandular presentations (conjunctival inflammation with reactive regional periparotid adenitis) include *Francisella tularensis* (tularemia), *Listeria monocytogenes* (listeriosis) and *Chlamydia trachomatis* (lymphogranuloma venereum).

A neoplasm in the superficial or lateral lobe of the parotid gland is removed by superficial parotidectomy. This involves dissection of the main trunk and branches of the peripheral facial nerve. Damage to this nerve, although possible, occurs infrequently during surgery. If malignancy is confirmed, the patient should be prepared for possible sacrifice of part or all of the facial nerve trunk. In some cases of high-grade malignancy, supplemental radiation therapy is recommended. If neck metastases are present or highly likely, neck dissection at the same time as parotidectomy may be indicated.

Inadequate resection of benign mixed tumor of the parotid gland will result in multiple recurrences within the parotid parenchyma and cutaneous incision line. Subsequent removal of recurrences may be difficult and carries a much higher risk of damage to the facial nerve.

The presence of a neoplasm in the submandibular gland requires removal of the gland. Removal of the submandibular gland carries a possible risk of damage to the ramus mandibularis branch of the facial nerve which innervates the depressor anguli oris. Loss of this nerve will result in loss of depression of the ipsilateral corner of the mouth and occasionally in some drooling while drinking liquids. Sacrifice of the ramus division may be necessary if malignancy is suspected or confirmed. Surgery for benign mixed tumor of the minor salivary glands originating in the oropharynx, most commonly in the soft palate, requires wide local excision.

17

Thyroid and parathyroid disorders

Gregory W. Randolph

Anatomy and physical examination
  Anatomy
  Physical examination of the thyroid
  Embryology
Work-up of the thyroid nodule
  Clinical assessment
  Testing algorithm
  Thyroid hormone suppression
Benign thyroid disease
  Thyroid function testing
  Hypothyroidism
  Hyperthyroidism
  Thyroiditis
    Hashimoto's thyroiditis
    Subacute granulomatous thyroiditis
    Lymphocytic thyroiditis
    Acute suppurative thyroiditis
    Riedel's struma
  Euthyroid goiter
Thyroid cancer
  Papillary carcinoma
  Follicular carcinoma
  Medullary carcinoma of the thyroid
  Lymphoma
  Anaplastic carcinoma
Parathyroid glands
  Parathyroid physiology
  Parathyroid anatomy
  Hyperparathyroidism
  Parathyroid surgery

ANATOMY AND PHYSICAL EXAMINATION

Anatomy

The thyroid and parathyroids are endocrine glands located in the base of the neck. The normal adult thyroid weighs between 15 and 25 g, and consists of two lateral lobes connected by an isthmus. The isthmus is attached to the trachea at the second to fourth tracheal rings. Laterally, the thyroid lobes are adjacent to the carotid sheath (carotid artery, jugular vein and vagus nerve), posteriorly to the prevertebral muscles and medially to the upper trachea and cricoid (Figure 17.1). The thyroid lobes are covered by the infrahyoid strap muscles. The thyroid is associated with an extensive lymphatic network draining to pretracheal (delphian), paratracheal, superior mediastinal and internal jugular lymphatic chains. The thyroid is attached to the laryngotracheal complex through both anterior and lateral suspensory ligaments. As a result, the thyroid elevates with the larynx and trachea with deglutition. A thyroid nodule, therefore, elevates with the larynx during deglutition, whereas a surrounding mobile lymph node does not.

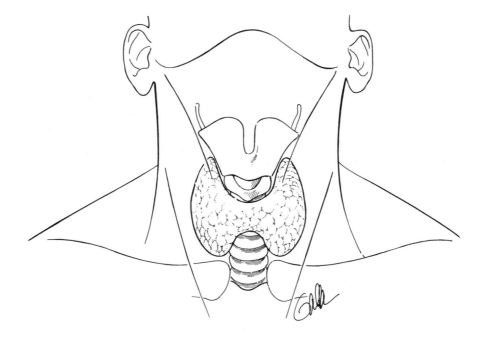

Figure 17.1 Normal thyroid anatomy

The recurrent laryngeal nerve branches from the vagus in the upper chest, traveling around the subclavian artery on the right and the aorta on the left, and ascending from the neck base to the larynx in the tracheoesophageal groove just behind the thyroid lobes. The recurrent laryngeal nerve brings motor fibers to all laryngeal intrinsic musculature, including vocal cords. Owing to the recurrent laryngeal nerve's position in the tracheoesophageal groove behind the thyroid lobe, it may be invaded by thyroid malignancy or injured during thyroid surgery. The resulting unilateral vocal cord paralysis presents with a spectrum of symptomatology. Classically, the immobile vocal cord produces a weak and breathy voice (as opposed to true hoarseness) and dysphagia, typically coughing with liquids. The degree of voice change and dysphagia varies with unilateral vocal cord paralysis, in part owing to varying degrees of contralateral vocal cord compensation, which evolves over time. As a result, a thyroid malignancy that slowly invades the recurrent laryngeal nerve over a period of time may lead to unilateral vocal cord paralysis that is completely asymptomatic. It is, therefore, prudent to check vocal cord function if the clinical examination in any way suggests malignancy, even in the setting of a grossly normal voice.

The superior laryngeal nerve's external division branches from the vagus in the superior neck and extends to the larynx along the inferior constrictor, innervating the cricothyroid muscle (see Chapter 13, Figure 13.4b). This muscle tenses the vocal cords. Its injury during thyroid surgery results in a loss of high vocal registers.

The dense vascularity of the thyroid gland led early physicians to hypothesize that the gland provided a vascular buffer to protect the brain from sudden increases in blood flow from the heart. The thyroid isthmus covers the first several tracheal rings, and can bleed significantly during emergency tracheotomy. Cricothyroidotomy can be performed for emergency access to the airway. The cricothyroid membrane is a relatively avascular space between the cricoid ring and the lowest aspect of the thyroid cartilage in the midline above the thyroid isthmus. A cricothyroidotomy accesses the airway at a relatively high level, and risks laryngeal injury and the development of subglottic stenosis.

Physical examination of the thyroid

The thyroid examination can be quite difficult unless one relates the position of the thyroid to the adjacent laryngeal cartilages. The isthmus of the thyroid is directly below the cricoid cartilage. The thyroid cartilage can be identified in the superior midline at the thyroid notch ('Adam's apple'). The position of the thyroid cartilage can be confirmed by palpating the relatively large and flat bilateral thyroid cartilage lamina. Just below the thyroid cartilage, the cricoid cartilage can be easily identified as a prominent, horizontally oriented ring-like structure in the midline. Directly below the cricoid ring lies the upper cervical trachea. On the first several rings of the trachea, the thyroid isthmus can often be palpated as a soft tube-like prominence running horizontally. Once the isthmus is identified, the bilateral lobes can be identified by placing the examining thumb between the trachea medially and the sternocleidomastoid muscle and carotid sheath laterally. It is useful when identifying the isthmus and the thyroid lobes to have the patient swallow. This elevates the thyroid and allows any abnormality within the thyroid to roll underneath the examining finger. It is probably best to examine the thyroid standing in front of the patient, using the pad of the thumb, palpating the isthmus, left and right lobes separately. It is sometimes useful to provide the patient with a glass of water, should repetitive swallowing be needed. Thyroid nodules of 1 cm or greater may be identified by palpation.

Embryology

The thyroid arises as a small diverticulum from the posterior tongue, and descends from this region through the hyoid bone down the anterior neck midline during gestation. If embryologic thyroid migration is completely arrested, a lingual thyroid results. Such patients may present with respiratory embarrassment, dysphagia or hemoptysis. Rests of thyroid tissue may remain anywhere along the thyroid migration path. If this occurs only at the inferiormost portion of the path, a pyramidal lobe results. Higher up in the neck, such remnant tissue can often cystify and present in an adult as a thyroglossal duct cyst. Such lesions are typically in very close association with the hyoid bone.

WORK-UP OF THE THYROID NODULE

Thyroid nodules are very common, occurring in about 5% of the normal adult population. When sonographic criteria are used, approximately one-third of the normal adult population has thyroid nodular abnormalities. Only about one in 20 newly discovered nodules are expected to be due to carcinoma. The task, then, is to identify those few patients requiring treatment. The vast majority of thyroid nodules are colloid nodules, adenoma, cysts, focal thyroiditis or carcinoma (Table 17.1). A colloid or adenomatous nodule is a nodule within a gland affected by a multinodular goiter. It is a focal hyperplastic disturbance rather than a true clonal lesion. Follicular adenomas are true monoclonal neoplasms.

Clinical assessment

Certain factors in the medical history and physical examination will raise the suspicion for carcinoma (Table 17.2). Patients less than 20 years of age with thyroid nodules have an increased risk of malignancy. Patients more than 60 years of age have a significantly worse prognosis should thyroid malignancy be diagnosed. Although thyroid nodular disease is more common in women than men, the risk of malignancy is higher in men. A

Table 17.1 Differential diagnosis of the thyroid nodule

1. Colloid nodule/multinodular goiter nodule
2. True adenoma
3. Cyst
4. Focal thyroiditis
5. Carcinoma

Table 17.2 Degree of clinical concern for carcinoma in a thyroid nodule, based on history and physical examination. Reprinted from Lee KJ, ed. *Essential Otolaryngology*, 7th edn. Stamford, CT: Appleton & Lange, 1999, with permission

Less concern
Chronic stable examination
Evidence of a functional disorder (e.g. Hashimoto's thyroiditis, toxic nodule)
Multinodular gland without dominant nodule

More concern
Age < 20 or > 60 years
Males
Rapid growth, pain
History of radiation therapy
Family history of thyroid carcinoma
Hard, fixed lesion
Lymphadenopathy
Vocal cord paralysis
Size > 4 cm
Aerodigestive tract compromise (e.g. stridor, dysphagia)

family history of medullary carcinoma increases the index of suspicion for this relatively rare form of thyroid cancer. Pain and rapid change in size may be associated with hemorrhage into a benign nodule or may represent carcinoma. Similarly, symptoms of airway distress, hoarseness, cough or dysphagia may be present in both benign and malignant disease. A history of exposure to low-dose radiation therapy increases the risk of development of benign and malignant thyroid nodules and increases the risk in a patient with a solitary nodule of thyroid malignancy. Such low-dose radiation therapy has been given in the past for adenoidal and tonsillar hypertrophy, thymic enlargement, facial acne, and head and neck tinea. Such treatment ended in approximately 1955, but benign and malignant nodules may develop with a latency of up to 20–30 years. Patients exposed to radiation therapy for Hodgkin's disease and scatter exposure from breast radiation have increased rates of thyroid nodular disease. Symptoms of hypo- or hyperthyroidism in general decrease the index of concern for malignancy. Thyroid malignancy in not generally associated with abnormal thyroid function testing.

During the physical examination, the thyroid nodule should be carefully scrutinized. It should be remembered that a dominant nodule in a multinodular gland has the same risk of malignancy as a solitary nodule. Size should be measured. The larger the thyroid nodule, the greater the risk of malignancy. Also, lesions that are larger than approximately 4 cm have an increased risk for false-negative results through inadequate sampling during fine needle aspiration. Firm nodules, nodules that are fixed to the laryngotracheal complex and nodules that are associated with lymphadenopathy have an increased risk of malignancy. Laryngotracheal deviation should be noted. In all patients with thyroid lesions vocal cord motion should be assessed. For large thyroid lesions, the degree of substernal extension can be assessed by relating the inferior aspect of the mass to the clavicle and sternal notch. With substernal goiters, the thoracic inlet may become obstructed, leading to a positive Pemburton's maneuver, i.e. the development of subjective respiratory discomfort or venous engorgement with arms raised over the head.

Testing algorithm

Few clinical chemistry tests are needed in the work-up of the thyroid nodule other than a sensitive test of thyroid stimulating hormone (TSH), which allows definitive diagnosis of hypo- or hyperthyroidism. In general, the identification of an abnormal TSH level requires a diagnosis of the underlying functional disorder. If the TSH level is normal, no further blood testing is warranted. If the TSH level is elevated, one may consider Hashimoto's thyroiditis, and test the level of thyroid peroxidase antibodies (TPO), which is elevated in 80% of cases. If the TSH level is low, one may consider Graves' disease or toxic goiter and consider I^{123} scanning. Thyroglobulin is a marker of well-differentiated thyroid carcinoma, but its concentration is elevated in a variety of benign as well as malignant thyroid conditions and it has no role as a screening test for the thyroid nodule. Calcitonin is a serum marker for medullary thyroid carcinoma. However, because of the rarity of medullary carcinoma, evaluation of calcitonin level is not recommended as a screening test in the work-up of the thyroid nodule.

Chest X-ray has no role in the work-up of the solitary nodule. If airway deviation is present, it can usually be identified on the chest X-ray of the tracheal air column. However, computerized tomography (CT) scanning with axial cuts is required for accurate assessment of the relationship between a large thyroid mass and adjacent cervical viscera (larynx, trachea, esophagus), and for assessment of the degree of substernal extension. CT scan contrast dye should not be used if thyroid functional status is unknown or if the patient is shown to be hyperthyroid or subclinically hyperthyroid. Chest X-ray and CT scanning have no role in the work-up of a routine thyroid nodule.

In the past, radionuclide scanning (I^{123} or technetium) was used in the work-up of the thyroid nodule. Approximately 95% of all nodules are 'cold' i.e. fail to take up radioisotope, on such scanning. The remaining 5% are 'hot'. Generally, it is considered that the risk of malignancy is very low in a hot nodule. The large group of nodules that are cold are primarily benign, although malignancies occur within this large, cold group. Such testing, therefore, adds little in the work-up of the thyroid nodule and is not currently recommended.

Thyroid sonography can accurately assess the size of the thyroid nodule and its characteristics (solid, cystic, mixed), and can identify contralateral nodular disease as well as perithyroid lymph nodes. Sonography does not allow identification of a given lesion as benign or malignant. The risk of malignancy is slightly higher in solid lesions, but certainly malignancies may result in lesions that are cystic. Sonography can, however, very accurately provide useful baseline information for nodules that will be followed clinically or suppressed. Sonography can identify contralateral nodules, which are important in making decisions regarding post-lobectomy suppression.

A key diagnostic test in the work-up of the thyroid nodule is fine needle aspiration (Figure 17.2). It is highly accurate, of low morbidity and inexpensive. Fine needle aspiration is typically performed with a 22- or 25-gauge needle on a syringe that can be held directly, or in a syringe gun-type holder. Approximately 1–2 ml of suction is applied after the needle is inserted into the nodule, and the needle is oscillated through the nodule repetitively, allowing cells within the nodule to lodge within the shaft of the needle. Although needle-induced hemorrhage is not a common problem, caution should be exercised when needling any large nodule or any nodule associated with airway compromise. Fine needle aspirations can be reported as malignant, suspicious, benign or non-diagnostic. Cytologic identification of malignancy is quite accurate, with false-positive rates being approximately 1%. Typically, false-positive results are due to co-existing Hashimoto's thyroiditis, Graves' disease or toxic nodules. Papillary carcinoma can usually be identified through characteristic nuclear features on cytology.

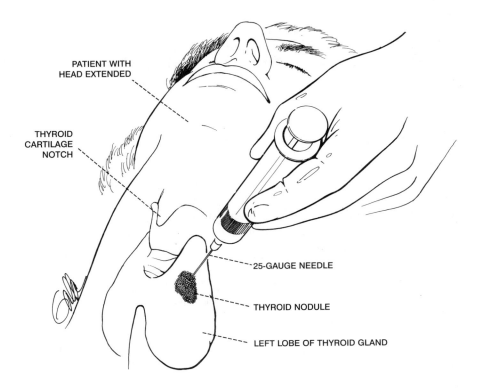

Figure 17.2   Fine needle aspiration

The principal diagnostic difficulty with fine needle aspiration in identification of malignancy is with follicular carcinoma. Follicular carcinoma can be distinguished from its benign counterpart, follicular adenoma, only by histologic evaluation of the lesion's capsule. Follicular neoplastic lesions that are found on fine needle aspiration to be hypercellular and to contain microfollicular arrays with minimal colloid, are described, therefore, as suspicious. Surgery is recommended for such lesions. Approximately 20% of such suspicious lesions will be found to be follicular carcinoma pathologically. Lesions identified as benign through fine needle aspiration cytology have a false-negative rate of approximately 1–10%. These relate primarily to sampling errors, which are more likely in small lesions (less than 1 cm) or lesions larger than 3 cm, as well as cystic lesions. Patients with benign pathology with fine needle aspiration may be managed by clinical follow-up, thyroxine suppression or surgical excision. Patients with non-diagnostic results should undergo repeat fine needle aspiration, usually with sonographic guidance. Thyroid cysts, when small, may completely resolve after successful fine needle aspiration. Cysts larger than 3–4 cm typically recur and should be surgically excised.

The thyroid nodule should be evaluated with a complete history and physical examination, followed by TSH assessment and fine needle aspiration. In some circumstances, sonography should be considered (Figure 17.3).

Thyroid hormone suppression

Treatment with thyroid hormone has been known to decrease goiter size and has been used to control nodular disease of the thyroid. Thyroid nodule suppressive therapy presupposes that benign nodules should respond to hormonal control and undergo reduction in size, while malignant nodules will grow. The goals (i.e. nodule stability, size reduction or complete disappearance of the nodule) and length of suppressive therapy have not been standardized. Randomized trials show unclear benefit of suppressive therapy. Further, it is known that only a small percentage of nodules that grow on suppressive therapy are malignant, and that a small percentage of malignant thyroid nodules shrink in the face of thyroxine therapy. Suppressive therapy should be used with caution in the elderly group, and can result in an increased rate of atrial fibrillation, as well a decrement in bone density. TSH should not be suppressed below 0.3 mU/l. Although there are no standard criteria, it seems reasonable that one should expect a decrease in size of the nodule through suppressive

History, physical examination
↓

TSH high → possible Hashimoto's thyroiditis → TFTs
↗   TPO
TSH assessment → TSH abnormal
(consider sonogram)   ↘

TSH low → possible Graves' disease → TFTs, I^{123} scan
Toxic goiter

↓

TSH normal

↓

FNA

↓

– Malignant → surgery
– Benign → follow, suppress or surgery
– Suspicious → surgery
– Non-diagnostic → repeat FNA
– Cyst > 4 cm → to surgery
        < 4 cm → reaspirate, consider suppression

Figure 17.3   Algorithm for evaluation of a thyroid nodule. TSH, thyroid stimulating hormone; TPO, thyroid peroxidase antibodies; TFT, thyroid function test; FNA, fine needle aspiration

therapy, and that suppression should be offered for a limited period of time (e.g. 6 months). All non-responders should have surgery. Re-biopsy of benign nodules managed non-surgically can be performed 1 year after initial biopsy.

BENIGN THYROID DISEASE

It is important, when evaluating a thyroid nodule or thyroid mass, to assess the associated functional status of the thyroid gland with an understanding that, in general, thyroid malignancy is not associated with functional disorder of the gland. Large benign masses (with or without an associated functional disorder) may impact significantly on adjacent structures and warrant careful work-up.

Thyroid function testing

The production of thyroid hormone (TH) by the thyroid gland is controlled by thyroid stimulating hormone (TSH) from the anterior pituitary. The anterior pituitary thyrotrophs, through monitoring plasma levels of TH, elaborate appropriate levels of TSH to keep thyroid hormone levels stable. As TH levels rise, a negative feedback is exerted primarily on the anterior pituitary, and TSH secretion is reduced. Conversely, as TH levels fall, anterior pituitary secretion of TSH increases in order to normalize TH levels. Two forms of thyroid hormone exist, T_3 (triiodothyronine) and T_4 (thyroxine). Most thyroid hormone exists as T_4, although T_3 is the more physiologically potent form of TH. Most circulating T_3 derives from peripheral conversion of T_4. Thyroid hormone stimulates calorigenesis, potentiates epinephrine (adrenaline), lowers cholesterol levels and has a role in normal growth and development. TH derives from iodinization of tyrosine residues. Such residues are stored on thyroglobulin in thyroid colloid and are cleaved off thyroglobulin and released into the circulation under the direction of TSH. The vast majority of circulating TH is bound to thyroid binding globulin. As a result, total T_4 and total T_3 measures vary in response to changes in thyroid binding globulin level. T_3 resin uptake allows for correction of total T_4 measure for thyroid binding globulin fluctuation. In states of thyroid binding globulin excess, such as pregnancy, T_3 resin uptake is low. In states of low thyroid binding globulin level, such as hypoproteinemic states, T_3 resin uptake is high. In true thyroid disease, total T_4 and T_3 resin uptake fluctuate in the same direction, whereas in protein binding abnormalities, total T_4 and T_3 resin uptake move in opposite directions. TSH measures are used routinely in the initial diagnosis of thyroid functional disorders, as well as in monitoring replacement of suppressive therapy.

Hypothyroidism

Hypothyroidism is characterized by increased TSH and decreased TH. Hypothyroidism can be associated with depressed mental function, cold intolerance, hoarseness, thickened tongue, changes in hair and skin, weight gain, constipation, menstrual disturbances, edema and, when occurring chronically and untreated in infancy, with mental retardation (cretinism). In the USA, hypothyroidism is most commonly caused by Hashimoto's thyroiditis (see below). Other common causes of hypothyroidism include iodine deficiency, radiation-induced (I^{131} or external beam) or postsurgical states. Treatment for hypothyroidism is through T_4 replacement and is typically started at a low dose, especially in elderly patients or patients with coronary artery disease.

Hyperthyroidism

Hyperthyroidism results from excess TH biosynthesis and secretion, and is usually associated with a reduced TSH level. Hyperthyroidism can be associated with weight loss, nervousness, tremor, palpitations, increased appetite, heat intolerance, diarrhea, menstrual disturbance and fatigue. Hyperthyroidism is typically caused by Graves' disease or toxic nodular goiter. Hyperthyroidism may also be associated with some acute phases of thyroiditis, in which case it is generally self-limiting.

In Graves' disease, hyperthyroidism results from thyroid gland stimulation by an autoantibody that stimulates the TSH receptor. The gland is diffusely enlarged and anodular. Patients may also have an infiltrative ophthalmopathy associated with exophthalmos. Patients with Graves' disease may also have an infiltrative dermopathy resulting in localized myxedema. Graves' disease is typically treated with radioactive iodine or antithyroid drugs and occasionally with surgery.

Hyperthyroidism can also occur as a result of a focal hyperplastic disturbance in the gland such as uninodular or multinodular toxic goiter. Here, one or more foci of hyperfunctional tissue arise and produce TH autonomously (i.e. without TSH regulation). Hyperthyroidism here presents without the eye or skin findings of Graves' disease. TH levels are high and the TSH level is low. On I^{123} scans, hyperfunctional areas appear hot, and normal regions of the gland may appear cold, since they have lost TSH stimulation as TSH levels have fallen. Toxic multinodular goiters may develop slowly. Many patients may initially present for evaluation with so-called subclinical hyperthyroidism, where TH is normal, but TSH shows evidence of early suppression (i.e. low to normal range). In such circumstances, exogenous iodine loads (e.g. iodine CT contrast) may result in the development of overt hyperthyroidism, the so-called Jod–Basedow phenomenon. Treatment for toxic nodules is either surgery or radioactive iodine. There is a high recurrence rate with the use of antithyroid drugs. When surgery is indicated for hyperthyroidism, whether Graves' disease or toxic goiter, it is important to render the patient euthyroid and asymptomatic preoperatively. This is typically performed through a combination of antithyroid drugs (propylthiouracil or methimazole), β-adrenergic blockers and administration of a short course of preoperative iodides (potassium iodide, Lugol's solution).

Thyroiditis

Hashimoto's thyroiditis

Hashimoto's thyroiditis is an autoimmune lymphocytic infiltration of the thyroid gland that results in hypothyroidism. It is associated with antithyroid peroxidase antibodies in 80% of patients. Hashimoto's thyroiditis usually presents as a painless, firm, symmetric goiter. Patients may be euthyroid or hypothyroid at the initial presentation. Hypothyroidism may develop with time, and so intermittent thyroid function assessment is warranted. Surgery is usually not necessary unless the goiter is large and unresponsive to thyroid hormone. Thyroid lymphoma may arise out of a Hashimoto's gland. Fine needle aspiration is warranted if a mass develops within Hashimoto's gland, but is otherwise usually unnecessary for patients with Hashimoto's thyroiditis.

Subacute granulomatous thyroiditis

Subacute granulomatous thyroiditis (DeQuervain's thyroiditis) is thought to be viral in etiology. Patients present with an enlarged and painful thyroid. Fifty per cent of patients present with hyperthyroidism that is considered to be associated with virus-induced follicular cell disruption. The pain and hyperthyroid phase resolves over about a month. About 50% of patients will enter a subsequent hypothyroid phase, which can last several months. Most ultimately return to euthyroidism.

Lymphocytic thyroiditis

Lymphocytic thyroiditis, also termed postpartum thyroiditis, is considered to be an autoimmune disease. Patients present with an enlarged but painless thyroid gland. The initial phase is characterized by hyperthyroidism, which is followed by hypothyroidism, similar to subacute granulomatous thyroiditis. Lymphocytic thyroiditis occurs frequently in the postpartum period and has a high incidence of recurrence with subsequent pregnancies.

Acute suppurative thyroiditis

Acute suppurative thyroiditis represents a rare suppurative thyroid infection with abscess formation. Acute suppurative thyroiditis is more common in children where it is associated with branchial cleft cyst abnormalities. Patients present with pain, fever and swelling, and are typically euthyroid. The treatment is the same as for any neck abscess.

Riedel's struma

Riedel's struma is a rare, inflammatory condition of the thyroid of unknown etiology, characterized by progressive and invasive fibrosis. Patients present with a non-tender goiter fixed to surrounding structures, with progressive regional symptoms of the upper aerodigestive tract.

Euthyroid goiter

Thyroid enlargement (i.e. goiter formation) may occur in a variety of clinical settings. Euthyroid thyroid enlargement may be diffuse (non-toxic diffuse goiter) or through multinodular growth. Goiter formation may be sporadic or associated with iodine deficiency. In non-toxic diffuse goiter, thyroid function tests are within normal limits. For multinodular goiter, thyroid function tests may be normal or may show subclinical hyperthyroidism (TSH low-normal with a normal T_3 and T_4). Over a period of years, subclinical hyperthyroidism may evolve into frank hyperthyroidism, especially with exogenous iodine loads. Large, diffuse non-toxic and euthyroid multinodular goiter can present clinical problems through esophageal or airway compromise or substernal extension. Such goiters may grow slowly over a period of time or may grow rapidly secondary to hemorrhage within a portion of the goiter. Such patients may be asymptomatic or may present with chronic cough, nocturnal dyspnea, choking episodes, positional respiratory distress, sensation of fullness or lump in the neck, or may describe the goiter as a cosmetic issue. The airway may be significantly compromised, as identified through radiographic or flow volume loop studies, yet the patient may be asymptomatic. Acute respiratory distress may occur in the setting of a chronic stable cervical or retrosternal goiter.

The physical examination should focus on accurate measurement of the goiter and determination of tracheal deviation, and should include a judgment regarding substernal extension. Pemburton's sign should be assessed, as should vocal cord mobility, which may be impaired secondary to recurrent laryngeal nerve stretch with benign goiter. Fine needle aspiration of dominant nodules within a multinodular gland should be considered, unless the airway is tenuous. Although chest X-ray provides a useful assessment of tracheal air column, axial CT scanning is necessary to delineate the relationship of the goiter to the adjacent cervical viscera, especially the esophagus and trachea, as well as to estimate the degree of substernal extension.

T_4 suppression may be effective in small diffuse goiters, but is generally not effective in large or multinodular goiters. Suppression should not be instituted if there is evidence of subclinical hyperthyroidism. Surgery is considered for large symptomatic goiters and for all substernal goiters. Substernal tissue is not available for routine monitoring or fine needle aspiration and, when progressive, impacts the airway at a mediastinal level. Subtotal thyroidectomy for large cervical or substernal goiters can routinely be performed through a cervical approach, and is generally tolerated quite well.

THYROID CANCER

Thyroid carcinoma overall represents between 1 and 2% of all new cancer cases in the USA each year. Papillary and follicular carcinoma (well-differentiated thyroid carcinomas) arise from the follicular epithelium and are the most common thyroid malignancies, followed by medullary thyroid carcinoma (arising from parafollicular C-cells), anaplastic carcinoma and thyroid lymphoma.

Papillary carcinoma

Papillary carcinoma has a tendency towards early spread through intraglandular and regional cervical lymphatic spread. The multiple foci of papillary carcinoma that can often be found within the gland are thought to represent this early intraglandular lymphatic spread.

Low-dose radiation exposure is associated with the development of papillary carcinoma, although the majority arise sporadically. Patients irradiated during childhood for Hodgkin's disease, patients receiving breast radiation and patients exposed to nuclear fallout, including those in Hiroshima and more recently Chernobyl, also have increased rates of papillary thyroid cancer.

Although patients presenting with papillary carcinoma have a low rate of distant metastasis, about 30% of patients will have involvement of regional cervical nodes. Cervical nodal disease is more common in the pediatric patient with papillary carcinoma. Despite their more advanced presentation, pediatric patients have a favorable long-term prognosis with papillary carcinoma. In general, most studies suggest that the presence of cervical lymph node metastasis does not significantly worsen the prognosis for papillary carcinoma.

Follicular carcinoma

Follicular carcinoma is a well-differentiated thyroid carcinoma with follicular differentiation typically seen as small groups or solid sheets of follicular cells. Morphologically, there is considerable overlap between the follicular adenoma and follicular carcinoma. Follicular carcinoma is diagnosed when histologic capsular invasion is identified. Cytologically, there is no way to distinguish adenoma from carcinoma. As cellularity increases on fine needle aspiration, the question of carcinoma is raised, and surgery to evaluate the nodule's capsule histologically is warranted. The degree of histologic invasiveness of a follicular carcinoma is strongly correlated with its clinical virulence. Little is known about the etiology of follicular carcinoma, although this occurs more frequently in iodine-deficient regions, presumably as a result of prolonged TSH stimulation. At presentation follicular carcinoma infrequently is associated with regional metastasis and has a higher rate of distant metastasis than papillary carcinoma. Hürthle cell carcinoma is considered a subtype of follicular carcinoma that is generally found to follow a slightly more aggressive course than follicular carcinoma, with poorer radioactive iodine uptake.

In general, the majority of patients with well-differentiated thyroid carcinoma have a favorable long-term prognosis. A number of prognostic procedures have been developed to segregate patients with well-differentiated thyroid carcinoma into a large group with a low risk of mortality and a small group with a high risk of mortality. The key prognostic factors include:

(1) Age (poor prognosis with advanced age, females over 50, males over 40);

(2) Degree of invasiveness/extrathyroidal extension;

(3) Presence of distant metastasis;

(4) Sex (males generally have poorer prognosis than females);

(5) Size (lesions larger than 4 cm have poorer prognosis).

Almost 90% of patients fit into the low-risk category, with an overall mortality rate of 1–2%. About 10% of patients fit into the high-risk category with a mortality rate of nearly 50%.

The extent of thyroidectomy for well-differentiated thyroid carcinoma is controversial. The segregation of patients with well-differentiated thyroid carcinoma into risk groupings allows appropriately aggressive treatment in patients in high-risk groups, and a more conservative approach with avoidance of undue complications in patients in the lower-risk group. For papillary carcinoma, occult microscopic disease, whether in the contralateral lobe or in the regional lymphatic bed, is of little clinical significance. Elective neck dissection and contralateral lobe surgery are generally considered unnecessary, despite the incidence of microscopic disease in these locations. In general, total thyroidectomy and other forms of bilateral thyroid surgery are associated with increased risk of complications of permanent hypoparathyroidism and vocal cord paralysis. Ablation of a thyroid remnant after less than total thyroidectomy can prepare the patient for whole-body scanning and allow use of thyroglobulin as a marker after surgery. The general principle in surgery for well-differentiated thyroid carcinoma is that all gross disease should be encompassed in both the thyroid and the neck. In general, patients at low risk will be well treated with conservative unilateral thyroid surgery, as long as the opposite lobe is negative to intraoperative palpation or preoperative sonography. Bilateral thyroid surgery seems, however, to improve survival in patients in high-risk groups, with near-total thyroidectomy being equivalent to total thyroidectomy. Neck dissection is offered for patients with gross nodal disease. Postoperatively, all patients with well-differentiated thyroid carcinoma should be offered TH suppression of TSH, which withdraws a potential stimulatory influence from any residual or microscopic thyroid carcinoma. In patients with well-differentiated thyroid carcinoma who are considered to be at risk for distant metastasis, radioactive iodine whole-body scanning can be performed. Prior to whole-body scanning, the thyroid must be completely ablated with a combination of either total thyroidectomy or conservative thyroid surgery with postsurgical remnant radioactive iodine ablation. When patients are rendered hypothyroid, whole-body scanning can be performed to detect distant metastases, which can then be treated with therapeutic-dose radioactive iodine treatment. Patients with well-differentiated thyroid carcinoma are followed with physical examinations, chest X-ray, sonography, intermittent thyroglobulin assessment and I^{131} whole-body scanning, depending on their risk for distant metastasis.

Medullary carcinoma of the thyroid

Medullary thyroid carcinoma (MTC) is a rare, but interesting form of thyroid carcinoma deriving from parafollicular C-cells, not from thyroid follicular cells. About 75% of MTC occurs as a sporadic neoplasm, with the remaining 25% occurring in three different inherited forms.

All inherited forms of MTC are inherited as autosomal dominant traits, and are associated with pre-malignant multifocal C-cell hyperplasia. In multiple endocrine neoplasia (MEN) IIa, MTC is associated with pheochromocytoma and hyperparathyroidism. In MEN IIb, MTC is associated with Marfanoid habitus, multiple mucosal neuromata and pheochromocytoma. In non-MEN familial MTC, medullary carcinoma occurs as an inherited neoplasm, without associated endocrinopathy.

The parafollicular C-cell secretes calcitonin. Calcitonin levels are elevated in C-cell hyperplasia and all forms of MTC. This tumor marker has been useful both in establishing the diagnosis of medullary carcinoma, and in postoperative tumor surveillance. Patients with normal basal calcitonin levels can be found to have elevated calcitonin levels with provocative infusion of calcium and/or pentagastrin. More recently, RET oncogene mutations have been identified in a large percentage of patients with inherited MTC. Currently, RET oncogene mutational analysis is available for familial screening. Sporadic MTC typically presents as a thyroid mass and has a high incidence of regional lymph node metastasis. Inherited forms (except for MEN IIb) may be detected quite early through familial screening programs, and may be identified before the development of a clinical mass. MEN IIb is the most virulent subtype of MTC, and typically presents as a new mutation with a thyroid mass with regional metastasis. Patients suspected of having MTC are preoperatively evaluated with urine testing to rule out coexisting pheochromocytoma. Total thyroidectomy is performed with a nodal sampling in the central neck compartment. Neck dissection is performed if nodal disease is present or suspected. Survival in MTC is intermediate between anaplastic carcinoma and well-differentiated thyroid carcinoma and improves with early detection through family screening. Basal and provocatively stimulated calcitonin levels are followed postoperatively.

Lymphoma

Thyroid lymphoma is a relatively rare form of thyroid neoplasia, which typically arises in the setting of pre-existing Hashimoto's thyroiditis. Thyroid lymphomas are typically of the B-cell type. The prognosis relates to degree of extrathyroidal extension and the presence of distant metastases. Treatment is usually with biopsy or limited surgery, followed by radiation therapy often combined with chemotherapy.

Anaplastic carcinoma

Anaplastic carcinoma occurs in older age groups, and is one of the most aggressive human malignancies, with average survival about 6 months. There can be diagnostic confusion between anaplastic carcinoma and lymphoma. Patients with anaplastic carcinoma typically present with a large, fixed thyroid mass, usually with ipsilateral vocal cord paralysis and cervical adenopathy, often with distant metastases at presentation. Surgical treatment is generally limited to isthmusectomy, often with tracheotomy. Postoperative treatment usually includes radiation therapy combined with adriamycin-based chemotherapy.

PARATHYROID GLANDS

Parathyroid physiology

The parathyroids secrete parathormone (PTH), which mobilizes plasma calcium through gastrointestinal absorption, bone calcium mobilization, inhibition of renal excretion and stimulation of renal vitamin D hydroxylase activity. Since 50% of plasma calcium is bound to albumin, total calcium measures vary with albumin. Total serum calcium levels can be corrected in the setting of abnormal albumin levels (the total serum calcium level is increased by 0.8 mg/dl for every 1 g/dl fall in albumin).

Parathyroid anatomy

Parathyroid glands are small (approximately 5 mm long), and have a varying position centered in the base of the neck. They have a characteristic yellow–brown color, often appearing as a flat bean- or leaf-like profile with a discrete capsule separating them as a discrete structure from the surrounding fat. The superior parathyroid arises from the fourth branchial pouch, and descends in the neck closely associated with the lateral thyroid, assuming its adult position on the posterolateral aspect of the thyroid lobe. The superior parathyroid is typically located at the level of the cricothyroid articulation, and is usually vascularized by a vessel that arises from both inferior and superior thyroid arteries. The inferior parathyroid arises from the third branchial pouch and migrates with the thymus anlage to assume its adult position adjacent to the inferior thyroid pole. Often closely associated with fat, the inferior parathyroid is supplied by the inferior thyroid artery.

Hyperparathyroidism

Primary hyperparathyroidism is caused by a single parathyroid's adenomatous change in about 80% of cases. About 15% of the remaining cases are caused by four-gland hyperplasia. Double adenomas account for about 2–3% of cases. Parathyroid carcinoma accounts for approximately 1% of primary hyperparathyroidism. Four-gland hyperplasia may occur in several clinical settings: sporadically; as familial hyperparathyroidism; and as MEN I (Werner's) or MEN IIa (Sipple's) syndromes.

Secondary hyperparathyroidism occurs as a hyperplastic parathyroid response typically to renal failure. When this response persists despite correction of the renal failure, as with renal transplant, it is termed tertiary hyperparathyroidism. Pseudohyperparathyroidism occurs when a nonparathyroid neoplasia results in a PTH-like paraneoplastic factor.

Although elevated calcium levels can occur in a variety of clinical entities (Table 17.3), the combination of elevated calcium, decreased phosphorous and elevated intact PTH help to confirm the diagnosis of hyperparathyroidism. Elevated calcium and PTH can occur in benign familial hypocalciuric hypercalcemia. This is an autosomal dominant disease characterized by abnormal renal calcium handling, resulting in stable lifelong serum calcium elevations and low urine calcium. A positive family history and low urinary calcium level helps to distinguish benign familial hypocalciuric hypercalcemia from hyperparathyroidism.

Table 17.3 Causes of hypercalcemia

Primary hyperparathyroidism
Secondary hyperparathyroidism
Tertiary hyperparathyroidism
Pseudohyperparathyroidism
Sarcoid
Granulomatous disease
Milk alkali syndrome
Benign familial hypocalciuric hypercalcemia
Malignancy
Excess calcium or vitamin D intake
Lithium and dyazide diuretics
Immobilization

In the past, patients with hyperparathyroidism presented symptomatically through 'painful bones, kidney stones, abdominal groans, psychic moans and fatigue overtones'. Most patients today with primary hyperparathyroidism are identified with minimal symptoms upon routine laboratory screening or surveillance bone density analysis.

Parathyroid surgery

Surgical exploration is the only curative option available for hyperparathyroidism. Most surgeons agree that patients with symptomatic hyperparathyroidism warrant surgical exploration. Asymptomatic patients are offered surgery if their calcium levels are significantly elevated (> 11.5 mg/dl) or if there is evidence of significant bone loss or renal dysfunction. Also, patients less than 50 years old are offered surgery because of the potential for development of symptoms if followed non-surgically (Table 17.4). In experienced surgical hands, hyperparathyroidism is cured through surgical exploration in over 95% of cases.

Preoperative localization studies are available to assist the surgeon in parathyroid localization and are especially helpful if unilateral exploration is planned. Most modalities are about 80% sensitive for detecting single adenomas. A variety of modalities have been used including sonography, CT scanning, magnetic resonance imaging (MRI) and, most recently, sestamibi scanning. Localization studies should not be used to confirm the diagnosis of hyperparathyroidism.

During surgery for hyperparathyroidism, one must keep in mind that the gross size of the parathyroid glands cannot be the sole factor in deciding between single adenoma versus four-gland hyperplasia. The minimum requirement is resection of an enlarged gland and biopsy of one normal-appearing parathyroid. If the enlarged gland is hypercellular with decreased fat, and the normal gland biopsy is normocellular with normal fat complement, then the diagnosis of adenoma is made, and four-gland

Table 17.4 Surgical indications in hyperparathyroidism

Symptoms (e.g. nephrolithiasis, bone pain, peptic ulcer disease)

Calcium > 11.5 mg/dl

Significant bone loss

Renal dysfunction

Young patients (< 50 years)

---

hyperplasia excluded. If the normal-sized gland biopsy is hypercellular, then four-gland hyperplasia must be considered. When hyperparathyroidism is caused by a single adenoma, calcium levels normalize once the adenoma is resected. With four-gland hyperplasia, surgical treatment varies from resection of only enlarged glands versus three-and-a-half gland resection with preservation of the one-half gland remnant.

18

Radiology of the ear, nose and throat for the primary care physician

Alfred L. Weber

Conventional radiography
Computed tomography
Magnetic resonance imaging
Radiographic studies of anatomic regions of the head and neck or
    specific disease processes
  The paranasal sinuses
    Radiologic technique and indications
    Radiologic interpretation of sinus disease
  Cysts and polyps
  Tumors and dysplasia
Facial and orbital trauma
The nasopharynx
Parapharyngeal space
Temporal bone
  Jugular fossa lesions
  Trauma of the temporal bone
  Congenital malformations of the temporal bone
Skull base
Oral cavity and oropharynx
The neck
  Salivary glands
  Cervical esophagus
  The larynx
  The thyroid gland
  The parathyroid gland

The purpose of this chapter is to provide the otolaryngologist and primary care physician with practical information regarding radiology of head and neck diseases. A discussion of the radiological examinations and procedures for diagnosis, as well as practical instructions for interpreting these examinations will be provided.

CONVENTIONAL RADIOGRAPHY

The conventional radiologic studies utilized in the analysis of head and neck diseases consist of conventional sinus films for evaluation of sinus disease, including the nasopharynx and base of the skull and as a survey examination in facial trauma[1]. For assessment of the orbits, the conventional sinus films are supplemented with optic foramen views. The anteroposterior and lateral neck views depict the pharynx, larynx and cervical trachea and simultaneously delineate the cervical spine. Fluoroscopy is applied in conjunction with barium to investigate the swallowing mechanism, the pharynx, esophagus and remaining gastrointestinal tract. In addition, fluoroscopy is utilized to evaluate vocal cord motion and to monitor interventional studies, such as sialography, dacryocystography and fistulous injections.

COMPUTED TOMOGRAPHY

In computed tomography (CT) the majority of the X-ray beam is blocked and only a very narrow beam is allowed to penetrate the patient. The CT scanner provides cross-sectional images of objects deep within the body that are free of interference from images of overlying tissues. The CT axial images allow reconstructions in the coronal, sagittal and oblique planes. Iodinated contrast materials can be utilized to enhance different tissues, which is helpful in the differential diagnosis. Spiral CT is one of the newer modalities of computed tomography[2]. The advantages include minimal motion artifact, especially during swallowing and respiration, and ability to produce enhancement with smaller amounts of contrast material. Moreover, the scan time is about 3–5 min, as opposed to about 15–20 min with conventional CT. Spiral CT also allows three-dimensional reconstruction from the volumetric scan data. The scan is obtained with 1-mm axial sections, as opposed to the conventional 4–5-mm thick slices. Spiral CT, by virtue of its fast acquisition of data, demonstrates arteries and veins in the entire neck after the administration of iodinated contrast material. This allows evaluation of the vascular lumen of arteries and veins, and demonstration of the vascularity of tumors. Most recently, the Multi–Detector CT

(MDCT) with increased spatial resolution has been developed. It has a slice thickness as low as 0.5 mm and acquisition capabilities of eight images per second.

MAGNETIC RESONANCE IMAGING

Magnetic resonance images (MRI) are obtained by exposing the numerous hydrogen nuclei (protons) contained in a large amount of water found in the human body with a combined action of a high magnetic field and radiofrequency waves. The images generated are based on variable signal intensities related to the different T_1 relaxation times and T_2 relaxation times. By adjusting machine parameters, axial, coronal, sagittal and oblique views can be obtained without moving the patient. On the T_1-weighted images, fat, melanin and subacute hemorrhages show high signal intensity; cerebrospinal fluid, edema, fluid in cysts and necrosis, cortical bone and fibrosis are low; and proteinaceous fluid is low or high, depending on the protein concentration. On the T_2-weighted images, the signal intensities are as follows: fat is intermediate to high; free water and proteinaceous fluid are high; muscle is intermediate; cortical bone and fibrosis are low; and subacute hemorrhage is high or low depending on the stage of evolution of the blood degradation products (deoxygenated, low; methemoglobin, high).

The images can be further modified with the introduction of a contrast agent gadolinium-DTPA. This contrast material elicits shortening of the relaxation time of T_1 with consequent increase in signal intensities. Fluid within a cyst, sinus cavity, mucocele, or necrotic tissue reveals no enhancement. Solid tissue (including tumor tissue) shows a variable degree of enhancement with most carcinomas being of intermediate enhancement and schwannomas and vascular lesions revealing a marked degree of enhancement. These enhancement patterns of various abnormal tissues can be utilized in conjunction with the T_1- and T_2-weighted signal intensities to characterize a lesion and arrive at a definite or presumptive diagnosis. Furthermore, flowing blood emits no signal intensity and is indicated by a flow void with the blood being dark in the lumen of the vessels.

MRI is contraindicated in the presence of ferromagnetic foreign bodies in the eye and orbit. In suspected cases (e.g. metal workers), a conventional view of the orbit should be obtained as a screening examination. Other contraindications include patients with cardiac pacemakers and aneurysmal clips. Magnetic resonance angiography allows complete demonstration of imaging sequences of the arterial and venous systems in the head and neck area or in the intracranial cavity. It is useful for demonstrating stenoses, aneurysms, vascular malformations and tumor vascularity.

RADIOGRAPHIC STUDIES OF ANATOMIC REGIONS OF THE HEAD AND NECK OR SPECIFIC DISEASE PROCESSES

The paranasal sinuses

Radiologic technique and indications

Conventional sinus films consist of an upright Water's view (Figure 18.1), Caldwell view (Figure 18.2), base view (Figure 18.3) and lateral view (Figure 18.4).

CT in the axial and coronal planes with soft tissue and bone window algorithms provides detailed information on the soft tissue structures, including membrane thickening and fluid, along with bony abnormalities such as thinning, expansion, sclerosis and lytic destruction. CT is indicated

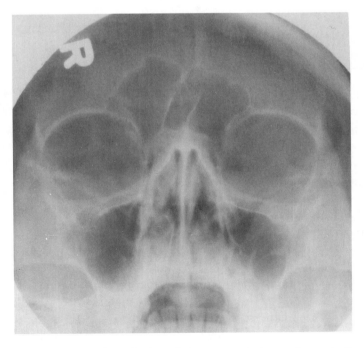

Figure 18.1 Normal Water's projection of the paranasal sinuses demonstrating normal maxillary antra, floor of orbits, inferior orbital rim, anterior ethmoid sinuses and frontal sinus

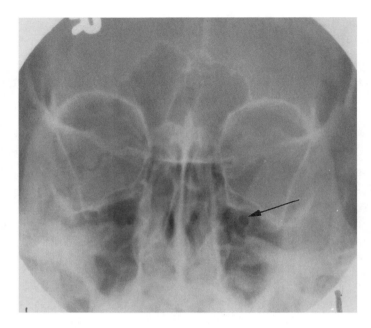

Figure 18.2   Normal Caldwell view of the paranasal sinuses and orbits demonstrating the frontal sinus, ethmoid sinuses, both orbits, including the superior orbital fissures, lesser wing of the sphenoid, innominate line, and posterior and anterior floor of both orbits. Note foramina rotunda projected into the upper maxillary antra (arrow). Most of the maxillary antra are obliterated by the petrous bones on this view

for evaluation of recurrent chronic sinusitis, suspected granulomatous and fungal diseases, mucoceles, and benign and malignant tumors, including calcifications and bony abnormalities. Iodinated contrast material is used in the assessment of orbital and intracranial extension of sinus disease, some benign tumors and malignant lesions.

MRI is performed with T_1-weighted images, proton density, and T_2-weighted images in the axial, coronal and sagittal planes. T_1-weighted images provide the best anatomic detail, while T_2-weighted images allow characterization of lesions and surrounding structures. Gadolinium is added for evaluation of malignant tumors and differentiation of solid from cystic lesions. Fat suppressed, T_1-weighted images with gadolinium are helpful when evaluating the orbits and skull base. MRI is the method of choice for evaluation of mucoceles, suspected malignant tumors and inflammatory processes that have extended outside the paranasal sinuses into the nasal cavity, pterygopalatine fossa, parapharyngeal space, infra-temporal fossa, masticator space, orbits and intracranial cavity. MRI is also

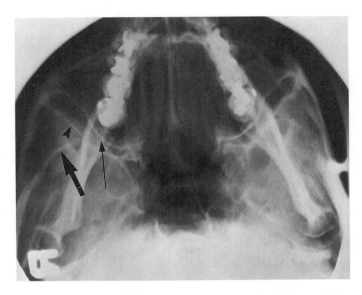

Figure 18.3 Normal base view of the paranasal sinuses and middle cranial fossa demonstrating the sigmoid-shaped posterior wall of the antrum (long arrow), posterior wall of the orbits (greater wing of the sphenoid; arrowhead), and curvilinear anterior wall of the middle cranial fossa (large arrow), pterygopalatine fossa, foramen ovale and foramen spinosum

useful when differentiation between a fluid-filled structure and solid tissue is needed.

Radiologic interpretation of sinus disease

In non-pathologic sinuses (conventional films and CT), the mucosa is not demonstrated and the bony walls are clear-cut and distinct. Infection causes swelling of the mucosa and increased density of the sinus cavity[3]. This may be associated with an air–fluid level, best demonstrated in the upright projection on the Water's and lateral views or on the CT study. When contrast CT is performed, the thickened inflamed mucosa enhances while the retained secretions or pus remain of water density. On MRI, the T_1-weighted images are low in signal intensity, while on the T_2-weighted images fluid and edema are characterized by high signal intensity. The enhancement pattern is the same as with CT in that the inflamed mucosa enhances, while secretions are non-enhancing.

In chronically obstructed sinuses with desiccated secretions, however, T_1 and T_2 relaxation times are variable. Chronic sinus disease is recognized by a combination of membrane thickening and bony sclerosis of the sinus

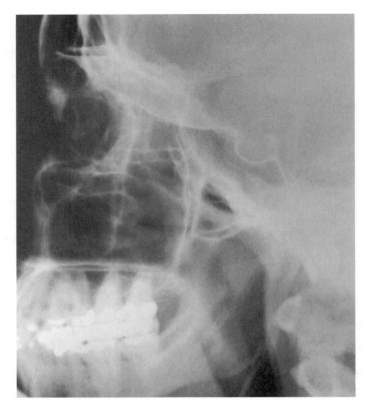

Figure 18.4   Normal lateral view of the paranasal sinuses demonstrating a normal sphenoid sinus, adjacent sella and nasopharynx. Both maxillary antra are superimposed. The anterior and posterior walls of the frontal sinus are also visualized

walls. In advanced cases, there may be complete opacification secondary to fibrosis with contraction of the sinus cavity. Increased density in the paranasal sinuses with sclerosis may also be caused by chronic granulomatous and fungus diseases of various etiologies, most commonly Wegener's granulomatosis and aspergillus infection. Acute sinusitis may lead to complications that affect the adjacent structures, such as the orbits and intracranial cavity. In orbital infection, subperiosteal exudate may be seen most commonly along the lamina papyracea. The inflammatory infiltrate is best demonstrated by CT and is reflected by a low attenuation area along the bony orbital wall (Figure 18.5). Displacement and enhancement of periorbita, displacement of the medial rectus muscle laterally, lid swelling, variable degree of proptosis of the globe and intracranial complications can be visualized with contrast CT or MRI (Figure 18.6).

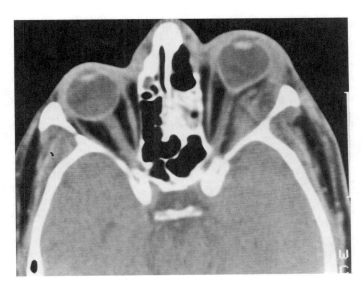

Figure 18.5   Left orbital cellulitis from sinus disease. Axial contrast CT section through the mid-orbits demonstrating an ill-defined, slightly heterogeneous inflammatory mass in the lateral orbit with swelling of the lids. Note anterior displacement of the left globe, stretching of the optic nerve with tenting of the posterior portion of the globe

Mycotic and granulomatous sinonasal diseases are characterized by non-specific membrane thickening, sclerosis and/or bone destruction and calcification (e.g. aspergillosis) (Figure 18.7). On MRI, in the acute stage, the findings are similar to inflammatory disease and are reflected by low T_1 and increased T_2 signal intensities[1]. In the chronic, non-invasive, stage, the presence of concretions and desiccated mucosal secretions result in hypointensity on the T_2-weighted MRI.

Cysts and polyps

Gadolinium is useful to differentiate a solid tumor from a mucocele. In the mucocele, there is no enhancement of the cyst content with gadolinium, but there is usually peripheral wall enhancement, especially if an inflammatory reaction is associated with the mucocele. In the frontal sinus, a mucocele causes loss of the scalloped margin with enlargement of the sinus cavity. Ethmoid sinus mucoceles occur predominantly in the anterior and mid-third of the sinus and commonly extend into the adjacent nasal cavity and orbital cavity. Sphenoid sinus mucoceles are associated with erosion and expansion of the sphenoid sinus with extension to the cavernous

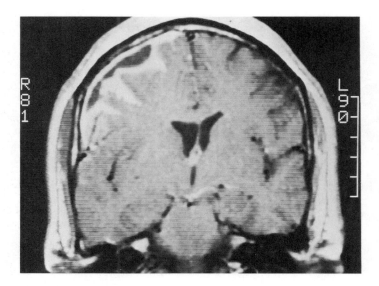

Figure 18.6 Subdural and extradural empyema of the right intracranial cavity after endoscopic sinus surgery. Coronal contrast T_1-weighted image at the level of the middle cranial cavity demonstrating diffuse contrast enhancement of the dura and meninges within the sulci of the brain. An area of low signal intensity demonstrates non-enhancing pus in a subdural location

sinuses, adjacent clivus, apex of the orbits (including optic canals), middle cranial fossa and pterygopalatine fossa.

On CT, polypoid masses are composed of an admixture of low density areas reflecting edematous mucosa with high density regions caused by inspissated secretions. Commonly, the bony ethmoid trabeculae are thickened.

Tumors and dysplasia

CT and MRI are the modalities of choice for assessment of malignant tumors within the sinuses and nasal cavities. These modalities provide detailed information of the origin and extent of these tumors. In the advanced stage, these tumors extend into adjacent structures, including the nasal cavities, pterygopalatine fossa, infratemporal fossa, nasopharynx, orbits and intracranial cavity. CT is the modality of choice for detailed assessment of bone destruction and bony remodeling. On MRI, malignant tumors are usually low to intermediate in signal intensity on T_1-weighted images and intermediate to high in signal intensity on T_2-weighted images with moderate enhancement following the introduction of gadolinium

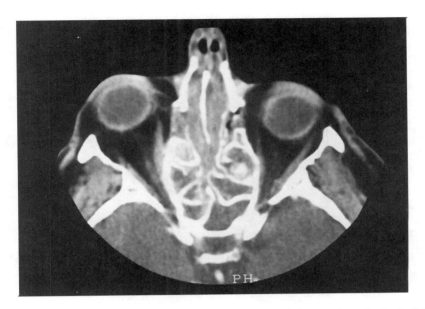

Figure 18.7 Nasal and paranasal sinus allergic polyposis. Axial CT study at the level of the ethmoids demonstrating complete heterogeneous opacification with low and high density areas representing edematous polypoid tissue (low density) and desiccated secretions (high density). Note the thickened bony trabeculae and involvement of the sphenoid sinus

(Figure 18.8a and b). Contrast MRI with fat suppression is mandatory for assessment of tumor extension outside the sinonasal cavities, including orbits, intracranial cavity, along cranial nerves, pterygopalatine fossa, parapharyngeal space and masticator space[4]. Contrast MRI with fat suppression is mandatory for

CT demonstrates the various components of fibrous dysplasia. Fibrous tissue results in a low attenuation value, while osteoid and woven bone are of increased density. On MRI, fibrous dysplasia is low in signal intensity on the T_1- and T_2-weighted images and there is moderate to marked heterogeneous enhancement of the dysplastic process.

FACIAL AND ORBITAL TRAUMA

For assessment of facial trauma, conventional films comprised of a facial bone series (Water's, Caldwell, lateral and base projections, zygomatic arch view and optic foramen view) are indicated[5]. These plain films may suffice in the assessment of a trauma patient if no significant comminution and displacement resulted from the impact. In everyday practice, this applies

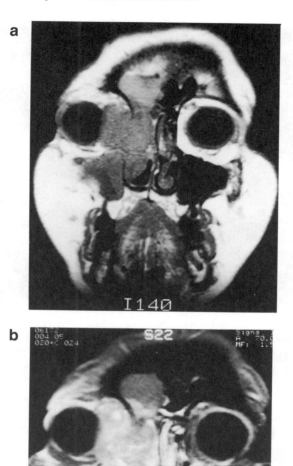

Figure 18.8 Squamous cell carcinoma of right antrum – ethmoid sinus. (a) Non-contrast T_1-weighted image displaying low intensity tumor in the right ethmoid sinus with extension to the right orbit and right maxillary antrum. (b) Contrast T_1-weighted image demonstrating moderate enhancement of the tumor mass, but no enhancement of the fluid in the right frontal sinus and lower lateral portion of the right antrum. Linear enhancing densities in the right antrum represent enhancing mucosa. Note enhancing tumor in the lowermost portion of the right frontal sinus adjacent to the fluid

predominantly to isolated or trimalar fractures. Fractures of the floor of the orbit (blow-out fractures) represent the most common type and occur following a blow to the globe. These fractures can be demonstrated in 95% of cases by Water's and Caldwell projections.

Nasal fractures may be encountered singly or in combination with other facial bone fractures. The roentgenographic examination of the nasal bones consists of a lateral view, Water's and hyperextended Water's projections, and a superoinferior projection of the nasal bones with an occlusal dental film. For fractures with comminution, displacement and rotation of fragments, CT is the modality of choice[5]. MRI is reserved for soft tissue injuries, principally those affecting the globe, optic nerve and orbit, brain hematoma, shearing injuries and extra-axial fluid collection.

The optimal modality for the assessment of frontal sinus fractures is CT demonstrating the fracture lines in the anterior and posterior walls along with posterior displacement of the anterior wall and possible intracranial complications, including collection of blood in the extradural space or brain. Le Fort fractures should be evaluated with CT and for injuries of the orbital soft tissues, the visual pathway (optic nerve, chiasm) and intra-cranial cavity. CT demonstrates to best advantage the multiple fractures encountered in nasoethmoidal complex fractures (Figure 18.9), but MRI is more useful in evaluating injuries within the orbit and adjacent intra-cranial cavity.

THE NASOPHARYNX

Conventional examination (lateral and base views) are commonly utilized for the assessment of enlarged adenoid tissue in the pediatric age group[6]. For angiofibromas and malignant tumors, CT is the modality of choice for demonstration of the tumor mass and any bony changes in the base of skull. MRI is the preferred mode to outline tumor extension outside the nasopharynx, especially to the parapharyngeal space and intracranial cavity. Gadolinium-DTPA is utilized in vascular (angiofibroma) and malignant tumors, especially when intracranial extension is suspected. For vascular lesions, represented by juvenile angiofibroma, angiography is often per-formed prior to embolization of this very vascular tumor.

PARAPHARYNGEAL SPACE

The parapharyngeal space is shaped like an inverted pyramid with the base at the skull and its apex at the greater cornu of the hyoid bone. It is

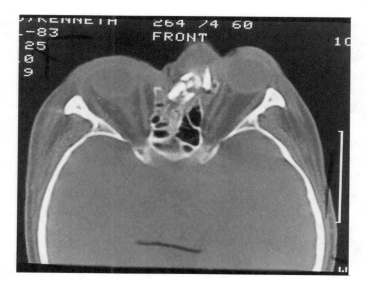

Figure 18.9 Nasoethmoidal complex fracture. Axial CT view (bone window setting) through the mid- to upper orbits, demonstrating comminuted fractures in the nasal bones, medial wall of orbits and ethmoid sinuses, with marked posterior displacement (telescoping) and splaying. Note the soft tissue swelling in both orbits, predominantly around the left and right globes

bounded laterally by the medial aspect of the medial pterygoid muscle (including intrapterygoid fascia; the deep lobe of the parotid gland including the parotid fascia), posteriorly by the belly of the digastric muscle and carotid sheath (prevertebral fascia), medially by the buccopharyngeal fascia (middle layer of the deep cervical fascia) and anteriorly by the pterygomandibular raphe and masticator space. The parapharyngeal space may be involved by infections, cysts, and benign and malignant tumors.

TEMPORAL BONE

Radiologic evaluation of the temporal bone consists of conventional radiography, high resolution CT and MRI[7]. Conventional radiography has had limited application since the introduction of CT. The only projection utilized most commonly consists of the lateral oblique projection (Schuller's view) to determine the pneumatization of the mastoid and assessing the position and integrity of cochlear implant electrodes and outline of fracture lines extending from the skull table into the temporal bone. For detailed assessment, high resolution thin section (1 mm) CT in the axial and coronal planes is the method of choice and allows simultaneous evaluation of the bony structures of the temporal bones and soft tissue densities within and outside the temporal bones (Figure 18.10a, b and c). MRI with contrast (gadolinium-DTPA) is indicated for assessment of acoustic neuromas, complications of infections and tumors extending outside the temporal bones such as glomus jugulare tumor. Conventional angiography is utilized for the assessment of vascular tumors, including glomus tympanicum and glomus jugulare tumors, commonly in conjunction with embolization of the tumor matrix to diminish blood supply prior to surgery.

The CT findings in cholesteatoma consist of erosion of the spur, the lateral wall of the epitympanic recess and ossicles. The glomus tympanicum tumor on CT appears as a sharply defined enhancing mass within the middle ear cavity, most frequently along the promontory. Contrast CT and MRI are indicated for delineation of the extent of malignant tumors. CT defines bone destruction, while the matrix of the tumor is preferably evaluated with contrast MRI. Acoustic neuromas reveal marked enhancement on MRI after gadolinium introduction[8]. Facial nerve neuromas should be suspected in a patient with gradual onset and progression of facial nerve paresis[9]. The most common site of involvement is the geniculate ganglion region, which manifests as a sausage-shaped bony defect in the area of the ganglion (Figure 18.11). On CT and MRI, they manifest as a localized, homogeneous, well-defined mass, or may grow along the course of the facial nerve causing diffuse enlargement of the nerve. Facial nerve neuromas reveal low signal intensity on the T_1-weighted images, but high signal intensity on the T_2-weighted images, along with marked enhancement (Figure 18.11).

Jugular fossa lesions

CT delineates to best advantage the bone destruction and the extent of the tumor within the temporal bone and adjacent base of the skull. The appearance on MRI is characterized by a low to intermediate signal intensity on the T_1-weighted images with increased signal intensity on the T_2-weighted images and moderate to marked enhancement after gadolinium introduction (Figure 18.12)[10]. The addition of magnetic resonance venography has been recommended when seeking tumor invasion of the jugular vein. On conventional angiography, there is an intense tumor blush.

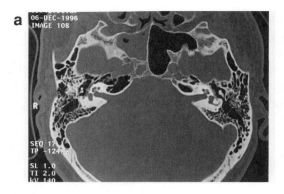

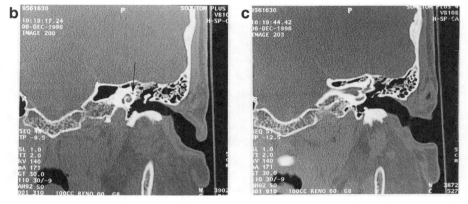

Figure 18.10 Normal CT study of the temporal bones. (a) Axial high resolution CT study through the temporal bones demonstrating normal cochleas, vestibules, ossicles and pneumatization of the mastoids. (b) Coronal CT study at the cochlear level demonstrating a normal cochlea, geniculate ganglion (arrow), malleus, spur, epitympanic recess, mesotympanum and external canal. (c) Coronal CT study at the vestibular level showing a normal internal auditory canal, vestibule, semicircular canals, incus, lenticular process, spur, epitympanum and mesotympanum

Trauma of the temporal bone

Fractures of the temporal bones are evaluated with preliminary mastoid films (Schuller's view) and high resolution CT (1-mm slices) in the axial and coronal planes with bone window settings[7]. If there is a suspicion of intracranial injuries, MRI is indicated.

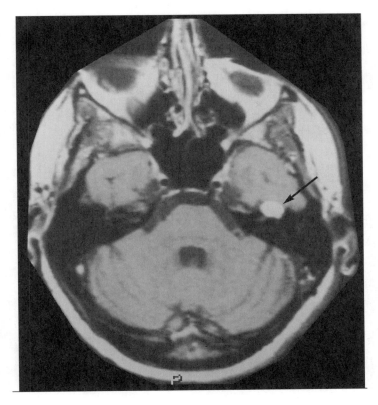

Figure 18.11 Geniculate ganglion neuroma. Axial contrast T_1-weighted image demonstrating an enhancing neuroma in the geniculate ganglion region (arrow)

Congenital malformations of the temporal bone

Congenital malformations of the temporal bones are evaluated by CT with 1-mm axial and coronal sections (Figure 18.13). CT assessment of the ear anomalies includes:

(1) Pneumatization of the mastoid;

(2) Size of the external auditory canal and its spectrum from slight narrowing to complete aplasia;

(3) Thickness of the atresia plate;

(4) Size of the middle ear cavity;

435

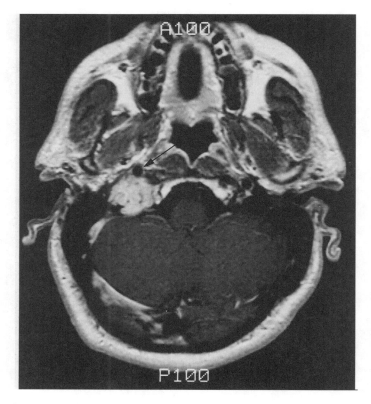

Figure 18.12   Glomus tumor of the right jugular fossa. Axial contrast magnetic resonance image showing moderate to marked enhancement of the mass in the right jugular fossa. Note anterior displacement of the right internal carotid artery, which is characterized by a signal void (arrow) and the tube-like areas of low signal intensity, representing increased vascularity within the tumor

(5)   Malformation of ossicles and the presence of fusion between ossicles and atresia plate;

(6)   Position of the vertical portion of the facial nerve canal;

(7)   Status of the inner ear structures;

(8)   Position of the jugular vein[7].

The most common suspected anomaly of the inner ear investigated by radiologic means is the Mondini malformation. In this condition, the cochlea is malformed with diminution or absence of the cochlear turns. The Mondini malformation is characterized by a sac-like appearance of

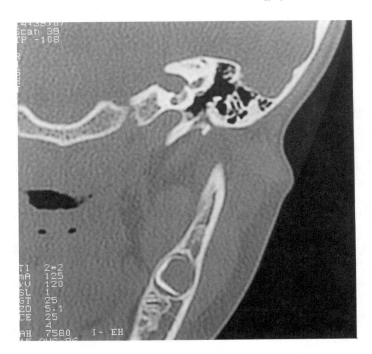

Figure 18.13 Aural atresia. Coronal high resolution CT section through the left temporal bone at the vestibular level demonstrating a thick atresia plate superiorly, and a thinner atresia plate inferiorly. There is deformity and fusion of the malleus and incus to the atresia plate. There is slight compromise of the tympanic cavity and no visible external auditory canal

the cochlea on the CT or MRI. This anomaly may be associated with enlargement of the vestibule and semicircular canals, especially the horizontal semicircular canal.

SKULL BASE

CT and MRI, with contrast material, are indicated for base of skull lesions[11]. Fat suppression with gadolinium is useful for malignant tumors infiltrating fatty compartments below the skull base. Epidermoid cysts are usually congenital lesions that arise from ectodermal cell rests and occur in the petrous apex and cerebellopontine angle cistern. On CT, they present as a sharply defined, bony defect within the petrous apex, adjacent clivus and middle cranial fossa. These cysts approach cerebrospinal fluid density and do not enhance following the introduction of contrast material (Figure 18.14a). On MRI, epidermoids tend to be relatively homogeneous, isointense, or slightly hyperintense to cerebrospinal fluid on T_1-weighted images and hyperintense on T_2-weighted images with no contrast enhancement (Figure 18.14b). The cholesterol cyst causes a sharply defined, round to oval, expansile, bony defect that is isodense to brain on CT. On MRI, these lesions are hyperintense on both T_1- and T_2-weighted images with no enhancement. Chordomas cause lytic bone destruction with no associated significant sclerosis. They are isodense with brain and show slight to moderate enhancement. The MRI appearance of chordoma is reflected by isointensity relative to brain on T_1-weighted images, moderate to marked increased signal intensity on the T_2-weighted images[12] with moderate to marked contrast enhancement. Chondrosarcomas arise in the petroclival fissure area. On CT, they demonstrate lytic bone destruction and show areas of calcification in 45–60% of cases. They reveal contrast enhancement following the administration of iodinated contrast material. Chondrosarcomas are low to intermediate in signal intensity on T_1-weighted images and reveal markedly increased signal intensity on T_2-weighted images and marked heterogeneous contrast enhancement.

The most common base of skull lesions are caused by metastatic disease. The lesions are lytic, sclerotic or mixed, with or without an associated soft tissue mass.

ORAL CAVITY AND OROPHARYNX

The location, extent and characterization of these lesions are optimally evaluated by radiologic means, which include CT and MRI. For malignant lesions, iodinated contrast agents are utilized to demonstrate the tumor margins more distinctly. MRI is performed with the head and neck coil or an anterior surface coil. Gadolinium-DTPA with optional fat suppression is added to delineate benign and malignant tumors[13]. Sagittal images provide valuable information for lesions of the tongue base and posterior pharyngeal wall.

On CT, cysts are hypodense (water density) and reveal no contrast enhancement. On MRI, they are hypointense on T_1- and hyperintense on T_2-weighted images with no enhancement after introduction of gadolinium. The ranula, a unilocular cyst, typically is located in the lateral oral cavity in the sublingual space. The dermoid cyst is located in the mid-sagittal plane and frequently arises in the sublingual or submental space. The dermoid manifests as a unilocular, cystic structure and may reveal increased signal intensity on T_1-weighted images from fatty tissue. Among the solid

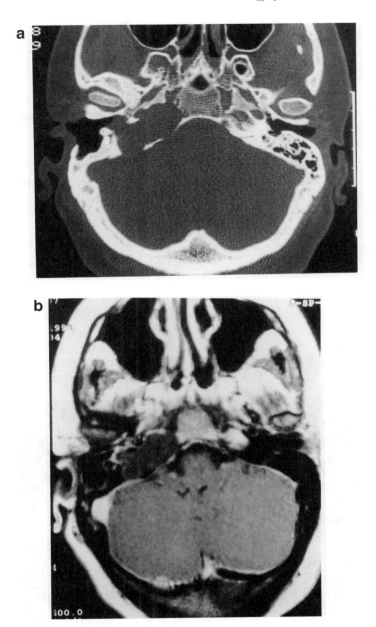

Figure 18.14 Primary epidermoid of the right petrous apex. (a) Axial CT study through the skull base demonstrating an expansile, sharply defined, lesion in the right petrous apex. (b) Axial contrast T_1-weighted image demonstrating the epidermoid to be of low signal intensity with no enhancement. Note the slight enhancement of some parts of the wall of the epidermoid

lesions located in the posterior tongue in the region of the foramen cecum is the lingual thyroid. Because of the high iodine content, this lesion demonstrates a well-defined mass with high attenuation values on CT (Figure 18.15). On MRI, the lesion is low on T_1- and high on T_2-weighted images.

CT and MRI optimally demonstrate the exact location and extent of carcinomas thereby providing important information for staging[13,14]. Advanced lesions, especially arising from the floor of the oral cavity, invade the adjacent mandible (Figure 18.16). Carcinomas are usually invasive with poorly defined borders. The tumor is usually low in signal intensity on T_1-weighted images, reveals moderate to increased signal intensity on T_2-weighted images, and there is usually slight to moderate enhancement of the tumor after gadolinium introduction.

THE NECK

The conventional examination consists of a lateral and frontal anteroposterior views of the neck. These conventional views are indicated to survey the neck and depict the pharynx, posterior tongue, larynx, trachea, precervical soft tissues, and cervical vertebrae, including the cervical spinal canal. The anteroposterior view is obtained with a high kilovoltage

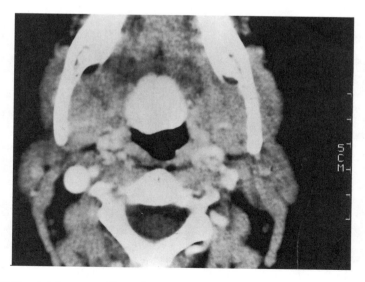

Figure 18.15 Axial contrast CT study revealing a sharply defined mass of high density in the posterior tongue, consistent with a lingual thyroid

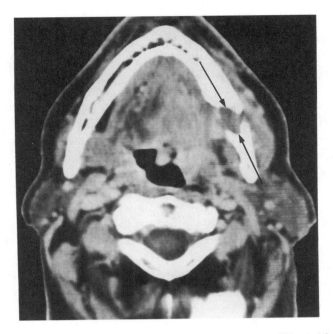

Figure 18.16 Carcinoma of the left tongue with erosion of the mandible. Axial contrast CT study through the mandible (soft tissue window) demonstrating a tumor in the left tongue with lytic destruction of the body of the left mandible (arrows)

technique, which defines the air and soft tissue interfaces optimally and lateralizes disease processes. For delineation of the pharynx and cervical esophagus, barium studies are performed. The barium swallow is conducted with fluoroscopy and acquisition of spot films to demonstrate anatomic abnormalities including luminal stenosis, outpouchings, filling defects and irregularity of the pharynx and cervical esophagus. For functional abnormalities, suggested by dysphagia, motility studies with fluoroscopy and simultaneous tape recording are indicated. CT in the axial plane delineates in detail different pathologic entities within the soft tissue structures of the neck, adjacent pharynx, larynx and trachea. The introduction of contrast material provides opacification of the vascular structures, which is mandatory to differentiate pathologies, especially enlarged lymph nodes from vessels and, furthermore, optimally enhances vascular lesions. CT is the preferred modality for the evaluation of neck pathology, such as inflammatory processes, cysts, and benign and malignant tumors. MRI defines vascular structures that are reflected by flow voids (vascular structures are dark) on T_1- and T_2-weighted images. These flow voids allow demonstration of stenosis, aneurysms and pathological vessels in hypervascular lesions, such as glomus tumors[15].

On CT, an abscess cavity is reflected by a low density collection of pus centrally surrounded by an enhancing rim reflecting the abscess wall. A retropharyngeal abscess is indicated by bulging of the posterior pharyngeal wall with widening of the retropharyngeal soft tissue space from an inflammatory infiltrate (Figure 18.17a and b). Cysts are characterized by low attenuation value (water density) with a sharply defined cyst wall. On MRI, the cyst fluid is low in signal intensity on T_1-weighted images and high in signal intensity on T_2-weighted images (Figure 18.18a and b). On CT, benign tumors are isodense with muscle with the exception of the lipoma which is low in density. On MRI they are low in signal intensity on T_1-weighted images and reveal increased signal intensity on the T_2-weighted images with variable enhancement after introduction of contrast material. On CT, paragangliomas reveal marked enhancement after introduction of contrast material. On MRI, they are low in signal intensity on T_1-weighted images and high signal intensity on T_2-weighted images and reveal marked heterogeneous enhancement after introduction of gadolinium (Figure 18.19a)[15]. On angiography, paraganglioma are supplied by branches from the external carotid artery and reveal an intense tumor blush in the capillary phase (Figure 18.19b). Lipomas are low in attenuation value on CT and on MRI reveal a high signal intensity on T_1-weighted images and intermediate signal intensity on T_2-weighted images.

Normal lymph nodes vary in size from about 5–15 mm. Lymph nodes are optimally evaluated by CT with introduction of iodinated contrast material and acquisition of contiguous 4–5-mm sections[16]. Enhancement of blood vessels is important for differentiation of lymph nodes from vessels. Lymph nodes are round to oval in shape and are isodense with muscle on CT. On MRI, lymph nodes are low in signal intensity on T_1-weighted images and contrast against the high intensity fat. They are of intermediate signal intensity on T_2-weighted images. They demonstrate moderate enhancement, which is optimally seen with fat suppression. For the most part, differentiation by CT or MRI of various pathological lymph node entities is not possible. Among enlarged lymph nodes, sinus histiocytosis and Castleman's disease are two entities with markedly enlarged lymph nodes. Lymphoma of the neck may be the first manifestation or part of a generalized lymphomatous process. These lymph nodes are frequently sharply defined and isodense with muscle on CT. Necrosis is

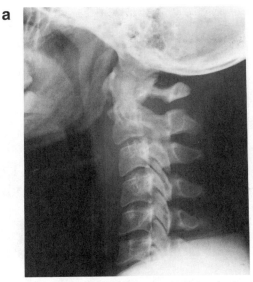

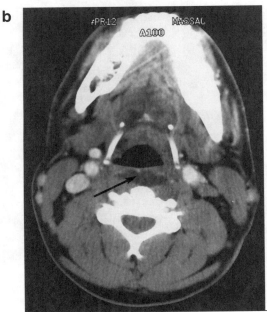

Figure 18.17 Retropharyngeal abscess. (a) Lateral view of the neck revealing diffuse soft tissue thickening of the retropharyngeal structures with anterior displacement of the pharynx. Note flexion deformity of the cervical spine from muscle spasm. (b) Axial CT study demonstrating a slightly irregular low density area within the enlarged retropharyngeal soft tissues consistent with an abscess cavity (arrow)

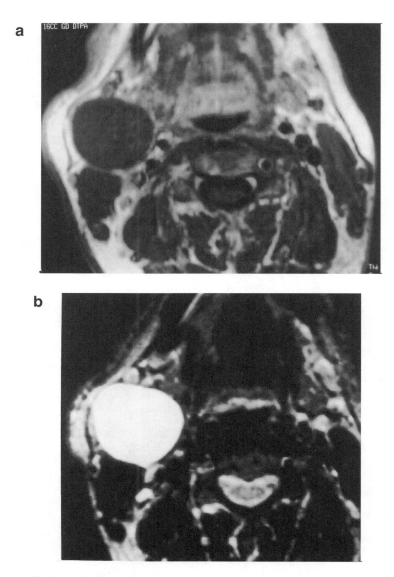

Figure 18.18 Right branchial cleft cyst. (a) Axial T_1-weighted image demonstrating a homogeneous, low intensity mass in the right neck at the angle of the mandible. (b) Axial T_2-weighted image demonstrating the cyst to be of high signal intensity

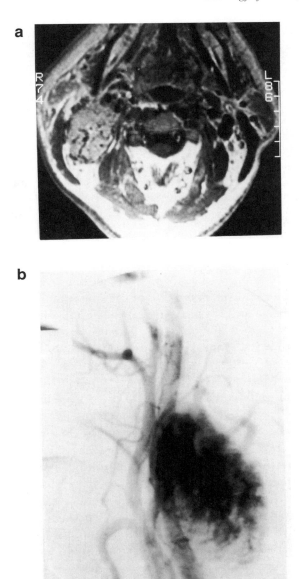

Figure 18.19 Right carotid body tumor. (a) Axial T_1-weighted image demonstrating a large mass in the right neck at the level of the carotid bifurcation with multiple flow voids reflecting the increased vascularity of the paraganglioma. (b) Carotid angiogram (different patient) representing a marked tumor blush of a right carotid body tumor

rarely encountered in lymphomatous lesions with the exception of Hodgkin's disease after treatment. Lymphomas are reflected by isointensity on T_1- and hyperintensity on T_2-weighted images. They frequently demonstrate slight to moderate enhancement after introduction of gadolinium. Nodes larger than 1.5 cm in diameter in the submandibular and jugulodigastric region along the internal jugular vein should be considered abnormal. There is, however, an overlap between enlarged metastatic lymph nodes and reactive lymph node hyperplasia with a 15–20% false-positive rate. Any lymph node, however, with a central lucency (excluding fat density in the hilum) regardless of size is abnormal. For evaluation of metastatic lymph nodes, helical CT is the most sensitive and accurate technique.

Salivary glands

Plain films provide a survey view for the presence and location of stones. Sialography, is indicated for evaluation of the duct system in the parotid and submandibular glands in patients with suspected stones and inflammatory swelling[17]. CT is the optimal modality for the assessment of inflammatory processes, stones and masses. MRI is applied for location and characterization of mass lesions. Because of the greater contrast resolution, tumors in dense salivary glands, tumors arising in the deep portion of the parotid gland and malignant tumors are better defined on MRI.

Sialolithiasis can be demonstrated by sialography (Figure 18.20a) or CT (Figure 18.20b). On CT, the pleomorphic adenoma is isodense with muscle and is often well delineated within the fatty parotid gland. On MRI, most pleomorphic adenomas are hypointense on T_1-weighted images and hyperintense on T_2-weighted images revealing moderate enhancement (Figure 18.21). Warthin's tumor (papillary cystadenoma lymphomatosum), on CT, is heterogeneous revealing low attenuation areas, representing fluid-filled cysts of variable size within the solid component of the tumor. On MRI, heterogeneous signal intensities are elicited reflecting the solid and cystic components. The low grade mucoepidermoid and adenoid cystic carcinomas are commonly well-defined and have similar imaging features as benign tumors. On imaging studies, the more aggressive salivary gland tumors demonstrate ill-defined, irregular borders, and often extend outside the boundaries of the salivary glands into the adjacent soft tissue structures (Figure 18.22). Their density and signal characteristics, however, are not specific.

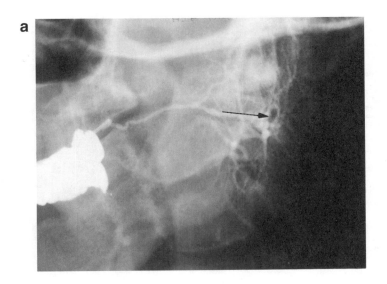

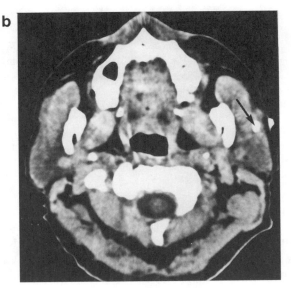

Figure 18.20 Left parotid duct stone. (a) Left parotid sialogram revealing a filling defect in the hilus of the left parotid gland (arrow). (b) Axial CT section through the mid- to upper parotid glands, revealing the stone in the left parotid duct (arrow) corresponding to the filling defect in the parotid sialogram

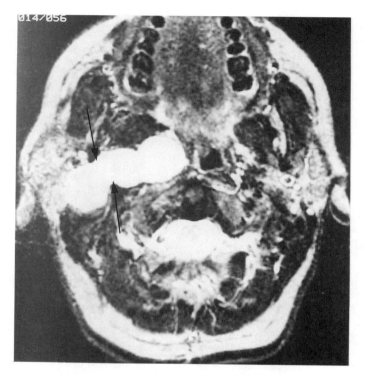

Figure 18.21   Pleomorphic adenoma of the deep lobe of the right parotid gland. Axial T_2-weighted image demonstrating a lobulated, longitudinally shaped pleomorphic adenoma arising from the deep lobe of the right parotid gland. Note indentation of the adenoma at the stylomandibular canal (arrows)

Cervical esophagus

Investigation of the cervical esophagus consists of a preliminary film of the lateral neck and barium swallow with fluoroscopy (including spot films and videotape recording). These studies allow evaluation of morphological and motility changes. For extension of disease processes, chiefly malignant tumors outside the esophagus and assessment of metastatic lymph nodes, CT and MRI are the modalities to be utilized.

A preliminary film of the neck in the lateral projection can easily identify foreign bodies, which are most commonly located in the lower hypopharynx and cervical esophagus (Figure 18.23). On the barium swallow, there is evidence of a filling defect in the esophagus and, in cases of perforation, evidence of a fistulous tract.

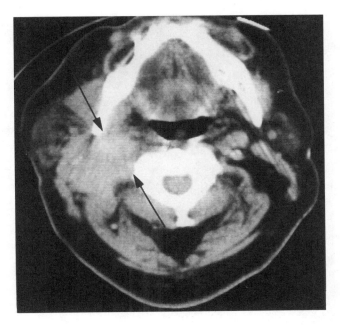

Figure 18.22 Carcinoma of the right parotid gland. Axial contrast CT section, demonstrating a mass in the medial posterior aspect of the right parotid gland, with extension of tumor into the paraoropharyngeal space (arrows) and posterior right neck medial to the sternocleidomastoid muscle

The barium swallow is the optimal modality in diagnosing and defining malignant tumors. A classical finding on the barium swallow is irregularity of the lumen of the esophagus associated with narrowing (Figure 18.24). The extra-esophageal component of the carcinoma can only be evaluated with CT and MRI[18]. Tracheal displacement, indentation or invasion is well delineated on CT study. Simultaneously, enlarged lymph nodes are identified in the neck and mediastinum. The most common post-laryngectomy complication is a sinus tract or fistula immediately after surgery. These fistulas are ideally demonstrated with barium or gastrografin. The tract may extend from the neopharynx anteriorly and connect with the adjacent skin. Some fistulas, however, extend inferiorly over a variable distance along the neopharynx.

The benign stricture is of variable length, has a smooth wall, and is often tapered at the inferior and superior margins. The marked dilatation of the pseudovallecula is secondary to an elongated, vertically oriented soft tissue shelf created after laryngectomy.

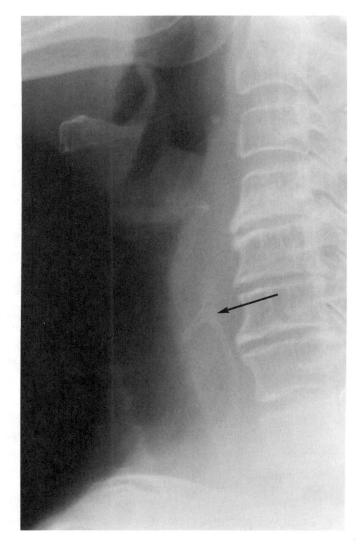

Figure 18.23 Lateral view of the neck revealing a chicken bone (scapula) in the cervical esophagus (arrow) with slight swelling reflected by a slightly increased anteroposterior diameter of the precervical soft tissues

The larynx

The first radiologic evaluation of the larynx consists of lateral and antero-posterior views of the neck. The lateral film demonstrates to best advantage

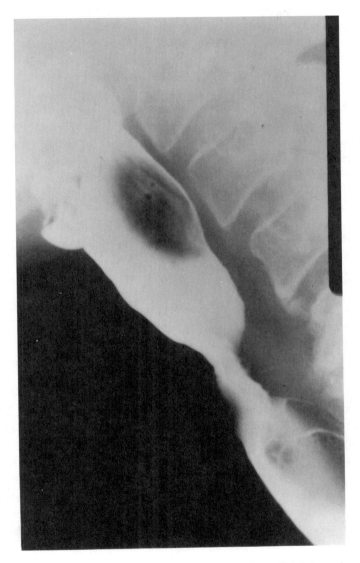

Figure 18.24   Barium swallow after laryngectomy demonstrating a slightly irregular narrowing in the neopharynx consistent with a recurrent carcinoma

the larynx, upper trachea, posterior portion of the tongue, vallecular area, precervical soft tissues and cervical spine. The anteroposterior view (high-kilovoltage technique) delineates lateral dimensions of the larynx and cervical trachea[19]. To study the dynamics of the larynx, particularly the motion of the vocal cords, fluoroscopy is used in conjunction with spot films. The barium swallow is part of the fluoroscopic examination of the larynx and hypopharynx when a patient has difficulty swallowing and a supraglottic hypopharyngeal tumor or esophageal tumor is suspected. CT (axial plane with 3–5-mm sections) is useful for assessment of the para-laryngeal soft tissue structures, pre-epiglottic space, anterior and posterior commissures and the cartilaginous laryngeal structures. MRI with its multiplanar capability (coronal, sagittal and axial planes) characterizes lesions on the basis of different signal intensities, such as high intensity fat from low intensity solid lesions and fluid from solid tissue. Gadolinium-DTPA may be added to delineate optimally enhancing benign and malignant tumors.

Acute supraglottitis (epiglottitis) shows a swollen epiglottis, aryepiglottic folds and arytenoid area (Figure 18.25). This swelling may completely obliterate the normal laryngeal airway. On CT, laryngoceles manifest as a low attenuation circumscribed air sac that may, on occasion, contain an air–fluid level or, rarely, polypoid tissue within the wall. On occasion, a laryngocele may be completely filled with fluid simulating a soft tissue mass or fluid-filled retention cyst.

Malignant tumors of the larynx are optimally evaluated by CT and MRI. The principal indication for imaging studies is to assess invasion of carcinoma from the mucosal surface into the deeper structures, such as the paralaryngeal space and pre-epiglottic space. On CT, squamous cell carcinomas are characterized by their isodensity with muscle. The para-laryngeal fat space is obliterated (Figure 18.26a) and there may be erosion of the adjacent cartilaginous structures[20]. The only definite sign of tumor invasion of the cartilage is extension outside the larynx. On MRI, the tumor is characterized by hypointensity on T_1-weighted images (Figure 18.26b), intermediate signal intensity on T_2-weighted images, and moderate enhancement after gadolinium administration[20]. The high intensity fat of the paralaryngeal and pre-epiglottic spaces becomes obliterated by tumor. Extension into the pre-epiglottic space is easily recognized on sagittal T_1-weighted images, as well as invasion of the tongue. On MRI, cartilaginous tumor invasion is reflected by loss of the normal signal void of the ossified cartilaginous cortex and obliteration of the high intensity fatty marrow. CT is the modality of choice in imaging abnormalities related to trauma in the larynx[21]. There may be swelling and hematoma formation within the larynx associated with vertical or horizontal fractures of the thyroid or cricoid cartilages (Figure 18.27). In addition, avulsion of the epiglottis or arytenoids may occur.

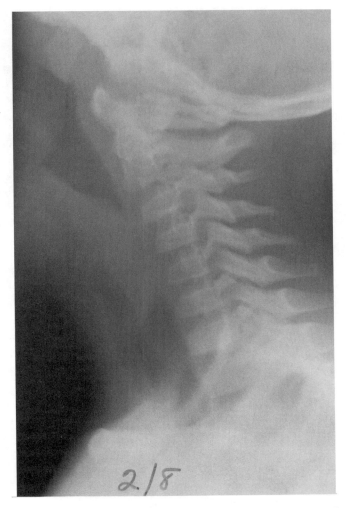

Figure 18.25 Lateral view of the neck, including larynx and trachea, revealing marked supraglottic swelling of the epiglottis, aryepiglottic folds and arytenoids, with marked compromise of the laryngeal lumen. Note the bulging of the edematous mass into the hypopharynx

The examination of laryngeal stenosis should be carried out with preliminary anteroposterior and lateral neck films followed by fluoroscopy to assess vocal cord motion. For assessment of the entire circumference of the stenotic lesion, CT or MRI may be performed (Figure 18.28). Foreign

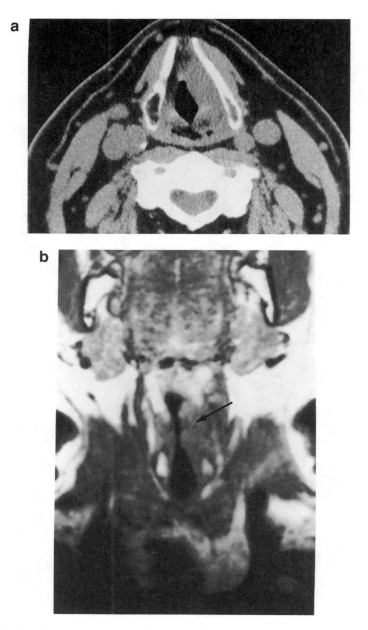

Figure 18.26 Carcinoma of left vocal cord and false cord with subglottic extension. (a) Axial CT section demonstrating a mass in the left false cord (arrow) with extension into the paralaryngeal space. The adjacent thyroid cartilage is intact. (b) Coronal T_1-weighted image demonstrating a tumor in the left false cord and left true cord, with obliteration of the left ventricle and left subglottic extension

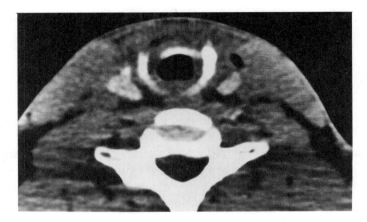

Figure 18.27 Fracture of the cricoid cartilage. Axial non-contrast CT section demonstrating a fracture in the anterior portion of the cricoid cartilage with slight posterior displacement and circumferential edema in the subglottic larynx

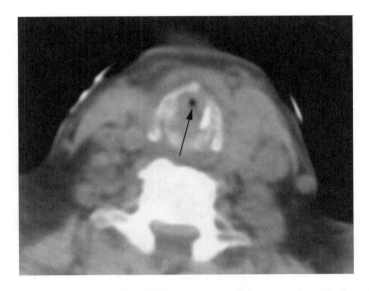

Figure 18.28 Subglottic stenosis. Axial non-contrast CT section through the subglottic larynx demonstrating marked narrowing secondary to fibrosis with a small remaining lumen of the subglottic larynx anteriorly (arrow)

bodies in the food, and less commonly air passages, present as emergency problems requiring endoscopy and/or radiologic investigation.

The thyroid gland

Ultrasound is indicated for evaluation of small thyroid nodules (< 2 cm) and differentiation of cystic from solid lesions[22]. Nuclear medicine studies are utilized to assess the function of thyroid nodules (hot or cold) and the functional status of the thyroid gland (hypo- or hyperthyroidism), and search for metastases in malignant thyroid tumors, principally papillary carcinoma of the thyroid. CT is indicated for large thyroid masses or differentiation of a thyroid mass from an adjacent neck mass (metastatic lymph nodes) and to investigate compression or invasion of the larynx and trachea by benign and malignant tumors (Figure 18.29)[22]. Contrast CT, however, delays nuclear scintigraphy and radioactive iodine application in tumors by 4–8 weeks because of the presence of the iodinated material within the gland. MRI is indicated in the evaluation of mass lesions and is

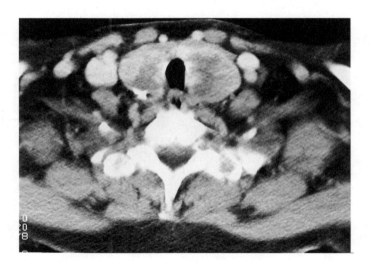

Figure 18.29 Multinodular goiter. Axial contrast CT section through the thyroid gland revealing diffuse, heterogeneous enlargement of the gland with some compression of the trachea. Note an area of calcification in the posterior portion of the goiter on the right

the preferred method for assessment of large, malignant tumors, substernal goiter and the postoperative neck for question of recurrent tumor[23]. Solid, homogeneous lesions usually reveal low signal intensity on T_1- and high signal intensity on T_2-weighted images.

Calcification, including peripheral, eggshell-like calcifications and large, multiple, globular calcifications suggest a benign lesion (Figure 18.29); whereas fine, punctate calcifications are more in keeping with malignancy (papillary carcinoma). Multiplicity of nodules in an enlarged thyroid is usually suggestive of benign processes, or more remotely, metastases. The presence of lymphadenopathy or infiltration of adjacent tissues suggests malignancy.

On CT, adenomas are usually solid and enhancing. Most thyroid cysts represent degenerated adenomas. They have low attenuation on CT and appear anechoic with enhanced through-transmission on ultrasound. The MRI signal intensity depends on the cyst content with colloid cysts characterized by homogeneous, high signal intensity on T_1-weighted images.

Multinodular goiter is composed of solid and cystic lesions with hemorrhagic foci. On MRI, the signal intensities vary on T_1- and T_2-weighted images reflecting the heterogeneity of the lesion.

The parathyroid gland

Imaging methods include ultrasound, CT, MRI and scintigraphy[22,23]. The major indications for imaging studies represent localization of parathyroid hyperplasia, adenoma and carcinoma in the clinical setting of hyperparathyroidism. Diagnostic evaluation includes ultrasound, CT or MRI, angiography and nuclear medicine scintigraphy. At ultrasound, parathyroid adenomas are oval, oblong or bulbous lesions with echogenecity less than that of the thyroid gland. The sensitivity of ultrasound is about 60–70% and the specificity is 90–96%. CT approaches the same sensitivity and specificity when compared with ultrasound, although other authors found CT to be more accurate (by more than 10%). By combining ultrasound and CT studies, the yield or detection rate was 89%. On MRI, the detection rate is about 80–85%. Adenomas are isointense to muscle on T_1-weighted images (Figure 18.30a), hyperintense to muscle on T_2-weighted images and reveal moderate enhancement after gadolinium introduction. Most centers have embraced technetium-99m sestamibi imaging without subtraction as a technique of choice for localization of parathyroid adenomas (Figure 18.30b).

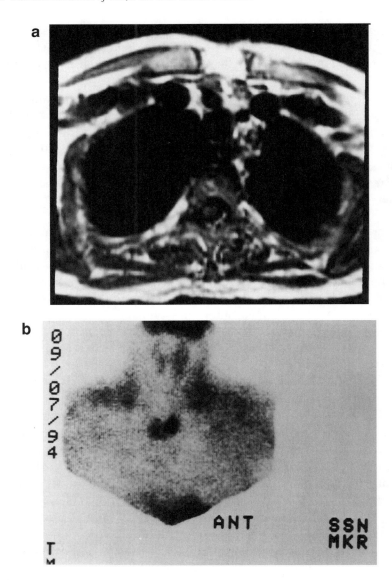

Figure 18.30 Two parathyroid adenomas below the lower pole of each thyroid gland. (a) Axial T$_1$-weighted image demonstrating a soft tissue mass isointense to muscle beneath the medial end of the right clavicle and another smaller mass adjacent to it. (b) Technetium-99m sestamibi scan of anterior neck and upper chest at 3.5 hours after injection, demonstrating increased uptake of the two parathyroid adenomas. There was diminished activity in the thyroid gland when compared with earlier scan (not shown)

Bibliography

1. Hudgins PA. Sinonasal imaging. *Neuroimaging Clin North Am* 1996;6:319–31
2. Heiken JP, Brink JA, Vannier MW. Spiral (helical) CT. *Radiology* 1993;189:647–56
3. Hesselink JR, Weber AL. Infections of the sinuses and face. In *Textbook of Diagnostic Imaging*, 2nd edn, vol 1. Philadelphia: W.B. Saunders Co., 1994:375–88
4. Som PM, Dillon WP, Sze G, Lidov M, Biller HF, Lawson W. Benign and malignant sinonasal lesions with intracranial extension: differentiation with MR imaging. *Radiology* 1989;172:763–6
5. Weber AL. Radiologic evaluation of facial and orbital trauma. In Taveras JM, Ferrucci JT, eds. *Radiology: Diagnosis, Imaging, Intervention*. Philadelphia: J.B. Lippincott Company, 1993:1–12
6. Weber AL. Anatomy of the nasopharynx, pterygopalatine fossa, and infratemporal fossa. In Taveras JM, Ferrucci T, eds. *Radiology: Diagnosis, Imaging, Intervention*. Philadelphia: J.B. Lippincott Company, 1991
7. Swartz JD, Harnsberger HR. *Imaging of the Temporal Bone*, 2nd edn. New York, NY: Thieme, 1992
8. Lhuillier FM, Doyon DL, Halimi PM, Sigal RC, Sterkers JM. Magnetic resonance imaging of acoustic neuromas: pitfalls and differential diagnosis. *Neuroradiology* 1992;34:144–9
9. Weber AL, McKenna MJ. Radiological evaluation of the facial nerve. *Isr J Med Sci* 1992;28:186–92
10. Weber AL, McKenna MJ. Radiologic evaluation of the jugular foramen. Anatomy, vascular variants, anomalies, and tumors. *Neuroimaging Clin North Am* 1994;4:579–98
11. Laine FJ, Nadel L, Braun IF. CT and MR imaging of the central skull base. Part 2. Pathologic spectrum. *Radiographics* 1990;10:797–821
12. Weber AL, Liebsch N, Sanchez R, Sweriduk S. Chordomas of the skull base. Radiologic and clinical evaluation. *Neuroimaging Clin North Am* 1994;4:515–27
13. Vogl T, Bruning R, Grevers G, Mees K, Bauer M, Lissner J. MR imaging of the oropharynx and tongue: comparison of plain and Gd-DTPA studies. *J Comput Assist Tomogr* 1988;12:427–33
14. Cooke J, Parsons C. Computed tomographic scanning in patients with carcinoma of the tongue. *Clin Radiol* 1989;40:254–6
15. Vogl T, Bruning R, Schedel H, Kang K, Grevers G, Hahn D, Lissner J. Paragangliomas of the jugular bulb and carotid body: MR imaging with short sequences and Gd-DTPA enhancement. *Am J Roentgenol* 1989;153:583–7
16. Nyberg DA, Jeffrey RB, Brant-Zawadzki M, Federle M, Dillon W. Computed tomography of cervical infections. *J Comput Assist Tomogr* 1985;9:288–96
17. Rabinov K, Weber AL. *Radiology of the Salivary Glands*. Boston: G.K. Hall Medical Publishers, 1985
18. Quint LE, Glazer GM, Orringer MB. Esophageal imaging by MR and CT: study of normal anatomy and neoplasms. *Radiology* 1985;156:727–31
19. Weber AL. Radiology of the larynx. In Fried MP, ed. *The Larynx: a Multidisciplinary Approach*, 2nd edn. St. Louis: Mosby, 1996:101–14
20. Curtin HD. Imaging of the larynx: current concepts. *Radiology* 1989;173:1–11
21. Schaefer SD. Use of CT scanning in the management of the acutely injured larynx. *Otolaryngol Clin North Am* 1991;24:31–6

22. Freitas JE, Freitas AE. Thyroid and parathyroid imaging (review). *Semin Nucl Med* 1994;24:234–45
23. Hopkins CR, Reading CC. Thyroid and parathyroid imaging. *Semin Ultrasound CT MR* 1995;16:279–95

Appendix 1

Common medications used in otolaryngology

The information shown on the following pages is intended as a basic guide to the prescribing of medications to patients with a wide variety of ear, nose and throat complaints.

Every effort has been made to ensure that the information contained in this appendix is both accurate and up-to-date. However, it is intended to be used as a general guide, not a definitive prescribing manual, and it in no way replaces the official prescribing information supplied by the manufacturers of the medications listed.

Purpose	Generic name	Commercial name	Advantages	Disadvantages
Otic drops				
For bacterial infections				
	Polymyxin B + hydrocortisone	Pyocidin-Otic®	Non-ototoxic Rare skin sensitivity	Poor Gram(+) coverage
	Neomycin + polymyxin B + hydrocortisone	Cortisporin® Otic Solution, Cortisporin® Otic Suspension, and others	Covers Gram(+) & (−) bacteria	Neomycin potentially ototoxic if tympanic membrane perforation Neomycin has potential for skin sensitization Solution causes discomfort if contacts middle ear mucosa
	Ciprofloxacin	Cipro®		
	Ofloxacin	Floxin® Otic	Covers Gram(+) & (−) aerobes Non-ototoxic	
	2% acetic acid (+) hydrocortisone	VoSol® Otic VoSol® HC Otic	Broad coverage	Depends upon the antibacterial effects of low pH solution Middle ear irritant
	Tobramycin + dexamethasone solution, 0.3%	Tobradex®		
	Tobramycin solution, 0.3%	Tobrex®		
For fungal infections				
	Tolnaftate	Tinactin solution		'Off-label' use
	Clotrimazole	Lotrimin® 1% solution		'Off-label' use
For cerumen removal				
	Carbamide peroxide	Debrox® Murine ear®	Non-sensitizing Effective	
	Hydrogen peroxide, 3%		Readily available	
For swimmer's ear prevention				
	Isopropanol + 2% acetic acid	Swim Ear® Domeboro® Otic VolSol® Otic		Cannot be used with perforation of ear drum

continued on following page

continued

Purpose	Generic name	Commercial name	Advantages	Disadvantages
P.O. Antibiotics for acute otitis media and sinusitis				
Penicillins (sensitivity common)				
	Amoxicillin	Polymox® Amoxil®	Affordable	*Moraxella catarrhalis*, *Streptococcus pneumoniae* and *Haemophilus influenzae* often resistant
	Amoxicillin clavulanate	Augmentin®	Effective against ß-lactamase-producing bacteria Broad spectrum	Poor for some *Pseudomonas* and resistant *Pneumococcus*
Cephalosporins (occasional cross-sensitivity with penicillin)				
	Cefaclor	Ceclor®		Poor for *H. influenzae*; serum sickness
	Cephalexin	Keflex®	Good for strep, staph, *Escherichia coli*, klebsiella; better for sinusitis than acute otitis media	Poor for *H. influenzae*, *Baci fragilis*, resistant *Pseudomonas*
	Cefprozil Cefuroxime	Cefzil® Ceftin®	Both good for . *H. influenzae*, *M. catarrhalis*, *S. pyogenes*	Both poor for *B. fragilis*, some *Pseudomonas*, some *Staphylococcus*, drug-resistant *Pneumococcus*
	Cefixime	Suprax®	Good for *H. influenzae*, *M. catarrhalis*, *Neisseria gonorrhoeae*, *E. coli*, some *Klebsiella* Once daily dosage	Poor for some *Pseudomonas*, some *Staphylococcus*, *B. fragilis*
	Cefpodoxime	Vantin®	Good for *H. influenzae*, *N. gonorrhoeae*, *Streptococcus pyogenes*, *M. catarrhalis*	Poor for *B. fragilis*, some *Pseudomonas*, drug-resistant *Pneumococcus*
Macrolides/azalides				
	Erythromycin	E-mycin®	Inexpensive; good for many strains of *Staphylococcus*, *Streptococcus*, *Mycoplasma*, *Bordetella pertussis*	Frequent gastric irritation. *H. influenzae* often resistant; inhibit the metabolism of other drugs oxidized by P-450 cytochrome (e.g. theophylline, warfarin, digoxin, carbamazepine)
	Erythromycin ethylsuccinate	Erythromycin ES®	Absorbed well with food	

continued on following page

continued

Purpose	Generic name	Commercial name	Advantages	Disadvantages
	Azithromycin	Zithromax®	Well tolerated Once a day treatment	
	Erythromycin ethylsuccinate + sulfisoxazole	Pediazole®	Overcomes *H. influenzae* resistance	
	Clarithromycin	Biaxin®	B.i.d. treatment	Frequent gastric irritation, 'metal' taste in mouth
P.O. antibiotics for chronic otitis media and sinusitis				
	Amoxicillin clavulanate	Augmentin®	Broad spectrum	Poor for some *Pseudomonas* and drug-resistant *Pneumococcus*
	Floroquinolones Ciprofloxacin Ofloxacin	Cipro® Floxin®	Covers most *Pseudomonas*, many *Streptococcus*, *Staphylococcus*, *H. influenzae*, *M. catarrhalis*	Should be used only for known *Pseudomonas* infections as resistant strains develop
				Frequent drug interactions
Medications for vertigo				
	Diazepam, 2 mg	Valium®	One tablet p.r.n. up to q.i.d.	
	Meclizine, 25 mg	Antivert®		
	Lorazepam, 0.5 mg 1.0 mg	Ativan®	One tablet sublingual q. 6h p.r.n., Rapid acting	
Medications for allergic rhinitis				
	Mucolytics Guaifenesin	Humibid LA®	Tolerated well when taken with fluids	
	Antihistamines			
	Fexofenadine	Allegra®, 60 mg	Non-sedating	B.i.d. dosing
	Fexofenadine + pseudoephedrine	Allegra D®	Decongestant added	
	Diphenhydramine	Benadryl®	Sedating, a good night-time antihistamine	
	Loratadine + pseudoephedrine	Claritin® Claritin® D12hours Claritin® D24hours	Q.d. dosing Most adaptable decongestant dosing	

continued on following page

continued

Purpose	Generic name	Commercial name	Advantages	Disadvantages
	Chlorpheniramine	Chlor-Trimeton®	Effective, over-the-counter Timed release available	Somewhat sedating
	Clemastine	Tavist®	Over-the-counter	
	Cetirizine	Zyrtec®, 10 mg	Q.d. dosing	
	P.O. decongestants			
	Pseudoephedrine	Sudafed®		Short duration of action, multiple dosing
Nasal sprays				
	Azelastine	Astelin®	Antihistamine	
	Oxymetazoline	Afrin® and others	Long-acting decongestant	Reactive mucosal edema if over-used
	Cromolyn sodium	Nasalcrom®	Well tolerated, best when started before allergic exposure	
	Ipratropium bromide	Atrovent®	Reduces rhinorrhea (anticholinergic)	
	Steroid preparations (may increase ocular pressure in patients with glaucoma, may lead to drying and epistaxis)			
	Budesonide	Rhinocort®	Q.d. dosing	
	Beclomethasone	Beconase® Vancenase®		
	Fluticasone	Flonase®	Q.d. dosing	
	Flunisolide	Nasarel® Nasalide®		
	Mometasone furoale monohydrate	Nasonex®	Q.d. dosing	
P.O. antibiotics for acute pharyngitis and tonsillitis				
	Clindamycin	Cleocin®	Effective against ß-lactamase-producing bacteria, many *Streptococci*, most *Pneumococci*, most penicillin-resistant *Staphylococcus*, many anaerobes (including *B. fragilis*)	

continued on following page

continued

Purpose	Generic name	Commercial name	Advantages	Disadvantages
	Penicillin V	Pen-Vee K®	Good for many strains of *Pneumococcus*, *Streptococcus*, anaerobes, actinomycosis	Poor for ß-lactamase organisms (e.g. *H. influenzae*, *M. catarrhalis*, *Staphylococcus aureus*) Gastric acid destroys. Therefore given 1/2 hour before or 2 hours after meals
	Erythromycin ethylsuccinate	EES®		

Appendix 2

Common instruments used in otolaryngology

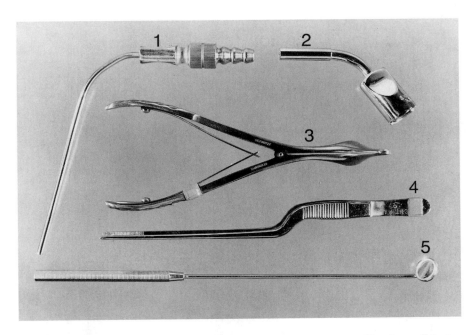

Figure 1 Nasal instruments. 1, Ferguson–Frazier nasal suction; 2, transilluminator light for use with Welch–Allyn battery handle; 3, nasal speculum, Vienna type; 4, Jansen–Gruenwald bayonet forceps; 5, nasopharyngeal mirror

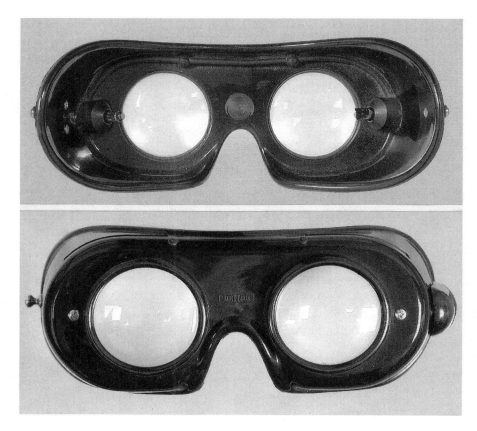

Figure 2 Frenzel's glasses. A, Internal view with small lamp and 20+ diopter lenses; B, external view

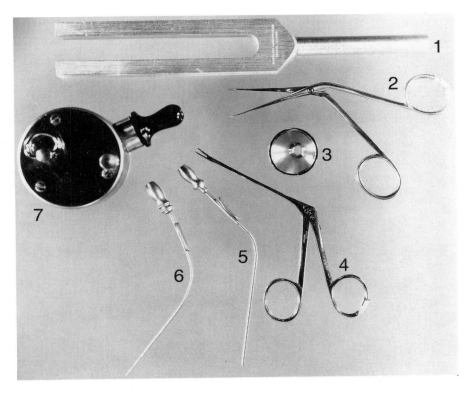

Figure 3 Ear instruments. 1, 512-Hz tuning fork; 2, Hartmann ear forceps; 3, ear speculum; 4, alligator forceps; 5, no. 5 ear suction; 6, no. 20 Schuknecht ear suction; 7, Bárány noise box

Index

abscess
  Bezold's 71
  brain 75
  neck 258, 442
  peritonsillar 280
  septal 224–225
acoustic neuroma 54–55, 102
  facial paralysis and 128
acoustic reflex decay (ARD) 25–26
acoustic reflex threshold (ART) 25–26
acoustic trauma 53, 157
Actinomyces 251–252, 281
acute necrotizing ulcerative gingivitis 274
acute suppurative otitis media *see* otitis media
acute suppurative thyroiditis 408–409
Adam's apple 235, 301, 399
adenitis, acute cervical 248–249
adenoidal hypertrophy 177
adenoma
  parathyroid gland 457
  salivary glands 391–392
  thyroid gland 457
ageusia 181
aging
  dysequilibrium of 103
  presbycusis 45–48
AIDS, sinusitis in 200
  see also HIV
airway
  acute laryngeal angioedema 364
  chronic respiratory obstruction in a child
    366–369
    congenital laryngeal webs 368
    foreign body 367
    laryngeal cysts and laryngoceles 368
    laryngeal papillomatosis 368
    laryngomalacia 366
    subglottic hemangioma 369
    vascular compression of the trachea 368
  emergency, initial assessment 355–358
  infections 360–364
    acute spasmodic croup 362–363
    bacterial tracheitis 363
    diphtheria 364
    epiglottitis 360–362
    pertussis 363–364
  management 358–360
  neoplastic obstruction 369–370
    laryngocele 370
    lingual thyroid 370
    malignant lesions 369
  respiratory obstruction in the newborn 366
  stenosis 370–371
  thyroid disease and 372–373
  trauma 373–375
allergic rhinitis 188–191
alternate binaural loudness balance test
  (ABLB) 21
angina

atypical 296
  Ludwig's 282–283, 386
  Vincent's 274
anosmia 181
anterior inferior cerebellar artery syndrome
  56, 106
antibiotic treatment
  acute suppurative otitis media 69
  external otitis 64–65
    systemic antibiotics 64
    topical antibiotics 64–65
  Ménière's disease 98
  ototoxicity 102
  septal abscess 225
  sialadenitis 385
  sinusitis treatment 194
antihistamines, allergic rhinitis treatment
  188–189
aphthous stomatitis 271–272
arytenoid cartilage 304–305
arytenoid granuloma 315
Aschan classification of positional nystagmus
  27
aspergillosis 206–207
aspiration 346, 367
auditory function tests 16–26
  auditory evoked response testing 22–23
  behavioral audiometry 17–21
    special behavioral tests 21
  otoacoustic emissions 23
  tests for functional hearing loss 26
  tuning fork and whisper tests 16–17
  tympanometry 23–26
auditory nerve pathology 21
auricle 3
  chondritis 67, 152
  hematoma 149
  lacerations 151–152
  perichondritis 152

bacterial meningitis 52
bacterial tracheitis 363
barium swallow 441, 448–449
barotrauma 34, 99, 156
basilar membrane 9
behavioral audiometry 17–21
  special behavioral tests 21
Behçet's syndrome 287
Békésy audiometry 21
Bell's palsy 126–127
  therapy 129
benign paroxysmal positional vertigo (BPPV)
  100
Bezold's abscess 71
blastomycosis 322
bony otic capsule 7–9
brain abscess 75
brain stem evoked response (BSER) 22–23
brain stem tumors 107

branchial cleft cyst 257–258, 392
buccal mucosa 270
  benign lesions 285
bullous myringitis 67
burning tongue syndrome 297

calculi, salivary 387, 446
Caldwell–Luc procedure 201
caloric tests 26, 91–92
candidiasis 273–274
  laryngeal 320
carcinoma
  laryngeal 330–334, 452
    carcinoma *in situ* 331
      glottic carcinoma 331–332
      subglottic carcinoma 334
      supraglottic carcinoma 332
    metastasis 262–263
    nasopharynx 177–178, 262–263
    oral cavity/oropharynx 289–290, 291–293,
      440
    salivary gland 293, 391, 392, 446
    thyroid gland
      anaplastic carcinoma 414
      follicular carcinoma 404, 411–412
      medullary carcinoma 412–413
      papillary carcinoma 403, 410–411,
        456
  upper aerodigestive tract 355, 369
carotidynia 143, 295
Castleman's disease 254–255, 442
cat scratch disease 250, 281
Cawthorne–Cooksey exercises 96, 108–111
cerebellar infarction 106
cerebellopontine angle tumors 54–55
  diagnosis 54–55
  facial paralysis and 128
  treatment 55
cerebrospinal fluid (CSF)
  leakage 221, 222–223
  otorrhea 161
cerumen 35
cervical lymph nodes 242–243
  central 242–243
  deep 242
  superficial 242
chemodectoma 261
choanal atresia 187
cholesteatoma 73–74, 79
chondritis, auricle 67, 152
chondroma 262
chondroradionecrosis 322
chondrosarcoma 262, 438
chorda tympani nerve 3
chordoma 438
chronic fibrosing external otitis 67–68
chronic otitis media *see* otitis media
coccidioidomycosis 321
cochlea 7–9
cochlear implants 59
cochlear Ménière's disease 96
Cogan's syndrome 104–105

colds 185–186
computed tomography (CT) 421–422
  cervical esophagus 448–449
  facial and orbital trauma 431
  larynx 452–456
  lymph nodes 442–446
  nasopharynx 431
  neck 441–446
  oral cavity and oropharynx 438–440
  paranasal sinuses 423–424, 425–426
  parathyroid gland 457
  polyps 428
  salivary glands 446
  skull base 437–438
  temporal bone 433–437
  thyroid gland 456–457
  tumors and malignancy 428–429
conductive hearing loss 34–45
  external canal obstruction 35–37
    cerumen 35
    developmental defects 36
    exostoses and osteomas 37
    external otitis 36
    foreign body 35–36
  middle ear disorders 39–45
    effusions 39–41
    incus resorption 41
    malleus fixation 41
    mass lesions 41
    stapes fixation 43–45
  tympanic membrane disorders 37–38
    hyalinization and tympanosclerosis 37
    perforation 37–38
cortical evoked response 22
corticosteroids, rhinitis treatment 190, 192
cough 309
cranial nerve VII *see* facial nerve
cricoarytenoid arthritis 317–318
cricoarytenoid muscle 304–305
cricothyroidotomy 337, 359, 398
cristae ampullares 9–12
Crohn's disease 289
croup 320
  acute spasmodic 362–363
Crouzon's disease 7
cupulolithiasis 100–101
cystic hygroma 259
cysts 442
  branchial cleft 258–259, 392
  epidermoid 437–438
  laryngeal 316–317, 368
  nasopharynx 178
  oral cavity 438
  parotid gland 392
  radiographic studies 427–428
  salivary glands 446
  thymic 260
  thyroglossal duct 260
  thyroid gland 404, 457

deafness *see* hearing loss
dental pain 139–140, 145

DeQuervain's thyroiditis   408
dermatitis herpetiformis   289
dermoid   259, 438
diphtheria   276, 364
    laryngeal   320
discrimination testing   20, 21
Dix–Hallpike maneuvers   90, 100
dizziness *see* vertigo
dry mouth   296
dysgeusia   182
dysphagia   343–352
    differential diagnosis   348–351
    examination   346–348
    history   345–346
    treatment   351–352
dysphonia
    muscle tension   313
    spasmodic   323–324

Eagle syndrome   144, 295
ear   3–16
    anatomy   3–13
        auricle   3
        external auditory canal   3
        facial nerve   12–13
        inner ear   7–12
        mastoid cell system   6
        middle ear   6
        ossicles   7
        tympanic membrane   3–6
    examination   14–16, 136–137
        inspection and cleaning   14
        otoscopy   14–16
        see also auditory function tests; hearing
            loss
    headache and   145
    pain *see* otalgia
    sensory innervation   139
eardrum *see* tympanic membrane
electrocochleography   22
electromyography   124
electroneuronography   124
electronystagmography (ENG)   26, 92–94
endolymph   9
endolymphatic sac operation   97
epidemic vertigo   98
epidermoid cysts   437–438
epiglottis   301, 452
epiglottitis   276, 360–362
epistaxis   211–220
    anterior septal bleeding   211–212
    arterial   213–214
    rare disorders   212–213
        treatment of   220
    treatment for persistent nasal bleeding
        214–220
        anterior and posterior nasal packs
            215–219
        nasal balloons   214–215
        nasal tampons   214
        surgical treatment   219–220
Epley maneuver   101

Epstein–Barr (EB) virus, nasopharyngeal
    carcinoma and   177–178
epulis   286
erythema multiforme   286
erythroplakia   290
esophagus
    masses   262
    otalgia and   141–142
    radiographic studies   448–449
ethmoid sinuses   168–169
    functional endoscopic sinus surgery   203
    mucocele   427
    see also paranasal sinuses
ethmoidectomy   201–202
ethmoiditis
    acute   198
    chronic   199–200
eustachian tube   6
    dysfunction, serous otitis media and   39–40
    functional evaluation   15–16, 39–40
evoked otoacoustic emissions (EOAE)   23
exostoses, ear canal   37
external auditory canal   3
    atresia   36
    obstruction   35–37
        cerumen   35
        developmental defects   36
        exostoses and osteomas   37
        external otitis   36
        foreign body   35–36, 153
    otalgia and   135
    trauma   154
    vertigo and   87–88
external otitis   36, 63–68
    bullous myringitis   67
    chondritis of the auricle   67
    chronic fibrosing external otitis   67–68
    diagnosis   63
    herpes zoster oticus (Ramsay Hunt
        syndrome)   67
    malignant external otitis   65–67, 128
    treatment   64–65
        analgesia   65
        systemic antibiotics   64
        topical antibiotics   64–65
    see also otitis media

facial laceration repair   227–228
    through-and-through lip lacerations   230
facial lymph nodes   241
facial nerve   12–13, 269, 343, 344
    disorders   123, 125–128
        iatrogenic injury   126
        physiology of degeneration   116–117
        site-of-lesion testing   28, 124–125
        trauma   125–126
        see also facial nerve paresis/paralysis
    functional anatomy   115–116
    imaging of   125
    neurophysiologic tests of neuronal viability
        28
    regeneration evaluation   117–118

facial nerve paresis/paralysis   71, 74
  bacterial disorders   127–128
  Bell's palsy   126–127, 129
  central causes   128
  cerebellopontine angle neoplasms and
    128
  congenital/genetic facial paralysis   126
  functional tests   122–125
    electrical excitability   124
    electromyography   124
    electroneuronography   124
    topognostic testing   28, 124–125
  history   119–121
  Lyme disease and   126
  Melkersson–Rosenthal syndrome   127
  physical examination   121–122
  sites and subtypes of   118–119
  traumatic   125–126
  treatment   128–131
    cross-facial nerve grafting   131
    eye protection   129
    hypoglossal facial anastomosis   130–131
    nerve decompression and exploration
      130
    static and dynamic facial slings   131
    surgical repair of facial nerve   130
  viral disorders   127
  see also facial nerve
facial pain, referred   144–156
facial trauma   429–431
familial hereditary telangiectasia   212
Fick operation   97
fine needle aspiration   255–257
  thyroid gland   403–404
fissured tongue   284
fistula
  labyrinthine   74
  neopharynx   449
  perilymph   99–100
fistula test   27, 87–88
foreign body
  airway   367
  external auditory canal   35–36, 153
  hypopharynx   294–295
  nasal obstruction   187
frontal sinuses   169
  acute sinusitis   196–197
  chronic sinusitis   198–199
  functional endoscopic sinus surgery   203
  mucocele   427
  osteoplastic obliteration   202
  see also paranasal sinuses
furunculosis, nasal   185

geniculate neuralgia   143
gentamicin, Ménière's disease treatment   98
gingival hyperplasia   286
glomerulonephritis   277
glossitis   284–285
glossopharyngeal nerve   269, 343–344
glossopharyngeal neuralgia   142–143, 295
goiter   407, 457

eurythroid   409–410
gonococcal pharyngitis   276
gout   387
Gradenigo's syndrome   74, 136
granulomas
  arytenoid   315
  epistaxis and   212
  midline   206
  salivary gland infiltration   389
Graves' disease   402, 407

hairy tongue   284
halitosis   297–298
Hand–Schüller–Christian disease   255
Hashimoto's thyroiditis   402, 408
hay fever   188–190
head
  lymph nodes   238–243
    metastasis   262–263
  lymphoma   263–264
head injury
  repair of soft tissue lacerations   225–230
    evaluation   226
    facial lacerations   227–229
    mucosal lacerations   229–230
    through-and-through lip lacerations
      230
    wound preparation for closure   227
  skull fracture   158–161
  vertigo and   105
  see also trauma
headache   144–145
  migraine, vertigo and   107
  referred pain   144–146
  see also sinusitis
hearing aids   58–59
hearing loss, diagnostic strategy   33–34
  see also conductive hearing loss; sensorineural
    hearing loss (SNHL)
hearing tests see auditory function tests
Heerfordt's syndrome   389
hemangioma   259
  laryngeal   316, 369
hematoma
  auricle   149
  septal   220
hemilaryngectomy   339
hemorrhage, vocal cords   315
  see also epistaxis
hemotympanum   40–41, 156
Hennebert's sign   88
hereditary deafness   48–51
  diagnosis   48–51
  treatment   51
herpangina   273
herpes zoster (varicella)
  herpes zoster oticus   67, 99
    facial paralysis and   127
  oral vesicles   273
herpetic stomatitis   272–273
histiocytosis X   255
histoplasmosis   321

HIV
 benign lymphoepithelial salivary gland
   lesion and   388–389
 lymphadenitis in   249–250
 sinusitis in   200
hoarseness   308–311
 hyperfunctional voice disorders   312–313
 laryngotracheal bronchitis   320
 laryngotracheal diphtheria   320
 polypoid corditis   313–314
 reflux and   312
 vocal cord hemorrhage   315
 vocal cord nodules   314
 vocal cord polyps   314
hyalinization, tympanic membrane   37
hyoid bone   305
hyperfunctional voice disorders   312–313
hyperosmia   182
hyperparathyroidism   415–416
hyperthyroidism   407–408, 409
hypogeusia   181
hypoglossal facial anastomosis   130–131
hypoglossal nerve   343, 344
hyposmia   181
hypothyroidism   406–407

incus   3, 7
 resorption   41
infectious mononucleosis   281
inner ear   7–12
 blood supply   105
 trauma   157–158
internal auditory canal   7–12
intubation   359, 361

jerk nystagmus   88, 89, 90–91
Jod–Basedow phenomenon   407
juvenile nasopharyngeal angiofibroma   220

Kaposi's sarcoma   286, 293
Kawasaki's disease   255, 286, 289
Kikucki disease   254
Kobrak test   26

labyrinth   7–9
labyrinthectomy   97
labyrinthine fistula   74
labyrinthine infarction   106
labyrinthitis   98–100
 perilymph fistula   99–100
 Ramsay Hunt syndrome (herpes zoster
   oticus)   99
 sudden idiopathic sensorineural hearing loss
   with vertigo   99
 vestibular neuritis   98–99
labyrinthotomy   97
lacrimation test   28
laryngeal conversion disorders   316
laryngeal surgery   334–340
 cricothyroidotomy   337, 359
 laryngectomy   337–340
   hemilaryngectomy   339

near-total   340
 supracricoid   339–340
 supraglottic   339
 total   337–339
microlaryngoscopy   334
tracheal cannulation   336–337
tracheostomy   334–335
tracheotomy   334–335, 359, 361,
   373–374
laryngitis   311–312
 acute   311
 chronic   311–312
 systemic lupus erythematosus and   318
 see also hoarseness; laryngopharynx; larynx
laryngocele   258, 316–317, 368, 370
laryngomalacia   366
laryngopharynx   306
 clinical evaluation   308–311
 inflammatory lesions   289
 neurologic disorders   323
 otalgia and   141–142
 reflux   312
 see also hoarseness; laryngeal surgery; larynx;
   vocal cords
laryngoscopy   310
laryngospasm   319
laryngotracheal bronchitis   320
larynx
 acute laryngeal angioedema   364–365
 anatomy   301–306
 arytenoid granuloma   315
 cancer   329–334, 452
   carcinoma *in situ*   331
   glottic carcinoma   331–332
   leukoplakia   330
   subglottic carcinoma   334
   supraglottic carcinoma   332
 chondroradionecrosis   322
 congenital laryngeal webs   368
 cysts   316–317, 368
 diphtheria   320
 hemangiomas   316, 369
 mycotic infections   321–322
   blastomycosis   322
   candidiasis   320
   coccidioidomycosis   321
   histoplasmosis   321
   paracoccidioidomycosis   321–322
 papillomatosis   317, 368
 radiographic studies   450–456
 sarcoid   318
 spasmodic dysphonia   323–324
 stenosis   370–371, 453
 superior laryngeal nerve paralysis   328
 trauma   328–329, 373–375
 tuberculosis   320
 Wegener's granulomatosis   318
 see also hoarseness; laryngeal surgery;
   laryngitis; laryngopharynx; vocal cords
lateral medullary syndrome   55–56, 106
lateral venous sinus, phlebitis and thrombosis
   76

Lermoyez's syndrome 96
Letterer–Siwe disease 255
leukemia 263–264
leukoplakia 290, 330
lichen planus 288
light reflex 5
lingual nerve 343
lingual thyroid 293–294, 370, 440
lingual tonsillitis 280–281
lipoma 442
loudness recruitment 21
Ludwig's angina 282–283, 386
Lyme disease 126, 252
lymph nodes 238–243, 442
  central cervical nodes 242–243
  deep cervical chains 242
  facial nodes 241
  metastasis 262–263
  occipital nodes 240
  parotid nodes 240–241, 393
  preauricular nodes 240
  radiographic studies 442–446
  retroauricular (mastoid) nodes 240
  retropharyngeal nodes 241–242
  submandibular nodes 241
  submental nodes 241
  superficial cervical nodes 242
lymphadenitis 248–255
  infectious 249–253
    Actinomyces 251–252
    cat scratch disease 250
    HIV 249–250
    Lyme disease 252
    Mycobacteria 251
    syphilis 252
    toxoplasmosis 250–251
    tularemia 252
  non-infectious inflammatory 253–255
    Castleman's disease 254–255
    histiocytosis X 255
    Kawasaki's disease 255
    Kikucki disease 254
    Rossi–Dorfman disease 254
    sarcoid 254
    system lupus erythematosus 254
lymphadenopathy 245–248
lymphocytic thyroiditis 408
lymphoepithelioma 178
lymphoma 263–264, 293
  neck 442–446
  thyroid gland 413
  upper aerodigestive tract 355, 369

macula 12
magnetic resonance imaging (MRI) 422–423
  cervical esophagus 448–449
  cysts and polyps 427–428
  facial and orbital trauma 431
  larynx 452–456
  lymph nodes 442
  nasopharynx 431
  neck 442

oral cavity and oropharynx 438–440
  paranasal sinuses 424–427
  parathyroid gland 457
  salivary glands 446
  skull base 437–438
  temporal bone 433, 434, 437
  tumors and malignancy 428–429
malignant external otitis 65–67, 128
  diagnosis 66
  treatment 66–67
malleus 3, 7
  fixation 41
  manubrium 3, 7
mastoid cells 6
mastoid lymph nodes 240
mastoidectomy 71, 76–79
mastoiditis, acute suppurative otitis media and 70–71
maxillary sinuses 169
  acute sinusitis 197–198
  chronic sinusitis 199
  functional endoscopic sinus surgery 203
  see also paranasal sinuses
median rhomboid glossitis 284
medullary thyroid carcinoma (MTC) 412–413
melanoma 293
melanosis 286
Melkersson–Rosenthal syndrome 127, 284
Ménière's disease 56, 94–98
  treatment 96–98
    antibiotics 98
    surgery 97
  variants of 95–96
meningioma 54–55
meningitis 52, 75
meningoencephalocele 187
metastatic lesions
  brain stem 107
  head and neck nodal metastasis 262–263, 393
  parotid lymph nodes 393
  skull base 438
  temporal bone 54
microlaryngoscopy 334
middle ear 6–7
  effusions *see* otitis media
  trauma 155–156
midline granuloma 206
migraine, vertigo and 107
Mikulicz disease 388
Mondini malformation 436–437
mononucleosis 281
mouth 267–269
  benign oral lesions 284–286
    buccal mucosa 285
    gingiva and floor of the mouth 286
    palate 285
    tongue 284–285
  burning tongue syndrome 297
  dry mouth 296
  examination 270–271, 291

halitosis 297–298
inflammatory lesions 286–289
  Behçet's syndrome 287
  erythema multiforme 286
  lichen planus 288
  mucositis 287–288
  necrotizing sialometaplasia 288–289
  pemphigus and pemphigoid 286–287
  Reiter's syndrome 287
  systemic lupus erythematosus 288
medical history 269
oral cancer 289–294
  leukoplakia 290
  non-squamous cell neoplasia 293–294
  physical examination 291
  work-up 291–293
pigmental oral lesions 286
see also oral cavity; tongue
mucocele 199, 427–428
mucormycosis 206
mucositis 287–288
multiple endocrine neoplasia (MEN) 413, 415
multiple sclerosis 54, 103
mumps 385
muscle tension dysphonia 313
Mycobacterium 281–282
  lymphadenitis and 251
  see also tuberculosis
myringoplasty 38
myringotomy 40

nasal balloons 214–215
nasal cycle 169–170
nasal fractures 220–224
  examination 220–223
  radiographic studies 431
  treatment 223–224
nasal mucus 170–171
nasal obstruction
  bilateral 188–193
    allergic rhinitis 188–191
    polypoid rhinosinusitis 192–193
    rhinitis medicamentosa 192
    vasomotor rhinitis 191–192
  chronic 177
  unilateral 177, 186–188
    choanal atresia 187
    foreign bodies 187
    meningoencephalocele 187
    trauma 188
  unusual causes 204–207
    aspergillosis 206–207
    midline granuloma 206
    mucormycosis 206
    rhinoscleroma 205
    rhinosporidiosis 205
    sarcoidosis 204
    syphilis 205
    tuberculosis 204
    Wegener's granulomatosis 206
nasal septum 168
  anterior septal bleeding 211–212

septal abscess drainage 224–225
septal hematoma 220
  drainage 224
nasal tampons 214
nasopharyngitis 178
nasopharynx
  adenoidal hypertrophy 177
  anatomy 174–176
  carcinoma 177–178, 262–263
  cysts 178
  examination 173
    radiographic examination 173–174, 431
  otalgia and 140–141
  tumors 141
neck
  anatomy 233–243
    contents of the cervical triangles 235, 236–237
    lymph nodes 238–243
    skeletal landmarks 235
    triangles of the neck 233–235
  examination 243–244
  injury, vertigo and 105
    see also trauma
  lymphoma 263–264
  nodal metastasis 262–263
  radiographic studies 440–446
  referred pain from 142, 145
  repair of soft tissue lacerations 225–227
    evaluation 226
    wound preparation for closure 227
neck masses 233
  abscess 258, 442
  blood vessel-associated tumors 261–262
  branchial cleft cyst 257–258
  cystic hygroma 259
  dermoid 259
  diagnostic strategy 244–255
    lymphadenitis 248–255
    lymphadenopathy 245–248
  esophageal lesions 262
  fine needle aspiration 255–257
  hemangioma 259
  laryngocele 258
  skin-associated masses 260
  teratoma 259
  thymic cysts 260
  thyroglossal duct cyst 260
    see also ranula; thyroid gland
  necrotizing sialometaplasia 288–289
  neural tissue-derived masses 260–261
  neuralgia
    carotidynia 143
    Eagle syndrome 144
    geniculate 143
    glossopharyngeal (tympanic) 142–143, 295
    otalgia and 142–144
    sphenopalatine 143
    trigeminal 143
  neuroblastoma 261
  neurofibroma 260–261

nose
  anatomy   167–172
    external nose   167–168
    internal nose   168–169
    neural supply   171
    upper respiratory tract   169–171
    vascular supply   171–172
  examination   172–173
    differential diagnosis   172–173
    radiographic examination   173–174
  infections   185–186
    nasal furunculosis   185
    recurrent nasal vestibulitis   185
    viral rhinitis   185–186
  referred pain from   140, 145
  see also epistaxis; nasal fractures; nasal
    obstruction
nystagmus   26–27, 88–89
  Aschan classification   27
  electronystagmography (ENG)   26, 92–94
  jerk nystagmus   88, 89, 90–91
  rotatory nystagmus   88, 90
  spontaneous vestibular nystagmus   89

occipital lymph nodes   240
olfaction   181
  disorders of sense of smell   181–182
oral cavity   267
  carcinoma   440
  examination   270–271
  infections   271–275
    acute necrotizing ulcerative gingivitis
      (Vincent's angina)   274
    aphthous stomatitis   271–272
    candidiasis   273–274
    herpangina   273
    herpetic stomatitis   272–273
    syphilis   275
    varicella   273
  radiographic studies   438–440
  see also mouth; tongue
orbit, referred pain from   145–146
orbital trauma   429–431
organ of Corti   9
oropharynx   267
  cancer   289
  otalgia and   141
  radiographic studies   438–440
Osler–Weber–Rendu disease   212, 285
ossicles   7
  trauma   155–156
osteoma, ear canal   37
osteoplastic frontal sinus obliteration   202
otalgia
  examination   136–137
  follow-up   144
  history   136
  neuralgia and   142–144
  primary   135–136
  referred   136–142
    dental pain   139–140
    laryngopharynx and esophagus   141–142

  nasopharynx   140–141
  neck   142
  nose and paranasal sinuses   140
  oropharynx   141
  salivary glands   140
  temporomandibular joint syndrome
    139–140
otitis media
  acute suppurative   68–71
    complications   70–71, 127–128
    diagnosis   68
    follow-up   69–70
    otalgia and   135
    role of paracentesis   68–69
    treatment   69
  chronic   72–76
    complications   74–76, 128
    otalgia and   135–136
    with cholesteatoma   73–74
    without cholesteatoma   72–73
  sensorineural hearing loss and   52
  serous   39–40
    drainage   40
  surgical treatment   76–82
    expectations of   79–82
    risks of   79
  see also external otitis
otoacoustic emissions   23
otolithic membrane   12
otologic crisis of Tumarkin   96
otosclerosis   43–45
otoscopy   14–16
ototoxicity   34, 51–52, 101–102
  vestibular toxicity   101–102
oval window rupture   157–158

palate   179
  benign lesions   285
papillomas, laryngeal   317, 368
paracentesis, acute suppurative otitis media
  68–69
paracoccidioidomycosis   321–322
paraganglioma   442
paralysis of Foville   119
paralysis of Millard–Gubler   118–119
paranasal sinuses
  anatomy   168–169
  examination   173
    radiographic examination   173–174,
      423–427
  referred pain from   140, 145
  sinus surgery   201–204
    Caldwell–Luc procedure   201
    ethmoidectomy   201–202
    functional endoscopic sinus surgery
      202–204
    osteoplastic frontal sinus obliteration   202
  see also sinusitis
paraneoplastic syndrome   107
parapharyngeal space   431–432
  infection   283
  masses   293

parathormone (PTH) 414
parathyroid glands
  anatomy 397, 414
  hyperparathyroidism 415–416
  physiology 414
  radiographic studies 457
  surgery 416–417
parosmia 182
parotid gland 379–380
  cysts 392
  metabolic disorders 390
  neoplasms 391, 393
  see also salivary gland disorders; salivary
    glands
parotid lymph nodes 240–241, 393
parotitis 386
pemphigoid 286–287, 319
pemphigus 286–287, 319
Pendred's syndrome 56
perichondritis, auricle 152
perilymph 7–9
  fistula 99–100
  leakage 53, 157–158
peritonsillar abscess 280
pertussis 363–364
petrositis 74–75
  otalgia and 136
pharyngeal pain 294–296
  atypical angina 296
  burns 294
  carotidynia 295
  Eagle syndrome 295
  foreign body 294–295
  glossopharyngeal neuralgia 295
  musculoskeletal cervical pain 295
pharyngitis 275
  gonococcal 276
  non-infectious 282
  pharyngotonsillitis 277–278
pharynx 267
  burns 294
  cancer 289–293
    non-squamous cell neoplasia 293–294
    physical examination 291
    work-up 291–293
  examination 361
  foreign body 294–295
  infections 275–284
    diphtheria 276
    epiglottitis 276–277
    infectious complications 282–284
    infectious mononucleosis 281
    lingual tonsillitis 280–281
    peritonsillar abscess 280
    pharyngitis 275, 276, 282
    rare pathogens 281–282
    scarlet fever 276
    tonsillitis 277–280
  swallowing physiology 343–345
  see also laryngopharynx; nasopharynx;
    oropharynx; pharyngeal pain;
    pharyngitis; throat

phlebitis, lateral venous sinus 76
pleomorphic adenoma, salivary gland 391,
  392, 446
Plummer–Vinson syndrome 285, 290, 351
polycythemia 286
polypectomy 193
polypoid corditis 313–314
polypoid rhinosinusitis 192–193
polysomnography 180
positional testing 26–27, 89–91
preauricular lymph nodes 240
presbycusis 45–48
  diagnosis 45–47
  mechanical 47
  metabolic 45
  neural 45
  sensory 45
  treatment 48
ptyalism 390
pure-tone average (PTA) 20
pyriform sinuses 302–303

radiography 421
  cervical esophagus 448–449
  facial and orbital trauma 429–431
  nasopharynx 173–174
  neck 440–441
  nose 173–174
  paranasal sinuses 173–174, 423, 425
  temporal bone 432
  see also computed tomography (CT);
    magnetic resonance imaging (MRI)
Ramsay Hunt syndrome 67, 99
  otalgia and 135
ranula 286, 438
recruitment 21
recurrent laryngeal nerve 398
reflux 312
Reinke's edema 313–314
Reiter's syndrome 287
relapsing polychondritis 104, 319
retroauricular lymph nodes 240
retropharyngeal infection 283–284
retropharyngeal lymph nodes 241–242
rheumatic fever 277, 279
rhinitis 205
  allergic 188–191
  vasomotor (VMR) 171, 191–192
  viral 185–186
rhinitis medicamentosa 192
rhinoscleroma 205, 282
rhinosporidiosis 205
Riedel's struma 409
Rinne test 16
Rossi–Dorfman disease 254
rotatory nystagmus 88, 90
round window rupture 157–158

saccule 7, 12
saliva 379
salivary flow test 28, 125
salivary gland disorders 140

acute inflammatory disorders 384–387
  acute bacterial sialadenitis 385–386
  chronic obstructive salivary gland disease 386–387, 446
  mumps 385
chronic progressive inflammatory disorders 388–390
  benign lymphoepithelial lesions 388–389
  granulomatous infiltration 389
  metabolic disorders 389–390
  xerostomia 390
history 382–383
neoplasms 390–393, 446
  carcinoma 293, 392, 393, 446
physical examination 383–384
salivary glands
  anatomy 379
  duct obstruction 386–387
  minor salivary glands 381
  parotid gland 379–380
  radiographic studies 446
  sublingual gland 381
  submandibular gland 380
  see also salivary gland disorders
sarcoid 254, 289, 318
sarcoidosis, nasal obstruction and 204
scarlet fever 276
Schirmer's test 28, 124–125
schwannoma 261
scrofula 251
semicircular canals 7, 9–12
sensorineural hearing loss (SNHL) 45–57
  congenital, non-hereditary deafness 51
  diagnostic strategy 33–34
  genetically determined SNHL 48–51
  ototoxicity 51–52
  presbycusis 45–48
  unilateral or asymmetrical SNHL 52–57
    acoustic trauma 53
    arterial disease 55–56
    bacterial meningitis 52
    collagen vascular diseases 56
    immune-mediated SNHL 57
    Ménière's disease 56
    neoplasms 54–55
    neurologic disorders 54
    otitis media 52
    perilymph leaks 53
    sudden idiopathic sensorineural deafness 57, 99, 161–163
    syphilis 53–54
    trauma 52
septal abscess drainage 224–225
septal hematoma 220
  drainage 224
serous otitis media *see* otitis media
Shrapnel's membrane 3
sialadenitis, acute bacterial 385–386
sialolithiasis 446
sinuses
  lateral venous 76
  pyriform 302–303

see also paranasal sinuses; pyriform sinuses
sinusitis 193–200
  acute 193–198
    ethmoiditis 198
    frontal sinusitis 196–197
    maxillary sinusitis 197–198
    sphenoid sinusitis 197
  chronic 198–200
    ethmoiditis 199–200
    frontal sinusitis 198–199
    maxillary sinusitis 199
    sphenoid sinusitis 199
  in HIV-positive patients 200
  see also paranasal sinuses
Sjögren's syndrome 296–297
  benign lymphoepithelial salivary gland lesions 388–389
  treatment 389
skull fracture 158–161
sleep apnea syndrome 179–181
  central (CSAS) 180
  obstructive (OSAS) 180
smell, sense of *see* olfaction
snoring 181, 357
spasmodic dysphonia 323–324
speech reception threshold (SRT) 17–20
sphenoid sinuses 169
  acute sinusitis 197
  chronic sinusitis 199
  functional endoscopic sinus surgery 204
  mucocele 427–428
  see also paranasal sinuses
sphenopalatine neuralgia 143
stapedectomy 44
stapedial reflex 28, 125
stapes 3, 7
  fixation 43–45
    diagnosis 44
    treatment 44–45
Stensen's duct 380
  obstruction 387
Stevens–Johnson syndrome 286
stomatitis 271
  aphthous 271–272
  herpetic 272–273
streptomycin, Ménière's disease treatment 98
stridor 357–358
Sturge–Weber syndrome 285
stylopharyngeus nerve 269
subacute granulomatous thyroiditis 408
subclavian steal 106–107
sublingual gland 381
  see also salivary gland disorders; salivary glands
submandibular gland 380
  neoplasms 393
  sialadenitis 386
  stones 387
  see also salivary gland disorders; salivary glands
submandibular lymph nodes 241
submental lymph nodes 241